BIOLOGY OF DESIRE

YOUR BRAIN AND BEHAVIOR

WILLIAM HASELTINE

KIM HAZEL

ACCESS
HEALTH INTERNATIONAL

Cover art by Kim Hazel

All author proceeds from the sale of this book will be donated to the nonprofit global think tank ACCESS Health International.

*Some of the stories shared here are true, while others are invented or embellished. However, all of them are rooted in the factual experiences of real individuals. Some narratives have been shortened for clarity. Please note that names and identifying details may have been altered to protect privacy, and certain events may have been condensed.

This work is supported by ACCESS Health International (www.accessh.org).

DEDICATIONS

WILLIAM HASELTINE

To all my friends and colleagues at ACCESS Health International.

KIM HAZEL

To my loving husband, Colin Purcell. To my bonus family, Ami and Kyle Phelps, Jennifer, Jake, and Natalie Tharp. To my support system, Emily Trout and John Andrick.

OTHER BOOKS BY WILLIAM A. HASELTINE

***Affordable Excellence**: The Singapore Healthcare Story; William A Haseltine (2013)*

***Improving the Health of Mother and Child**: Solutions from India; Priya Anant, Prabal Vikram Singh, Sofi Bergkvist, William A. Haseltine & Anita George (2014)*

***Modern Aging**: A Practical Guide for Developers, Entrepreneurs, and Startups in the Silver Market; Edited by Sofia Widén, Stephanie Treschow, and William A. Haseltine (2015)*

***Aging with Dignity**: Innovation and Challenge is Sweden-The Voice of Care Professionals; Sofia Widen and William A. Haseltine (2017)*

***Every Second Counts**: Saving Two Million Lives. India's Emergency Response System.The EMRI Story: William A Haseltine (2017)*

***Voices in Dementia Care**; Anna Dirksen and William A Haseltine (2018)*

***Aging Well**: Jean Galiana and William A. Haseltine (2019)*

***World Class**. Adversity, Transformation, and Success, and NYU Langone Health; William A. Haseltine (2019)*

***A Family Guide to Covid**: Questions and Answers for Parents, Grandparents, and Children; William A. Haseltine (2020)*

***A Covid Back To School Guide**: Questions and Answers for Parents and Students; William A. Haseltine (2020)*

***Covid Commentaries**: A Chronicle of a Plague, Volumes I, II, III, IV, V, and VI; William A. Haseltine (2020)*

***My Lifelong Fight Against Disease**: From Polio and AIDS to Covid-19; William A. Haseltine (2020)*

***Science as a Superpower**: My Lifelong Fight Against Disease And The Heroes Who Made It Possible; William A. Haseltine (2021)*

***Variants!**: The Shape-Shifting Challenge of Covid-19 Vaccine Evasion & Reinfection; William A. Haseltine (2021)*

***COVID-Related Post-traumatic Stress Disorder (CV-PTSD)**: What It Is And What To Do About It; William A. Haseltine (2021)*

Natural Immunity And Covid-19: *What It Is And How It Can Save Your Life; William A. Haseltine (2022)*

Omicron: *From Pandemic to Endemic; William A. Haseltine (2022)*

Monoclonal Antibodies: *The Once and Future Cure for Covid-19; William A. Haseltine and Griffin McCombs (2023)*

The Future of Medicine: *Healing Yourself: Regenerative Medicine Part One; William A. Haseltine (2023)*

Viroids and Virusoids: *Nature's Own mRNAs; William A. Haseltine and Koloman Rath (2023)*

CAR T: *A New Cure for Cancer, Autoimmune and Inherited Disease; William A. Haseltine & Amara Thomas (2023)*

Ending Hepatitis C: *A Seven-step Plan for a Successful Eradication Program: A Roadmap for Ending Endemic Disease Globally; William A. Haseltine and Kaelyn Varner (2023)*

Better Eyesight: *What You and Modern Medicine Can Do to Improve Your Vision; William A. Haseltine and Kim Hazel (2024)*

Fusion! *The Melding of Human and Machine Intelligence; William A. Haseltine and Griffin McCombs (2024)*

Checkpoint Inhibitors: *A Key to Curing Cancer; William A. Haseltine & Amara Thomas (2025)*

Live Longer: *What You Can Do, What Medicine Can Do; William A. Haseltine and Koloman Rath (2025)*

Destiny's Child No Longer: *Rewriting Genetic Fate; William A. Haseltine and Kim Hazel (2025)*

Recent Textbooks

The COVID-19 Textbook: *Science, Medicine and Public Health; William A. Haseltine and Roberto Patarca (2023)*

Molecular Biology of SARS-CoV-2: *Opportunities for Antivirus Drug Development; William A. Haseltine and Roberto Patarca (2024)*

PROLOGUE

WHAT IS *this power that can so easily unseat reason? Is it simply weakness, or does it reveal something more profound, a conversation as old as time itself, between the wildness of appetite and the yearning of the soul?*

You step into a bustling room, yet your mind is weighed down by the burdens of the day. As you navigate through the throng, your thoughts swirl in a fog of concerns. Suddenly, your gaze collides with a stranger's across the room.

In less than a heartbeat, far faster than you could form a conscious thought, something shifts inside you. Your pulse quickens. Your senses heighten, every sound and scent sharply defined, as if the world has come into sharper focus just for this moment. An unexplainable magnetism draws you toward them, igniting a flame inside you. It is as if some part of you has awakened and seized the reins, leaving your rational mind scrambling to catch up.

Science tells us that these first seconds are decisive. Studies reveal that attraction is often decided in less than a second before reason, logic, or conscious intention can intervene. It is not a rational process but something more fundamental, orchestrated by primal forces deep within our brains. Subtle signals, such as posture, scent, and the flicker of a smile, are processed instantaneously, triggering a cascade of emotions and desires that shape our choices before we even know we've made them.

Reason becomes a distant charioteer in that fleeting instant, struggling to maintain control as the unruly horses of desire gallop recklessly forward, heedless of the forthcoming consequences. This is not a trivial failing of will, but a drama as old as consciousness: a dance of tension between impulse and restraint, the primal instincts that swirl within, and the rational mind that precariously rides atop this chaos. It's the ceaseless interplay of impulse and restraint, instinct and intellect, chaos and control.

Philosophers have peered into this inner theater for centuries. Plato's chariot comes to mind: the soul, pulled by two horses. One noble, straining for wisdom, and the other wild, hungry for pleasure. The charioteer, our reason, strives for balance, but must accept that the horses will never be fully tamed. Zen sages often describe the mind as a restless monkey, constantly jumping from craving to aversion and never finding peace. The path they advocate is not about eliminating desire but rather embracing it, understanding its roots, and learning to hold onto it.

Desire is not a flaw to be cured, but a signature of our humanity: a legacy written deep into our bones. Before we reasoned, we felt. Emotion is not the adversary of thought, but its ancestor and companion. It is the fertile soil from which our ideas and intentions grow, the pulse beneath the surface of every choice we make.

The architecture of the brain tells its own story. The brain is not just a machine but a living manuscript where primal instincts resonate beneath the surface of reason. The limbic system quietly works deep inside, while the amygdala sends quick, powerful messages. The amygdala fires bursts of raw, electric code: hunger that gnaws, fear that freezes, joy that erupts in sunlit surges. They aren't just signals; they're ancient instincts, handed down over thousands of years, each one meant to help us survive.

The rational mind, the cortex with its delicate folds, does not draft this story. It interprets, translates, *survives.* It wrestles with storms of anger that crackle like lightning, clings to love's warm currents, trembles before longing's tidal pull. These forces are not aberrations. They are ancestral fires, banked and relit in the dark forge of evolution.

To understand this is to stand humbled before our own biology. The brain does not pit reason against instinct; it marries them. Our noblest aspirations rise not in spite of desire's heat, but because of it. The same neural pathways that once propelled our ancestors to flee predators or cradle their young now drive us to create, to connect, to reach for meaning. We are not fallen creatures, but living archives; walking testaments to the brutal, beautiful alchemy of endurance.

This drama of desire is not ours alone.

It echoes in the bonds we share with other creatures. To truly understand how biology affects our emotions, one only needs to consider the companionship of man's best friend: the dog. With their warm, expressive eyes and wagging tails, dogs demonstrate true joy and connection. Watch as a dog greets its beloved human: the tail becomes a metronome of joy, pure happiness in motion. Eye shine. Ears flatten. The body sways in a playful dance. In these gestures, we glimpse the raw language of longing, love, and belonging. It's a language older than words, expressed through movement and felt in the heart.

Charles Darwin, in his *The Expression of the Emotions in Man and Animals*, saw in the dog's exuberant welcome and mournful gaze a mirror of our own emotional lives. "Man himself cannot express love and humility by external signs, so plainly as does a dog," he observed. He was struck by how a dog's drooping ears, wagging tail, and shifting posture come together as a wordless display of affection and humility. These are not mere reflexes. They are the language of connection, shaped by evolution and deepened by every shared experience.

Reflecting on a dog's emotional world is a glimpse into something universal. Their capacity for joy, empathy, and even guilt is not a pale imitation of our own but proof that the roots of desire and feeling run deep. They cross the boundaries between species. You're drawn into a quiet understanding when a dog looks up at you, eyes shining with trust or sorrow. When staring into puppy-dog eyes, you can't help but feel a quiet connection. You realize that your longing and connection are not just your private feelings. They're part of who we are, handed down through generations, shaped by a world where being in tune with other people and animals was key to survival. They are the pulse of life itself, echoing through fur and flesh, memory and instinct.

In these moments, we are reminded that our urges and affections are not flaws to be tamed. They are our living inheritance, shaped by a world where survival once meant staying alert. The dog's wagging tail, the warmth of its body pressed against your side; these simple gestures pull us back to something essential.

Emotion is the ground of being. It's the foundation of our being, the deep well from which reason and reflection spring. In the company of dogs, we see ourselves more clearly. We are beings of longing, molded by biology, yet capable of deep connection and understanding. This emotional landscape is reflected in the brain itself. The brain is not a battleground of sin and virtue. It's more like a vast, tangled forest. Some trails bring us to glistening glades of fulfillment, while others lead us into shadowed thickets of frustration. Each path winds into the same vast ecosystem. This is the complex biology of desire.

To live contemplatively is to pause amid this tangled forest and truly listen to the pull of our longings and the gentle whisper of reason. It is to recognize that our struggles are not failures. They are invitations to understand ourselves. This is not merely introspection but a turning outward and inward at once, a receptivity to the world and the depths of our own being.

Within us, the limbic system's architecture and the dance of neurochemicals like dopamine and oxytocin shape our experience. These quick, primal signals do more than keep us alive. They give us raw glimpses into our deepest hopes and fears, lighting up the desires and worries that color our days. These offer raw insights into our innermost selves. They illuminate the desires and fears that define our lives. To see this, to truly feel the sequence, emotion first, reason after, is to be human.

Emotions are not obstacles. They are as essential as reason in shaping the arc of our days. They guide, they warn, they inspire. If you pay attention, you'll notice the pattern: emotion comes first, reason follows. That's the human way. Consider the following everyday dilemmas that reflect this.

Imagine an intense wave of jealousy that surges over you as you sit across from a friend who is gushing over their latest accomplishment. Every word seems to highlight what you haven't yet achieved, at least, not yet. Alternatively, think of the simmering annoyance as you creep forward in a suffocating sea of traffic. Every moment feels like an eternity. A jarring horn's blow pierces every inch forward. It turns what was once an everyday commute into a boiling cauldron of frustration.

We all wrestle with the gap between the person we want to be and the person we are in everyday life. This is the dichotomy between our ideals and our lived reality. It's a constant tug-of-war between what we think we should do and what we actually do. In these moments, shame has a way of sneaking in. It's a quiet, persistent voice in the back of our minds. It tells us we're not enough, weak, selfish, or somehow flawed. It can make us question our worth and wonder if we'll ever measure up to our expectations.

But what if we looked at these struggles differently? What if we reframed them not as moral shortcomings but as valuable opportunities?

Instead of seeing them as proof of failure, we could treat them as invitations to get curious about what's really going on inside us. They are invitations to look deeper. These moments encourage us to ask what's really driving us: what we want, what we fear, what we're hoping for.

This book advocates for a perspective grounded in understanding rather than judgment. It encourages us to abandon the outdated notion that our behaviors can define us as "bad." It invites more existential inquiries: *What underlying narratives shape my inclinations? What desires propel me toward these choices?*

This journey draws on what neuroscience has taught us. It offers a way to make sense of the colorful, tangled, and sometimes overwhelming experience of being human. It seeks to illuminate the stunning complexities of our thoughts and actions. Since the dawn of our species, desire has served as our navigational compass.

Our brains were shaped by evolution to help us survive in a world that was often harsh and unpredictable. This world was a place where food was scarce, and danger lurked around every corner. Yet, now we are ensnared in a contemporary world overflowing with abundance and incessant stimulation. The same neural pathways once ignited by the pursuit of survival, ripe fruit, or a secure refuge now blaze with excitement at the flickering lights of social media, the thrill of acquiring the latest trend, or the siren call of a sweet indulgence.

What lies ahead in these pages is a journey into the entangled roots and soaring branches of our emotional and biological existence. Each chapter peels back another layer of what it means to be human. The chapters reveal the interplay between our ancient instincts and the modern environment that shapes our choices and desires. As we move through this exploration together, you might begin to see the beauty in our complexity and realize that our struggles aren't signs of failure. They're simply part of what it means to be alive.

In the chapters that follow, we'll begin with the most intimate of urges: our longing for closeness and pleasure. We'll explore how the brain orchestrates intimacy, why we seek connection, and how stress colors our closest relationships. Then, we'll turn to the powerful forces of appetite and excess, seeing how the gut and brain conspire to drive us toward indulgence, and why modern abundance can send our pleasure circuits into overdrive.

From there, we'll navigate the labyrinth of decision-making, tracing how impulses, temptations, and the promise of reward can override reason and steer our lives in unexpected directions. We'll examine the emotional storms that follow when our desires are thwarted. Stress, frustration, and unprocessed feelings can ripple through our minds and bodies, impacting health, memory, and relationships.

We'll confront the universal urge to avoid discomfort, uncovering why motivation sometimes slips through our fingers and how the brain's chemistry shapes our willingness to act. We'll journey into the heart of selfhood and memory, asking how our brains construct identity, pride, and the stories we tell about who we are. The book will also reveal the social roots of our desires, from the need to belong and compete to how we empathize, compare, and find meaning in community. We'll discover just how deeply our brains are wired for connection. Even the sting of jealousy or the warmth of shared joy isn't random; it's written into our neural code.

We'll also look ahead, exploring how science and technology might help us change our habits, manage our cravings, and even reshape the very circuits that drive our desires. We'll grapple with the ethics of self-modification and what it really means to embrace our humanity.

With each chapter, you'll find stories, scientific discoveries, and practical insights illuminating your mind's inner workings. You'll learn how to harness the power of self-awareness, using knowledge of the brain to make wiser choices, nurture healthier relationships, and cultivate a more compassionate view of yourself and others.

So, as you turn the page, prepare to meet yourself anew-not as a battleground of sin and virtue, but as a wondrous, evolving being shaped by millions of years of biology, memory, and feeling. The journey ahead will show that understanding desire is not to tame or banish it, but to recognize its place at the heart of what it means to be alive.

PART ONE
A DESIRING BRAIN

CHAPTER 1
LOVE AT FIRST SIGHT: THE CHEMISTRY OF ROMANCE, LOVE AND LUST

IT WAS A TUESDAY EVENING, the kind where the sun began to dip below the horizon, bathing the coffee shop in a warm, golden glow. Anne curled into her favorite corner nook as if settling into a secret cocoon. She was halfway through her drink as she glanced around. Her gaze settled on the stranger seated at the next table. When their eyes locked for a fleeting second, it felt as though time paused. The world around her faded into a soft blur.

A sudden flutter in her chest took her by surprise, a sensation that spread like warmth from her heart to her fingertips. What Anne didn't realize was that this electric moment was more than just chance; it was her brain at work. In an instant, neural circuits in her limbic system fired, dopamine flooded her synapses, and adrenaline spiked her heart rate. The ancient machinery of lust and desire had been activated, setting off a cascade that neuroscience is only beginning to map fully.

Across the room, Jerry nursed his coffee, lost in thought, as he scrolled through emails on his phone. He was only vaguely aware of the gentle hum of conversation and the comforting warmth of the shop —until he looked up and saw her. She sat in the corner, half-shadowed by the fading light, her presence somehow magnetic. The sensation was primal, a surge of adrenaline and curiosity mixed with a sudden, inexplicable certainty that he needed to know her. He found himself straightening, his attention narrowing to a single, vivid point: her smile, the way she tucked a strand of hair behind her ear, the spark of recognition in her gaze.

For Jerry, too, this moment felt like magic, a collision of fate and chemistry. Yet, just as with Anne, the real story was unfolding within: a cascade of neurotransmitters, a symphony of brain regions firing in synchrony, orchestrating the rush of desire, the longing for intimacy, and the first stirrings of romance. Most of us have felt that unmistakable jolt of connection at some point in our lives, but *what is it that transforms a fleeting look into a cascade of emotion and anticipation?*

These moments are so universal and deeply ingrained in our brains that they've inspired entire genres of storytelling. Today, the world is in the grip of a new literary wave: *romantasy*. This blend of romance and fantasy, where love stories unfold amid dragons, magic, and epic quests, has taken both bookstores and social media by storm. On BookTok, TikTok's vibrant book-loving community, readers share their favorite tropes, swoon over fictional heroes, and debate the best "enemies-to-lovers" arcs, fueling sales and shaping trends in an instant.

Why this obsession? At its core, romantasy taps into the same neurobiological circuitry that fires when Anne's pulse quickens or Jerry's attention narrows to a single smile. These stories offer more than escapism; they deliver emotional catharsis, a sense of belonging, and the thrill of desire, mirroring the dopamine and oxytocin surges that make real-life attraction so intoxicating. The popularity of these books is proof: our brains are hardwired for connection, craving not just adventure but the electric charge of intimacy and romance, whether in a crowded coffee shop or a world of fae and fantasy.

This universal hunger for connection—so vividly captured in both fiction and real life—begins in the smallest of moments. In the breathless instant after a first glance, when desire flickers to life like a spark in the silent dark and reason trips and falls behind, the world seems to stand still. Yet, beneath this swirl of poetry and raw emotion, a hidden architecture is at work. Science reveals that these electric moments of attraction are not just whims of the heart but the result of neural activity deep within the brain.

~

'Love at first sight' rarely describes the slow burn of romance. Instead, it's the electric jolt of attraction, a thunderclap of desire. In the blink of an eye, your brain's limbic system—the sentinel of emotion—sounds the alarm. The limbic system is responsible for quickly assessing the emotional significance and potential reward or threat. It's older than conscious thought, wired for survival, and always on the lookout for signals that matter. These lightning-fast assessments are driven by instinct rather than logic. They are fueled by the primal need to survive and, just as urgently, to connect.

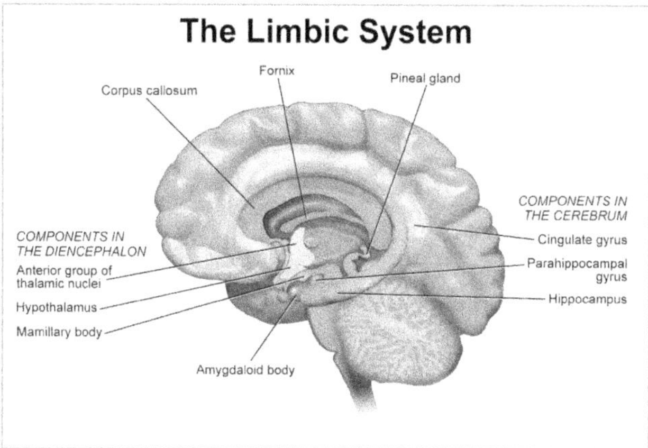

Figure 1. *The Limbic System.* Blausen Medical

Picture stepping into a lively party or scrolling through a dating app. In mere seconds, a blend of physical features, social cues, and your own background sets off an almost instant "maybe" or "not my type" response. Scientists have identified a key player in this process: the dorsomedial prefrontal cortex, a highly sophisticated brain region located near the front of the head. Research has shown that when people see the face of a potential match—even before any conversation —different parts within this region light up, busy sorting clues such as looks, body language, and other subtle signals. One segment focuses on classic signs of attractiveness; another tunes into the qualities that make someone personally appealing, striking a balance between universal traits and unique preferences.

When it comes to beauty and compatibility, the process involves more than just surface-level judgments. Features like symmetrical eyes or an "average" face tend to appeal to many and activate areas of the brain linked to reward—a gentle nudge to take a closer look. These universal signals, deeply rooted in human evolution, explain why some faces draw attention across cultures and generations. But a real connection isn't simply about meeting a checklist. Sometimes, it's a quirky laugh, a distinct style, or a shared hobby that stands out. Even if these traits stray from convention, the brain has circuits poised to respond when those personal quirks click. This explains why what's magnetic for one person might seem unremarkable to another; everyone's "type" is crafted by a blend of biology and lived experience.

True attraction, then, is a dance between broad appeal and authentic connection. What captures our interest—whether across a crowded room or in a digital profile—isn't just flawless looks. It's the mix of admired features and genuine individuality that brings someone into focus. The brain responds swiftly to symmetry and "average" faces, but it also gives special attention to uniqueness and authenticity—making it possible for sparks to fly in the most unexpected matches.

Yet, the brain's remarkable "social prediction engine" extends beyond romance. The same system helps us choose friends, decide whom to trust, and seek allies. When this circuitry encounters obstacles—such as social anxiety or certain neurodevelopmental differences —quick connections and social reading become tougher. Fortunately, science shows that these skills can be developed. New experiences, learning, and small acts of social courage help the brain become more attuned to picking up cues and making connections. Awkward beginnings can mature into deeper relationships as the mind adapts, refines its "gut feelings," and learns from each new interaction.

Lust, in its purest form, is sparked by a whisper of scent, the curve of a smile, or the confident tilt of a chin. These subtle cues trigger a cascade of sex hormones, such as testosterone and estrogen. They surge through your bloodstream. This process is almost instantaneous and largely subconscious, having been designed by evolution to identify potential mates quickly.

It is raw. It is urgent. It is primal. It is a powerful craving that pulses beneath the surface, pulling you toward connection with a mix of excitement and anticipation. It's the spark that electrifies your breath, sets your pulse galloping, and ignites your senses like a firework bursting in the night, often before your mind has a chance to catch up. It's the body's way of saying: *Pay attention. This matters.*

The neurobiological foundation of lust is centered in the hypothalamus. When lust takes hold, the hypothalamus sends signals that trigger the release of sex hormones. These hormones not only stir desire but also sharpen your senses. They heighten sensitivity, increase blood flow, and tune your senses to every subtle cue.

Of course, lust is more than just hormones racing through your veins. It's a dance of chemicals and neurons, with dopamine taking center stage. Often called the brain's "feel-good" chemical, dopamine lights up the brain's reward centers. This pathway floods your brain with waves of pleasure and reward. It's the reason your pulse quickens at a glance, why your thoughts might circle back to that person again and again.

At the same time this rush is happening, the part of your brain that usually keeps your impulses in check, the prefrontal cortex, quietly steps back. During these moments of intense sexual arousal, its activity diminishes, loosening the tether on your self-control.

Yet discoveries suggest the story is richer. The prefrontal cortex, once cast as a mere brake pedal, flexes with a subtler rhythm. In a series of breakthrough studies in mice, new circuits were traced within the layered folds. This is a network that listens to oxytocin and ovarian surges. It also calibrates the drive to seek connection. When these neurons fire in a fertile female, they paint the mind with longing; in males, the same electrical storm cools the urge.

All of this explains why lust can sweep away hesitation and caution. It's as if your brain, in a moment of wild abandon, hands the keys over to your deepest cravings. You're invited to surrender to the moment, to let yourself be carried away by the irresistible pull of what you want. Boundaries blur, and reason retreats, leaving you open to the thrill of acting on pure, unfiltered desire.

This interplay of hormones and brain activity brews the unmistakable rush of lust: a heady cocktail of craving, excitement, and anticipation. It can be as exhilarating as it is overwhelming. It may feel like standing at the edge of a precipice, heart pounding, breath quickening, caught between fear and longing. This is your body's biological invitation to connect and explore. At its core, lust is a profoundly human experience. It is a reminder that beneath the layers of civilization and restraint, we are still driven by the same primal forces that have shaped us for millennia.

Yet, while lust ignites this initial spark, it is only the opening act in a far more intricate and beautifully coordinated biological performance. Lust sets the pace, but sexual arousal is where the body fully joins the dance.

~

Once craving takes hold, your brain transforms those intense feelings into a cascade of physical reactions. Sexual arousal is a symphony of activation, an intricate partnership between your central nervous system, made of the brain and spinal cord, and the vast, winding highways of your peripheral nervous system. Together, they process every whisper of sensation, every electric touch, ensuring that your body responds in real time to the world around you. They create a seamless flow of sensation and reaction.

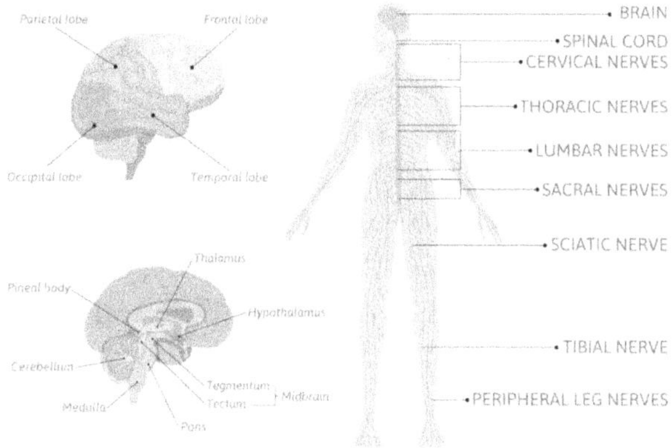

Figure 2. *The Central Nervous System.* Macrovector on Freepik

Your brain's emotional hubs, the amygdala and hippocampus, instantly scan fleeting moments, such as a gentle brush of fingers against your skin or the sparkle of a lover's smile. The amygdala acts like an emotional radar, scanning for signals of safety, excitement, or danger. Meanwhile, the hippocampus sifts through your memories, adding context and color to the present moment. When these regions give the green light, they trigger a chain reaction, initiating physiological changes that prepare the body for intimacy.

In this way, sexual arousal is much more than just feeling "turned on." It's a full-body experience. The symphony of neural signals and hormonal shifts heightens sensitivity, increases blood flow, and prepares the body to respond to desire. The leap from lust to arousal is the moment when emotion and biology collide, turning a flicker of attraction into a palpable, embodied experience.

When you see, hear, touch, or even imagine something sexually stimulating, the limbic system springs into action. The amygdala evaluates the emotional weight of the stimulus, while the hippocampus contextualizes it within your personal history. Together, they communicate with the hypothalamus, the brain's master regulator of bodily functions and primal drives.

The hypothalamus acts like a conductor, coordinating the release of hormones and activating neural pathways that prepare the body for sexual response. It signals the pituitary gland to release hormones that influence your reproductive organs. This sparks a surge of testosterone and estrogen. These hormones fan the flames of arousal, fueling your body's readiness for intimacy.

The brain's role is only part of the story. Arousal also depends on the autonomic nervous system. This system regulates involuntary bodily functions, including heart rate, breathing, and blood flow. This system has two main branches that work together during arousal.

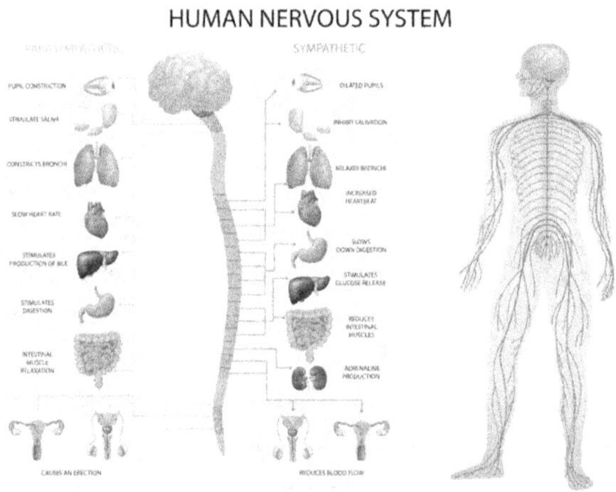

Figure 3. *The Parasympathetic & Sympathetic Nervous Systems.* Macrovector on Freepik

The parasympathetic nervous system is responsible for what are called "rest and digest" functions. During sexual arousal, it promotes the widening of blood vessels. This widening, also known as vasodilation, increases blood flow to the genital area. It leads to erections in men and sexual arousal in women, the physical signs that the body is responding to desire.

The sympathetic nervous system, often referred to as the "fight or flight" system, also plays a role in increasing heart rate, blood pressure, and respiration. This dual activation explains why sexual arousal involves such widespread physiological changes. It encompasses everything from flushed skin to increased breathing rate.

Another layer is the spinal cord, particularly in the sacral region, located near the lower back. This area contains neural circuits capable of generating basic sexual reflexes, such as genital responses, even in the absence of direct brain input. This means that some sexual responses can occur reflexively, independent of conscious thought. However, the brain continuously modulates and coordinates these reflexes, allowing sexual behavior to be both automatic and under voluntary control. This hierarchical system lets us respond instinctively while also integrating emotional, psychological, and social factors into our sexual experiences.

How does this wave of desire turn into action? Why do we sometimes act on impulse, even when reason tells us to pause? And what does this tell us about ourselves and our relationships?

With your reward system humming and your self-control taking a backseat, the stage is set. Motor regions in your brain coordinate movement, while your spinal cord handles reflexive responses like genital arousal or rhythmic contractions. The result? *You act*—sometimes before you've had a chance to think it through.

Research shows that only a small fraction of our decisions are truly rational; emotions, instincts, and the drive for reward shape most of them. This isn't a flaw—it's a feature of our biology, honed by evolution to help us survive and thrive. Emotions guide our attention, sharpen our memories, and drive us toward what feels good, even when it's not always the wisest choice. So, we leap, we let nature guide us, and as sexual arousal builds, the brain and body prepare for what comes next.

This journey of desire and arousal culminates in orgasm. This powerful, multi-sensory event stands as the peak of sexual pleasure and human connection. Often playfully called "the big O," orgasm is far more than a fleeting release. It's one of the most intense and widespread neural events known to science and one of the most misunderstood throughout history.

The orgasm is often poetically referred to as *"la petite mort,"* which translates to "the little death." It originated in 16th-century France and became a common metaphor for orgasm by the late 19th century. The term expresses the paradoxical nature of orgasm as a momentary "death" of the self, where consciousness and ego dissolve in a fleeting surrender, only to be reborn anew. Historically, the idea of orgasm as a "little death" was also deeply intertwined with medical beliefs that sexual climax drained a person's vital life force. This idea persisted across cultures and centuries.

In ancient Greece, for instance, Hippocrates and Aristotle both warned that excessive sexual activity could weaken the body, and the loss of seminal fluid was thought to deplete energy and shorten lifespan. In Traditional Chinese Medicine, orgasm was seen as "spending" Jing, the essential life energy stored in the kidneys, while Western medicine once blamed sexual pleasure for everything from exhaustion to infertility. What is perhaps little known and most fascinating is how these ancient beliefs still ripple through modern wellness and spiritual practices.

Today, certain spiritual traditions still caution against "losing" sexual energy through orgasm, advocating instead for channeling it toward creativity and vitality. Yet modern neuroscience reveals a dramatically different story. Rather than depleting life, orgasm is a life-affirming storm of neural fireworks. It illuminates vast networks throughout the brain. Reward centers blaze, emotional hubs pulse, and even regions controlling movement and automatic bodily functions join the celebration. The result is a cascade of feel-good chemicals—dopamine and oxytocin—that bathe the body in pleasure, deepen emotional bonds, and melt away stress.

As this cerebral light show unfolds, it gives orgasms a unique and subjective quality. The experience is shaped by a complex interplay of brain regions associated with euphoria, and those responsible for craving become activated simultaneously. This intricate connection results in the unmistakable erotic intensity that characterizes sexual climax. The widespread brain activation during orgasm also stimulates pain-inhibitory systems, transforming pleasure into a powerful pain reliever. This effect helps to explain why many people report feeling wonderfully relaxed, even blissfully numb, during and after moments of sexual ecstasy.

It turns out that all isn't fair in love. Research shows that there are differences in sexual brain activity between men and women, particularly in the ways they experience pleasure. These variations highlight how each sex processes pleasure differently, among other factors.

Sex hormones exert a profound influence on brain structure and function throughout development and into adulthood. Testosterone and estrogen affect the development of neural circuits involved in sexual behavior, creating sex differences in brain organization that persist throughout life. These hormonal influences help explain observed differences in sexual motivation, arousal patterns, and relationship behaviors between males and females.

The cyclical nature of female hormones creates dynamic changes in sexual motivation and behavior throughout the menstrual cycle. Estrogen and progesterone fluctuations influence the activity of neural circuits in the hypothalamus and limbic system, with peak fertility periods typically associated with increased sexual motivation and changed mate preferences. These hormonal cycles reflect evolved mechanisms for timing sexual behavior with reproductive opportunities.

Male hormonal patterns exhibit less dramatic cyclical variation but still significantly influence sexual behavior and bonding. Testosterone levels typically decrease during pair bonding and early parenthood, potentially promoting monogamous behavior and paternal investment. This hormonal shift explains the transition from pursuit-oriented mating behavior to maintenance-oriented relationship behavior in long-term couples.

The temporal dynamics of sexual arousal also differ between males and females. Males often exhibit more rapid and focused neural responses to sexual stimuli. At the same time, females typically display more distributed and sustained patterns of activation. These differences may contribute to the observed variations in sexual response patterns and relationship satisfaction between the sexes.

During sexual activity and the build-up to orgasm, what is called the plateau phase, women's brains show more activation in areas involved in touch and movement. This suggests that women are more attuned to the sensory and physical aspects of the experience. It may be possible that women integrate more of their body's sensations into the moment. Men, on the other hand, exhibit more activity in regions associated with visual processing and motor planning. This might mean that men are more visually stimulated or focused on the mechanics of the act during this phase.

Once orgasm arrives, though, most of the differences fade away. It is one of those rare moments where the brain's response is strikingly similar between the sexes. Neuroimaging studies reveal that during climax, both men and women experience a surge of activity in the anterior lobe of the cerebellum, a region crucial for coordinating movement and emotion.

Both sexes also experience a dramatic drop in activity in the orbitofrontal cortex, the brain's "brake pedal" for self-control and social judgment. This deactivation is thought to be what gives orgasm its sense of reckless abandon, the feeling of letting go and being swept away by pleasure. For both sexes, the experience of orgasm is marked by a flood of dopamine, oxytocin, and other feel-good chemicals, creating a sense of euphoria and connection that is hard to match.

Two central cores of the brain's reward system, the ventral tegmental area and nucleus accumbens, become overwhelmed by the dopamine flood that accompanies the orgasm. These two areas already exhibit high activity during sexual arousal. Once the dopamine hits, we are motivated to seek it out again and again. This pattern mirrors other intensely rewarding experiences, like savoring your favorite food.

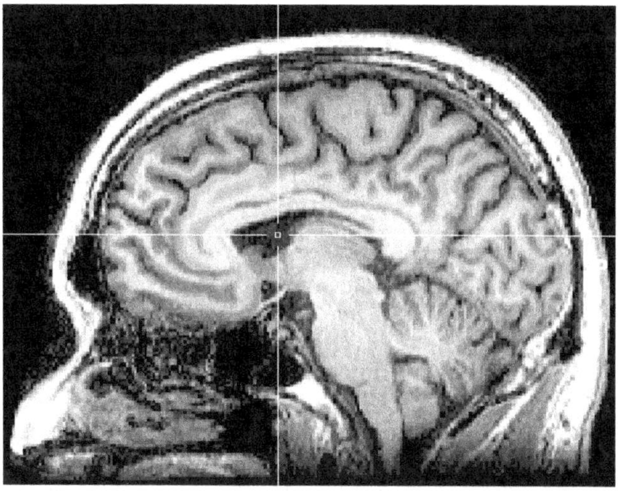

Figure 4. *Sagittal MRI slice with highlighting indicating the location of the anterior cingulate cortex.* Geoff B Hall

While the limbic and reward systems are busy generating pleasure and emotion, higher-order brain regions, such as the anterior cingulate cortex, play a more nuanced role in this process. This cortex processes the emotional significance of sexual experiences and is particularly active during the transition from arousal to orgasm. After orgasm, the brain releases prolactin, a hormone that promotes feelings of satisfaction and relaxation. This is part of the reason why we feel so content and calm after sex and why the experience can be deeply restorative.

For some, this peak of pleasure becomes a relentless, uncontrollable force. For a small subset of individuals, orgasm isn't a fleeting peak but an unending storm. Persistent Genital Arousal Disorder causes spontaneous, intrusive orgasms—sometimes hundreds daily—without sexual desire or stimulation. These episodes can last for hours, days, or even years, often triggered by mundane actions such as sitting or walking. Seventy percent of patients with the disorder report experiencing depression or anxiety; forty percent contemplate suicide due to feelings of shame and helplessness.

Many of us hear about the idea of multiple orgasms or persistent arousal and think... *"that doesn't sound so bad,"* but imagine, for a moment, being overwhelmed—not once, not twice, but over a hundred times a day and being stopped mid-sentence, mid-step, or mid-thought. How long before you would be begging, pleading, and wishing for a reprieve?

For Kim Ramsey, a woman from the United Kingdom, this became her relentless, exhausting reality. A reality that would change her life and challenge everything we think we know about sexual desire and the brain. For years, her life was hijacked by her own body. Her story began with a seemingly ordinary accident. In 2001, she took a fall down a flight of stairs—an event that, at the time, seemed like just another bump in life's unpredictable road. In the days that followed, she began to experience something profoundly unusual: spontaneous, uncontrollable orgasms that struck without warning, sometimes every few minutes, and often while she was sitting, standing, or walking.

The sensations were not pleasurable. Instead, they were overwhelming, exhausting, and deeply distressing. She found herself at the mercy of her own body, unable to predict or control the waves of arousal that washed over her day and night. She even described it as feeling like being electrocuted again and again and again.

In this case, the root cause was a Tarlov cyst, a fluid-filled sac that had formed on her spine after her fall. These cysts can press on or irritate the sacral nerves, which are responsible for transmitting sensations to and from the genital area. When these nerves are overstimulated, they can send false signals to the brain, tricking it into believing the body is experiencing sexual arousal. The brain's reward system becomes hyperactive, flooding the body with dopamine and other feel-good chemicals. In persistent genital arousal disorder, the system is stuck in overdrive, creating a cycle of unrelenting arousal that is anything but pleasurable.

She sought help from numerous doctors, but many were either unfamiliar with her disorder or dismissed her symptoms as psychological. She tried a variety of treatments, from medications to nerve blocks. Nothing brought lasting relief. The constant arousal severely impacted her mental health, leading to anxiety, depression, and a profound sense of isolation.

After years of struggle, Ramsey found hope when a specialist identified a connection between her Tarlov cyst and her symptoms. In 2008, she underwent spinal surgery to remove the cyst and relieve nerve pressure. Despite the risks, the surgery allowed her to regain control of her life. Her symptoms improved significantly; the frequency and intensity of her orgasms decreased, bringing her closer to normalcy. Although she still experiences some residual effects, the surgery marked a turning point in her journey.

Kim Ramsey's story is a powerful reminder of just how deeply the brain and body are entwined in matters of desire and pleasure. Her experience with persistent genital arousal disorder shows us what happens when the brain's delicate balance is disrupted—when the floodgates of arousal are forced open, and pleasure becomes a relentless storm. For most of us, though, sexual desire and arousal are fleeting and pleasurable, a natural part of being human.

What about romantic attraction? How does it fit into this picture?

Romantic attraction is both like and unlike lust, sexual arousal, and orgasm. It shares some of the same neural pathways and chemicals, but it is also something more. It involves a deeper emotional and psychological connection. While it can be sparked quickly, it usually develops over time as we learn more about a person's personality, values, and compatibility.

Romantic attraction often begins with something as simple as a glance, a conversation, or a shared moment of laughter. Like lust, it can ignite quickly, sparking the brain's reward centers and flooding us with dopamine that makes us feel excited, energized, and eager for more. While lust is rooted in physical desire and the pursuit of pleasure, romantic attraction quickly grows into something more profound: a longing to know someone's mind and heart, to share experiences, and to build a life together.

As we spend time with someone, learning about their personality, values, and unique quirks, romantic attraction tends to deepen. The same brain regions that light up during sexual arousal also become active during romantic love. Research shows that both passionate love and maternal love activate these areas, suggesting that our capacity for deep connection is a survival mechanism, hardwired to help us bond and cooperate.

Interestingly, romantic attraction isn't just about dopamine. Oxytocin, often called the "love hormone," plays a starring role as well. It's released during physical contact, sexual activity, and even affectionate conversation, promoting trust, empathy, and emotional closeness. In both men and women, oxytocin levels rise during arousal and peak at orgasm. Studies with prairie voles—small mammals known for their monogamous relationships—have shown that oxytocin receptor density is directly linked to pair-bonding behavior. When scientists activate these receptors, the animals form stronger attachments to their partners.

Oxytocin isn't the only hormone in the mix. Vasopressin is especially important in males. It works in conjunction with oxytocin to support long-term commitment and protective, mate-guarding behaviors. Together, these hormones create a robust neurochemical foundation for lasting romantic relationships.

Another chemical involved in romance and worth mentioning is serotonin. Serotonin is a neurotransmitter usually associated with mood regulation. It plays a more complex role in romantic love. During the early stages of attraction, serotonin levels drop, mirroring patterns seen in obsessive-compulsive disorder. This decrease may explain the obsessive thoughts and intense focus that often accompany new love. At the same time, norepinephrine levels rise, sharpening attention and energy and keeping us fixated on our romantic partner.

Neuroimaging studies reveal that simply looking at a photo of a loved one activates brain regions associated with motivation and reward, while reducing activity in areas linked to negative emotions and critical judgment. This neural shift helps explain the idealization and rose-colored glasses that often come with early romance. As relationships mature and move toward a more stable attachment, serotonin levels normalize, obsessive thinking fades, and emotional states become more balanced.

Initial sexual experiences trigger neuroplasticity—changes in brain structure and function, particularly in the medial prefrontal cortex and nucleus accumbens. These changes strengthen neural connections associated with partner-specific memories. This explains why certain relationships leave such a lasting impression. The degree of neural synchronization between these areas predicts the strength of pair-bonding behaviors. It suggests that successful long-term relationships depend on a delicate balance between reward, memory, and executive control.

Successful relationships are characterized by behavioral and physiological synchrony, where partners move, think, and even breathe in harmony with each other. In stable, loving relationships, research shows that baseline levels of oxytocin are often significantly elevated and consistently high over time. The mirror neuron system, which enables us to simulate and understand each other's actions and emotions automatically, is particularly active during intimate moments, fostering emotional attunement and deepening connections.

This synchrony manifests in various ways. Couples often find that their movements flow together effortlessly. Whether engaged in conversation or dancing, couples tend to mirror each other. Additionally, studies indicate that even heart rates can synchronize. Some couples experience similar physiological responses during shared moments of joy or stress. This intricate coordination nurtures and strengthens emotional bonds, creating a profound sense of shared experience and mutual support. As this synchrony deepens over time, it predicts greater relationship satisfaction and longevity.

In contrast, a breakdown in synchrony, reflected in decreased coordination and physiological alignment, may signal potential issues in the relationship. Therapeutic interventions, such as mindfulness or couples therapy, can help restore harmony. They've also been seen to reconnect partners who are struggling to feel connected.

From the initial spark of attraction to the deep synchrony of lasting love, emotion guides the way. Our brains are wired to feel before we think and to connect before we analyze. The neurobiological understanding of sexual behavior provides new frameworks for understanding and treating sexual dysfunction.

Many sexual problems stem from disruptions in neural circuits and neurochemical systems. For instance, erectile dysfunction often arises from impaired dopamine signaling to regions responsible for penile blood flow. At the same time, a decrease in sexual desire may indicate a disrupted reward system function.

Depression and anxiety often coexist with sexual dysfunction, mirroring interconnected neural pathways that influence both mental and sexual health. Given this multifaceted nature, it's clear that effective treatments must engage with multiple systems concurrently to achieve meaningful results. This insight has paved the way for holistic approaches in sexual therapy. These integrate psychological counseling, pharmacological treatments, and lifestyle modifications. Such comprehensive strategies aim to address the root causes of dysfunction, fostering a more integrated pathway to healing and enhanced sexual well-being.

Neuroscience also provides evidence-based strategies for enhancing relationship satisfaction. Interventions that encourage behavioral synchrony, such as participating in coordinated activities and practicing mindfulness, can strengthen the neural connections related to bonding and emotional attachment. These methods stimulate the same neurobiological systems that support the formation of successful relationships.

The future of relationship therapy increasingly integrates neurobiological insights into treatment. Techniques that promote oxytocin release, enhance dopaminergic reward responses, and improve neural synchrony between partners show promise in addressing relationship difficulties. This biologically informed approach complements traditional psychological therapies and may improve outcomes for couples facing relational issues.

Ultimately, this exploration highlights a profound truth: in the realm of sex, intimacy, and love, emotions frequently take the lead. Reason, on the other hand, often trails in their wake. Our brains instinctively prioritize swift, visceral reactions over the more painstaking processes of logic and detailed reflection.

As science delves deeper into this interplay, it gradually unveils the complexities of our ancient emotional dance. It sheds light on the biological foundations of our most intimate experiences. We come to understand that these emotions are not just fleeting impulses; they are complex phenomena that affect our survival, foster deep human connections, and define the essence of being alive.

CHAPTER 2
CRAVINGS UNLEASHED: EXPLORING EXCESSIVE DESIRE AND OVERINDULGENCE

YOU SIT HUNCHED at the kitchen table. Before you, the pint of ice cream sweats quietly. Your stomach is taut, distended with the ache of too much. Still, your mind spins in restless circles, haunted by the fleeting memory of sweetness. You can almost taste it still, the cold velvet on your tongue, the sugar dissolving into want. *Just one more bite,* the thought croons.

Most of us have wandered into this moment, if not with ice cream, then with chips, bread, chocolate—whatever form our longing takes. It is an all too common scene: the body signals fullness, a gentle protest rising from deep within, but desire lingers, bright and insistent, refusing to be soothed. There is a peculiar ache in this abundance, a paradox at the heart of plenty.

In a world where our cupboards overflow and supermarket aisles stretch endlessly, *why does "enough" slip through our fingers like water? Why does satisfaction, so close it seems we could almost hold it, dissolve into a gnawing urge for more?*

This is not just hunger but a yearning that lives in the marrow, a craving that is as much about memory and comfort as it is about taste. We eat not just to fill our bellies but to quiet the restless places inside us. Our bodies, sculpted by millennia of scarcity, are wired to seek, to store, to savor every calorie as if it might be the last. Survival mechanisms, once our shield against famine, now collide with a modern landscape of endless choice and convenience. The result is a cycle of overconsumption.

Most of us have felt that quiet sense of satisfaction that rises after a good meal. This sensation is not a simple switch. Your gut and brain are locked in a lifelong conversation. The dialogue is conducted not in words but in hormones, electrical impulses, and the whispers of 100 trillion microbes.

If we take a step back and listen closely, we see the conversation is conducted in two distinct languages. The first is the homeostatic pathway. It is the ancient and pragmatic voice of our biology. This pathway is concerned with survival and balance. It tells us when our bodies need nutrients, guiding us toward foods that replenish what we lack—vitamins, minerals, and fiber. It's the part of us that says, *"Eat the broccoli; it's good for you."* This system is grounded in necessity, a biological ledger keeping track of energy and nutrient demands.

Alongside this practical messenger runs a second, more seductive current: the hedonic pathway. This is the language of pleasure, desire, and reward. It speaks in dopamine-rich fireworks, lighting up the brain's pleasure centers and urging us to seek out indulgence. It's the voice that whispers, *"Eat the cake."* This pathway evolved to encourage behaviors that brought survival advantages, such as finding sweet fruits or fatty nuts. Yet, in today's world of hyper-palatable foods, its signals can become overpowering.

These two parallel circuits—one rooted in need, the other in delight—often pull us in opposite directions. They explain why it's possible to feel physically full, our stomachs stretched and hormones signaling satiety, yet remain psychologically ravenous, craving the next bite for the pleasure it promises rather than the nourishment it provides. Our biology is caught in a delicate tension between sustaining life and seeking joy, between the practical and the pleasurable.

This duality lies at the heart of why "enough" can feel so elusive. It is not simply a failure of willpower but a complex interplay of ancient survival systems and modern temptations, each speaking in its own language, each vying for our attention. This sets up a tug-of-war deep within the brain. On one side are the hormones and signals urging us to stop eating, each trying to restore balance. This is the satiety symphony, where leptin, GLP-1, and cholecystokinin, known as CCK, act as conductors. These three messengers orchestrate the delicate balance between hunger and fullness.

The first of these messengers, leptin, is a hormone produced by our fat cells—a kind of internal accountant, keeping a careful ledger of our energy reserves. When our fat stores are flush, leptin levels rise, sending steady updates to the brain: *"We're well-stocked. No need to go hunting for more."* In this way, leptin acts as a guardian, ensuring we don't waste precious energy searching for food when our pantry is already full.

Then there's cholecystokinin, or CCK, which steps in moments after we start eating. Released by the lining of the intestines, it's the conductor's baton in the symphony of satiety. As our stomach stretches with each bite, CCK signals to the brain: *"That's enough. Put down the fork."* It's a swift, decisive cue, helping us slow our eating and recognize fullness before we've gone too far. Where leptin manages the big picture, CCK is all about the present moment—an immediate, real-time check on our appetite.

If you've glanced at headlines, chatted with friends, or scrolled through social feeds lately, you've likely heard of the third messenger: GLP-1. This acronym is everywhere, the scientific secret behind a new wave of weight loss medications, such as Wegovy and Ozempic. GLP-1, or glucagon-like peptide-1, is another hormone produced in the gut. It slows the emptying of the stomach, allowing food to linger and prolonging the sensation of fullness. It also sends signals up the vagus nerve—our biological telephone line—directly to the brain's appetite centers, softly reinforcing the message: *"We're satisfied. The feast is over. Let's store this energy wisely."*

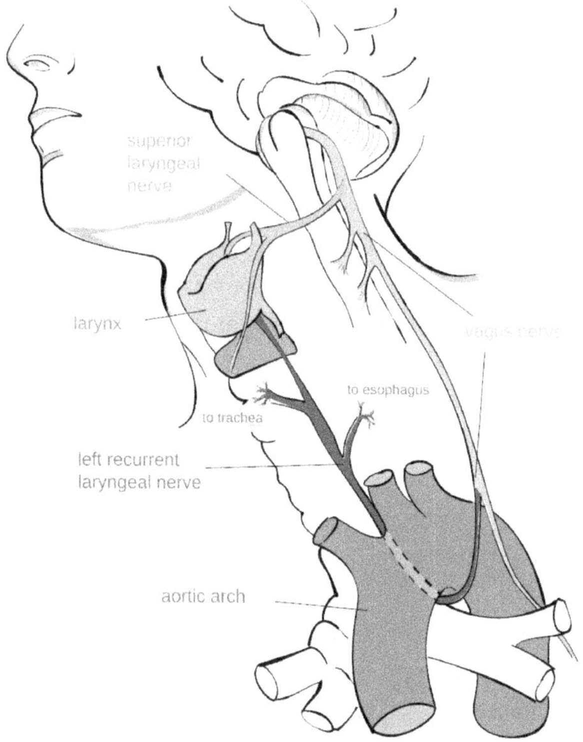

Figure 5. *A drawing of the left recurrent laryngeal nerve.* Jkwchui on Wikimedia Commons

GLP-1's influence extends even further. It stimulates the pancreas to release insulin, the hormone that helps shuttle sugar from the blood into cells. This ensures that the energy from our meal is stored or used efficiently. It is both a satiety signal and a metabolic guide, helping the body decide not only when to stop eating but also how to use the nutrients it has just received.

Why, then, do so many of us struggle to feel satisfied, even with such sophisticated systems in place?

First and foremost is stress. When life presses in, the body releases cortisol. This is our stress hormone. Cortisol's job is to marshal resources for survival. It sparks inflammation in the brain, clouding the signals that usually tell us we've had enough to eat. Stress can also weaken the protective barrier in our gut, letting tiny bacterial toxins slip into the bloodstream.

Imagine it as a mischievous locksmith, picking the gut's protective lock and allowing microscopic intruders—bacterial fragments and toxins—to slip into the bloodstream. This breach sets off a silent alarm. The immune system responds with inflammation, a low, persistent fire smoldering just below the surface. However, inflammation doesn't just make us feel run-down; it impairs the prefrontal cortex, the brain's executive center, weakening impulse control. It makes *"just saying no"* feel impossible.

A 2023 study found that mice fed a high-fat diet for six weeks developed inflammation in brain regions critical for decision-making. In this way, the foods we eat can slowly erode the very systems designed to regulate our desires. It's as if stress rewires our minds, making comfort foods not just appealing but almost irresistible. Brain scans using functional MRI support this.

When people are stressed, the amygdala—the brain's alarm center—lights up at the sight of high-calorie treats. At the same time, the prefrontal cortex, which helps us control impulses, grows quieter. The result? A perfect storm: our desire for tempting foods is turned up, just as our ability to say "no" is dialed down. In these moments, it's not just willpower we're fighting but a whole cascade of biological changes that make resisting comfort food feel nearly impossible.

Inflammation also interferes with leptin's message. This leaves the body in a perpetual state of perceived deprivation, even when energy stores are abundant. It's like static on a phone line. Proteins linked to this inflammation multiply, drowning out leptin's signal. Your brain, unable to hear the message, panics. It assumes the body is starving, even as fat stores sit full and untouched. This is why someone might feel ravenous after a sleepless night or during periods of stress: their body is swimming in energy, but their brain, deaf to leptin's reassurances, keeps sounding the alarm. *Eat. Now.*

GLP-1 and CCK, too, can lose their potency in the face of ultra-processed foods, which are engineered combinations of fat, sugar, and salt. These diminish the gut's responsiveness to these satiety cues. Such diets suppress GLP-1 release, delaying the onset of fullness and allowing desire to outpace need. The reward circuitry of the brain becomes hyper-responsive to these foods. It lights up in anticipation of pleasure and overpowers the quieter signals of homeostasis. Functional MRI studies confirm that, in those prone to overeating, the hypothalamus and insula—regions responsible for registering fullness—are less active. At the same time, the brain's pleasure centers remain ablaze, urging another bite, another taste, another fleeting reward. This tells us that not everyone walks this maze of hunger and satiety with the same compass.

For some, their neurons fire crisp satiety signals; their vagus nerve hums a steady refrain of *"done."* A single bite satisfies, and their biology dances in rare harmony with modernity. For others, the symphony is muddled. Which compass you navigate with is determined by genetics. Our genes quietly shape the way we experience hunger and fullness, sometimes tipping the scales before we even take a bite. For some, genetic variations act like a dimmer switch on the body's satiety signals. They make it harder to feel satisfied after eating.

One of the most studied examples is the fat mass and obesity-associated, or FTO, gene. Specific versions of the gene are associated with a higher risk of obesity. Individuals who carry these variants often exhibit weaker responses to hormones that signal fullness, such as leptin and GLP-1. Research shows that these individuals may not only feel less satisfied after a meal but also tend to consume more calories overall, especially from high-fat foods.

Some gene variants disrupt the brain's ability to register satiety, so the *"I'm full"* signal never quite arrives. This explains why roughly 6% of people either never feel full or feel perpetually content. People with these loss-of-function mutations are more likely to overeat and gain weight. Other genes influence people's tendencies toward specific cravings. Some forms of genes make fatty foods taste more appealing, which can lead to a stronger preference for rich, energy-dense meals.

Even genes involved in the production and action of our satiety hormones can influence eating patterns. Some variants are associated with larger meal sizes or more frequent snacking, suggesting subtle yet meaningful differences in how the body manages hunger and satisfaction. Large-scale studies have shown that children with a higher genetic risk for obesity often have lower satiety responsiveness, meaning they're less likely to feel full and more likely to gain weight in environments where food is plentiful.

Additionally, individuals with fewer dopamine receptors may require more intense stimuli, such as consuming more sugar, to experience the same level of joy. Ultimately leading them to chase satisfaction in a world of endless buffets. In an environment where high-fat snacks are everywhere, this push can make resisting temptation especially challenging.

Our modern food environment is a sensory minefield where every grocery aisle becomes a "temptation alley." Supermarkets don't just sell food—they choreograph desire, deploying strategies rooted in neuroscience and anthropology to keep hyper-palatable foods perpetually *"in sight, in mind."*

The architecture of craving begins right at the doors of the supermarket. Here, you stand at a crossroads. On one side, a gleaming apple sits atop a mountain of shiny fruit, promising crisp refreshment and the quiet pride of a healthy choice. On the other, a doughnut—golden, glossy, dusted with sugar—beckons from behind a glass case, sweet and impossible to ignore. For someone whose belly is comfortably full, the decision might be a gentle tug-of-war, a moment's pause before choosing virtue or indulgence. For a hungry brain, the doughnut doesn't just beckon, it blazes. It's as radiant as a neon sign flickering in the midnight dark, drowning out all other options.

This is the phenomenon psychologists call temporal discounting, a fancy term for a profoundly human tendency. When hunger gnaws at us, the promise of immediate pleasure eclipses the distant rewards of restraint. The future—six months of better health, a lower number on the scale—shrinks to a pinprick. All that matters is the now: the glaze, the sugar, the first bite.

Research reveals that food-deprived people are nearly 40% more likely to grab a snack rather than wait for a healthier meal, their brains locked in the present, blind to the horizon. This means that when you hear that age-old saying, *"Don't go to the grocery store hungry,"* there is actually something to that.

Everything in the store is arranged to catch the eye and trigger visual reward circuits, priming us for impulsive choices before we've even picked up a basket. As we move deeper, the traps multiply. Over sixty percent of products near the checkout are ultra-processed snacks positioned to exploit our decision fatigue. Here, when our willpower is frayed, we're three times more likely to reach for candy, the Skittles and chocolates beckoning from eye level beside glossy magazines. When we encounter these foods, our dopamine pathways light up like a constellation. They create what is known as *"incentive salience."* It is the neural basis of craving: the transformation of a simple food item into something irresistibly compelling.

A landmark 2019 study at the National Institutes of Health demonstrated this with startling clarity. When 20 participants were fed ultra-processed meals for two weeks, they consumed an additional 508 calories daily compared to when eating minimally processed foods. This was found despite both diets being matched for calories, macronutrients, fiber, and sodium. The participants gained an average of two pounds during the ultra-processed phase. The study showed these foods appear to bypass the brain's natural satiety mechanisms through multiple pathways. This turns abundance into a mirage. Your body has plenty, but your mind feels empty, urging you to eat and eat, searching for a fullness that never quite arrives.

Studies using functional MRI have shown that the brain's reward centers respond strongly to food cues, such as the sight or smell of palatable foods, even when individuals are physically full. For example, after eating to satiety, the brain's response to the specific food consumed drops sharply. Still, it remains responsive to other uneaten foods, illustrating the persistent allure of variety and the phenomenon of sensory-specific satiety.

The draw of variety explains why most aisles at the grocery are lined not with nourishing staples but with "variety packs" of chips and cookies. It's essentially a sensory reset button for brains wired to seek novelty. We naturally grow tired of eating the same food repeatedly, and our appetite resets when presented with new flavors, textures, or combinations. Studies show that people consume 44% more food when offered a variety of options compared to a single food item.

Our Stone Age brains, once elated by the rare discovery of a berry patch, now wander aisles of berry-flavored *everything*. We live in a world where "enough" is a maze designed to keep us craving. Portion distortion further warps our internal compass. Family-sized packages and oversized containers tap into scarcity mindsets, and neuroimaging reveals that merely seeing larger portions lights up pleasure centers in the brain, drowning out satiety signals. We consume up to 73% more from these bottomless packages, even when we're already full.

Distraction compounds the problem: eating while scrolling or watching TV hijacks our awareness, silencing the vagus nerve's gentle *"enough"* and leaving us adrift. Studies show we eat 45% more snacks when our minds are elsewhere. Even lighting conspires against us—warm spotlights on baked goods, cold LEDs on produce—subtly steering our choices, mimicking the cues our ancestors once used to find freshness and safety.

All these environmental cues, the endless buffet of flavors, the ever-present lure of variety, the engineered abundance, exploit our biological susceptibilities. Recognizing these environmental puppeteers is the first step toward reclaiming agency, toward advocating for spaces where nourishment, not manipulation, guides our choices.

Yet the influence of modern foods doesn't stop at the surface. These products rewrite the brain's script, exploiting neural pathways and feedback loops that once ensured survival but now fuel compulsion. To truly understand how modern foods take advantage of our brains, we need to look beneath the surface and examine the structures involved.

~

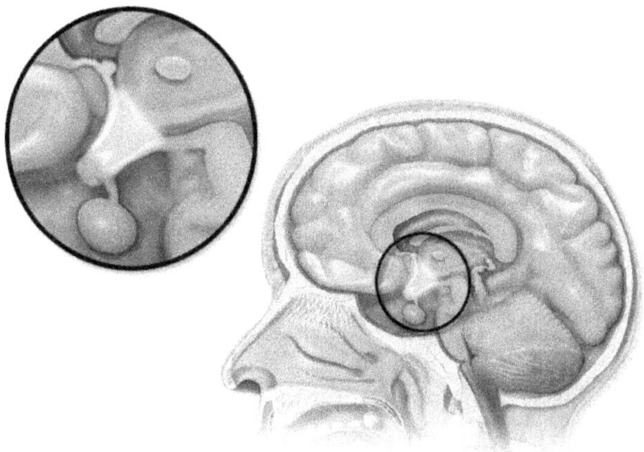

Figure 6. *The Hypothalamus*. Blausen Medical

Deep within the hypothalamus, a command center no larger than an almond, resides a cluster of neurons that serve as the body's vigilant sentries, constantly tracking our energy reserves. These POMC neurons act as gatekeepers of satiety. They send out signals that ripple through the brain, gently urging us to stop eating when we've had enough. Their quiet authority helps maintain balance, ensuring that our meals end before excess tips into discomfort.

Yet, these neurons are not simply guardians of restraint. Hidden among their many sensors are receptors exquisitely sensitive to sugar, transforming these sentries into double agents when sweetness enters the picture. This dual role helps explain the familiar "dessert stomach" phenomenon. Even after a hearty meal when fullness should reign, a sudden craving for pie or cake can emerge with surprising force. Functional MRI studies have shown that sugar, especially after a meal, activates the brain's thalamic opioid system—a pathway flooded with pleasure chemicals. It's as if the mind keeps a secret reserve, a hidden stomach always ready for a taste of sweetness.

This response is rooted in our evolutionary history. For early humans, sugar was a rare and valuable energy source worth seeking out even when other needs were met. In today's world, where confections are everywhere, this once-helpful adaptation can become a trap. Our neurons, caught between their roles as regulators and reward-seekers, illustrate the modern struggle. Ancient biology colliding with a landscape of constant abundance. Each slice of cake becomes a small battleground, a contest between the rational mind and the deep-seated drives of our past.

If sugar is the siren song—immediate, bright, and hard to resist—fat is the slow, enveloping tide: steady, comforting, and quietly powerful. Once, fat was a rare treasure, a vital reserve that could mean the difference between survival and starvation. Now, it saturates the modern diet, found in countless meals and snacks. While our bodies once celebrated its arrival, our brains are now grappling with the consequences of its constant presence.

Central to this story is the habenula, a tiny, often-overlooked region deep within the brain. The habenula acts like a circuit breaker, designed to temper the thrill of reward and signal when it's time to stop. It's the neural equivalent of a gentle hand on the shoulder, reminding us not to overindulge. However, when high-fat foods become a daily staple, this system becomes weakened. The circuit breaker grows less responsive, and the signals to stop become faint.

Animal studies reveal this shift in vivid detail. Rodents fed a steady diet of rich, fatty foods develop habenula dysfunction, leading them to seek out more fat even when it no longer brings pleasure and comes at a cost. This process, known as "hedonic habituation," is the gradual numbing of the brain's pleasure response. Satisfaction slips further away, and the threshold for feeling rewarded rises. The more we indulge, the more the brain adapts, demanding ever greater quantities for the same fleeting sense of pleasure. In this way, fat transforms from a precious lifeline into a subtle saboteur, quietly reshaping our neural circuitry and fueling a relentless cycle of craving and consumption.

Hunger and the desire for food extend far beyond a simple ache in the stomach. They seep into our moods, our decisions, and even our sense of self. It narrows our focus, making us concentrate on what is immediately in front of us. This reaction was once a clever adaptation, a survival mechanism developed by our ancestors during the difficult times when the next meal was uncertain and focusing on the present was essential.

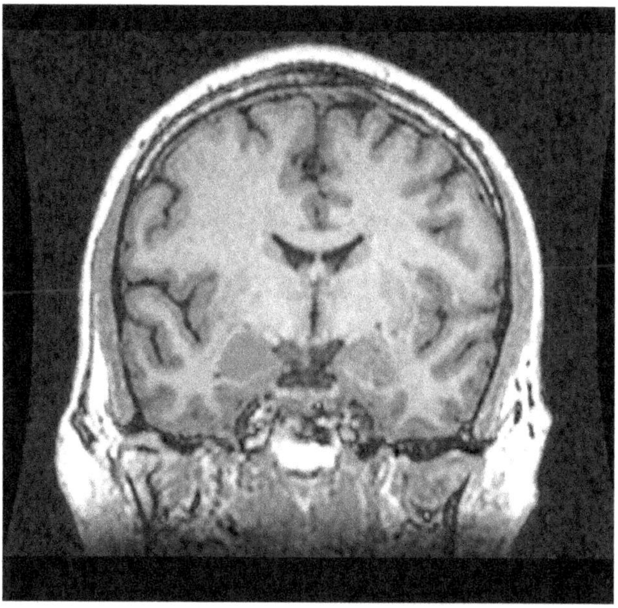

Figure 7. *MRI coronal view of the amygdala.* Amber Rieder, Jenna Traynor, Geoffrey B Hall

When we're hungry, the amygdala doesn't just wake up; it takes over. Its signals grow louder, more insistent, amplifying every feeling, every impulse. The world feels sharper, and our patience thinner. We snap at loved ones over minor annoyances and make decisions we later regret.

It's no wonder the term *"hangry"* has become a common cultural shorthand. This feeling is so familiar that candy commercials like Snickers' famous *"You're not you when you're hungry"* campaign have turned it into a punchline. Beneath the humor lies a very real truth: hunger doesn't just gnaw at our stomachs; it hijacks our mood, our choices, and even our sense of self.

Brain scans reveal this drama in vivid color. When hunger strikes, the amygdala lights up like a storm cloud, its electrical activity crackling across neural circuits. Our rational side drowned out. Whispers lost in the thunder. In these moments, we are not just hungry; we are primed for risk, for urgency, for the kind of choices that favor survival in the wild but leave us vulnerable in the supermarket aisle. This is why, for so many, *"just eat less"* isn't simple or helpful advice. When the body's signals go unheard, willpower alone is no match for the silent, persistent hunger that leptin resistance brings.

Hunger is only one part of the equation. Layer stress on top, deadlines looming, tempers flaring, the world spinning just a little too fast, and the chemistry of craving intensifies. Suddenly, the bag of chips in the cupboard isn't just a snack. It's a lifeline, a beacon in the storm. Most of us are familiar with this cycle intimately.

In fact, we all likely know this feeling so well that it's not difficult to envision a scenario. Imagine a nurse accustomed to the relentless rhythm of night shifts and the emotional weight of caring for others. The nurse swears to stop at one chip. By 2 a.m., the bag was empty, crumbs scattered like confetti on the breakroom table. The initial crunch brought a fleeting sense of calm, a hush in the chaos. As the last chip disappeared, guilt crept in—sharp, familiar, and unyielding.

This story is not unique. It's a portrait of the stress-eating feedback loop: stress leads to cravings, cravings lead to overeating, overeating breeds shame, and shame circles back to more stress. The brain, ensnared by its chemistry, becomes a captive. It chases solace in the very foods that deepen the trap. It's a cycle as old as humanity. In today's world of endless snacks and constant demands, it spins faster and tighter. Pulling us in with every anxious thought and every salty, sweet bite.

Escaping the cycle of stress, cravings, and regret is not a matter of sheer willpower; it's a process of gently rewiring both body and mind. One promising approach is time-restricted eating, a practice as simple as it is profound. By confining meals to a daily window, say, from 8 a.m. to 6 p.m., we give our bodies a chance to reset and recover. It's like pressing the "refresh" button on the brain's internal fullness detectors.

When we eat in sync with our natural circadian rhythms, the ancient clockwork that governs sleep and wakefulness, something remarkable happens: hunger signals become clearer, sharper, and more honest. Impulsive cravings, those sudden urges that once crashed through our resolve, begin to soften and fade. Consistency, eating at regular times, day after day, allows the brain to learn to recognize hunger and fullness rather than the static of habit or emotion.

Yet, even the most advanced medications, such as the much-discussed GLP-1 agonists, Wegovy, Ozempic, and their kin, have their limits. These drugs are remarkable in their ability to amplify the body's fullness signals, turning up the volume on satiety so that a person feels satisfied after less food. Unfortunately, they are not magic. In a 2023 clinical trial, patients taking GLP-1 medications still found themselves wrestling with cravings when surrounded by hyperpalatable snacks—chips, cookies, and candies engineered to be irresistible.

The lesson is clear: no pill or shot, no matter how powerful, can entirely silence the dopamine-driven drumbeat of the modern food environment. The world is awash in temptation, and biology alone cannot shield us from its pull. Actual change requires more than chemistry. It asks us to reshape our habits, curate our environments, and, perhaps most importantly, rewrite our relationship with food itself. It is a journey of awareness and intention, of learning to listen to the body's quiet wisdom amid the noise, and of finding satisfaction not just in what we eat but in how, when, and why we eat it.

The dance between hunger and choice is not a brute contest of willpower but an ongoing conversation—a delicate negotiation between the ancient circuitry that pulses beneath our skin and the dazzling, ever-present temptations of modern life. Each craving, each moment of weakness, is not a personal failure but a message from our evolutionary past, echoing through the corridors of our minds. When we recognize the amygdala's urgent alarms, the way stress and cortisol can twist a simple craving into a compulsion, and the subtle rhythms that can reset our biology, we begin to see ourselves with new eyes. These are not flaws to be conquered but signals to be understood.

Navigating a world of abundance with grace means letting go of rigid rules and harsh self-judgment. Instead, it calls for a gentler approach, one rooted in curiosity and compassion. We are, after all, creatures shaped by millions of years of hunger and hope, wired to seek pleasure and avoid pain, to survive and, when possible, to thrive. Our primal hunger is not an enemy; it is part of what makes us gloriously, vulnerably human.

So, as we stand before each meal—whether it's a hurried breakfast, a celebratory feast, or a midnight snack—we are offered a quiet moment of agency. Every bite is more than sustenance; it is a small act of self-definition. In choosing what, when, and how we eat, we are also choosing who we wish to become: someone who listens, learns, forgives, and moves forward, one mindful meal at a time. Yet the choices we make at the table echo far beyond the plate. The same impulses that shape our eating—our capacity for restraint, gratitude, or overindulgence—mirror deeper patterns in our lives.

CHAPTER 3
CRAVING, COVETING, AND THE NEUROSCIENCE OF NEVER ENOUGH

GREED IS a fire that feeds on itself. It begins as a spark, a simple wish for more, but soon grows into a blaze that is never quite satisfied. Neuroscientists have discovered that people who score high on measures of greed are not simply ambitious or driven; they are often less happy, more anxious, and more prone to anger and depression. Their psychological well-being erodes, replaced by a persistent sense of dissatisfaction.

At the center of our desires—whether for chocolate cake, a loving text, or a winning lottery ticket—lies the brain's reward system. Recall from earlier that this system is the brain's internal "pleasure highway," a network of roads that light up whenever something feels good or exciting. Whenever you anticipate or receive something pleasurable—say, a slice of your favorite cake or a compliment from a friend—these pleasure and reward regions work together. Part of the brain releases dopamine, a chemical messenger, which travels to other areas.

As we know and have discussed in detail, dopamine is our "feel-good" and "wanting" chemical. It doesn't just make you feel good; it makes you want more of whatever caused its release. It's the spark that gets you off the couch and into action, chasing after rewards. This reward system is crucial for survival. It encourages us to seek food when we are hungry, warmth when we are cold, and connection when we are lonely. In moderation, it's the engine behind motivation, learning, and even love.

Here's where things can go awry.

When greed takes the wheel, this pleasure highway gets jammed. The more we indulge, the more our brains crave. Over time, the reward system adapts. It's as if the city's residents become numb to the usual fireworks and demand bigger, louder displays to feel the same excitement. This is called "tolerance". It forces the brain to need more stimulation to achieve the same level of satisfaction.

The anticipation of gain—whether money, praise, or power—triggers a dopamine surge so potent that neuroscientists have likened its effect to the rush of addictive drugs. The more we indulge, the more the brain adapts, demanding ever-larger rewards to achieve the same fleeting thrill. This is the hedonic treadmill, and it leaves everyday joys dulled, the world drained of color, as we chase the next big thing. Always moving, never arriving.

Dopamine is only the beginning of the story. In the shadows of the reward system, other chemical actors play their parts. Serotonin, the regulator, tempers our retaliatory impulses and shapes our sense of fairness. When serotonin levels wane, research shows, we become more prone to lashing out at perceived slights and less able to accept the give-and-take of social life. Our ability to find satisfaction in fairness, to let go of small losses, is blunted. The result is a mind more vulnerable to envy, less anchored in contentment, a mind fertile for the growth of greed.

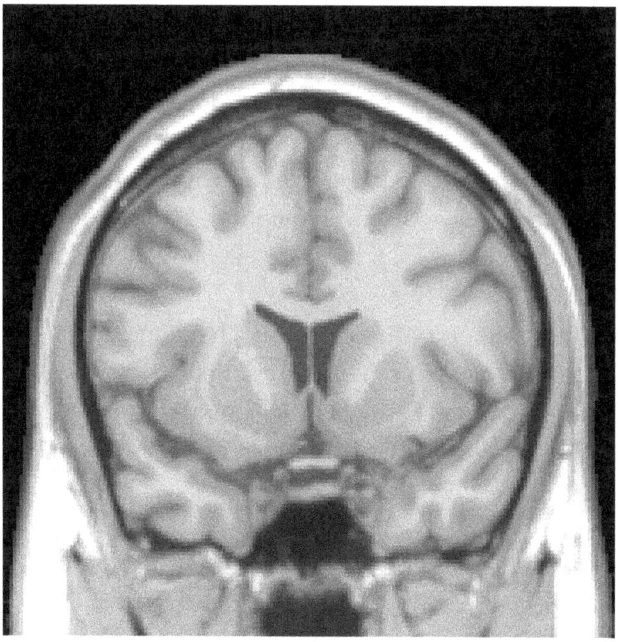

Figure 8. *Coronal MRI image showing the nucleus accumbens circled in red.* Genesis12 on Wikimedia Commons

The architecture of greed, like hunger, is as intricate as its chemistry. Within the brain, the nucleus accumbens and ventral striatum form the central nodes of the reward circuit, translating the promise of gain into motivation and action. These regions are the crossroads where emotion and reason meet. They are where the lure of a shiny reward can overpower the voice of caution. Magnetic resonance imaging reveals that for those prone to greed, these circuits are especially sensitive to the prospect of gain and curiously muted to the pain of loss. The usual neural brakes—signals that might warn, *"enough"*—are weakened, and the chase intensifies.

Greed isn't just about wanting more money or piling up shiny possessions. It isn't simply a dragon's urge to hoard gold, like Smaug from The Hobbit, lounging atop a glittering mountain of treasure yet still obsessing over the smallest missing trinket. Or the Niffler from the

Harry Potter universe, forever snuffling out coins and jewels, never satisfied, no matter how stuffed its pouch becomes.

Greed can be far more subtle—and far more familiar. It's the restless scroll through social media, searching for more likes or validation. It's the urge to buy the latest gadget, even when last year's model works just fine. It's eyeing a coworker's promotion, a neighbor's new car, or a friend's vacation photos and feeling that familiar itch: *Why not me? Why not more?*

We may not sleep on piles of gold or have magical pouches. Still, greed remains that little voice whispering that what we have isn't quite enough—that happiness is always just one shiny thing away. In a world overflowing with glittering distractions, it's all too easy to listen.

Why do we feel this? Why do we always want more and covet what others have?

The answer lies in the intricate wiring of our neurobiology. Humans are social creatures, and our survival has always depended on our place in the group. To help us keep track, the brain is equipped with a built-in "social radar." Two key regions are especially involved in social comparison. The first is the anterior cingulate cortex that acts as your brain's social scoreboard, tallying wins and losses—not just in games, but in life's endless comparisons: who's ahead, who's behind, who's fitting in. Meanwhile, another area serves as an emotional thermometer, registering how you feel about your social standing, as well as pride when you're ahead and embarrassment or envy when you're not.

When you notice someone else getting a promotion, posting glamorous vacation photos, or receiving public praise, these brain regions light up. If you feel you're falling behind, your brain doesn't just shrug it off. Instead, it interprets this as a kind of threat. It's almost as if your place in the tribe is at risk. This triggers a stress response. Your heart rate might quicken, your thoughts race, and you feel a renewed urge to "catch up."

This cycle—see, compare, crave, stress, repeat—can become a habit. Over time, it's like running on a treadmill that never stops. No matter how fast you go, there's always someone ahead, always something more to want. The result is chronic dissatisfaction. Even when you achieve something, the feeling of contentment is fleeting, quickly replaced by a following comparison.

Understanding this helps explain why social media can make us feel worse instead of better. There's that moment when the phone comes out—just for a minute, just to check. One swipe turns into ten, then twenty, and suddenly the world shrinks to a glowing screen filled with endless stories, photos, updates. Each flick of the thumb brings a new burst of someone else's good news: a friend's wedding, a coworker's marathon medal, another acquaintance's picture-perfect dinner. The scroll never stops; it's a conveyor belt of everyone else's best days.

The mind starts to race, quietly stacking up comparisons. There's a sense of falling behind, of missing out, even when nothing has changed in your own life. The more you scroll, the more it feels like everyone else is moving forward while you're standing still. It's a strange, hollow ache, familiar and persistent. The endless scroll isn't just a way to pass the time. It's a reminder that the scoreboard never resets, and the finish line keeps slipping further away. Every swipe is a new chance to feel a little less like you're measuring up, even when you know, deep down, that no one's life is really as perfect as it looks on the screen.

The story doesn't end there. When this cycle of comparison and craving becomes routine, its effects reach deeper than fleeting feelings of inadequacy. Over time, it can seep into your worldview and decision-making, clouding judgment and shifting your sense of what is enough. The desire for more, whether it's likes, recognition, or the next shiny thing, can start to steer your choices, often without you even noticing. It's as if your brain turns into a crowded boardroom, where the loudest voices are those urging you to chase more, faster, now.

At the head of this metaphorical boardroom table sits the prefrontal cortex, the CEO of your brain. This region, located just behind your forehead, is responsible for thinking in a big-picture manner. It helps you weigh the pros and cons, consider future consequences, and resist the urge to act on every impulse. When you decide to save money instead of splurging or to walk away from a tempting but risky deal, you're relying on your prefrontal cortex.

When greed takes over—when you're caught up in wanting more, more, more—the boardroom gets noisy. The reward regions start shouting for immediate gratification. The prefrontal cortex, usually calm and rational, struggles to be heard over the clamor. It's a bit like trying to perform heart surgery in the middle of a loud, crowded frat party.

Research shows that in moments of intense craving of any kind, the prefrontal cortex becomes less active. This means it's harder for you to think ahead or pause before acting. Instead, the impulsive, reward-seeking parts of your brain take the wheel. You're more likely to make snap decisions, choosing what feels good right now, even if you know it might hurt you later.

This is why unchecked greed is often associated with behaviors such as gambling, high-risk investments, or compulsive shopping. In these moments, the promise of an immediate reward, such as winning big, buying something new, or getting a quick thrill, overpowers your ability to consider the long-term costs. You might ignore warning signs, downplay risks, or convince yourself that *"just this once"* won't matter. This concept isn't new.

Centuries ago, long before brain scans or scientific journals, Buddhist philosophers looked inward and recognized a profound truth: greed, what they called lobha, is one of the three great poisons of the mind, alongside hatred and ignorance. In their teachings, greed wasn't just about wanting more things; it was a restless hunger that could never be satisfied, a force that kept people trapped in endless cycles of craving and regret. They saw how unchecked desire led to suffering, making it harder for people to find peace or contentment.

Today, neuroscience offers a fascinating echo of this ancient wisdom. Using brain imaging and careful experiments, we have discovered what happens when our desires run wild. When we're caught up in relentless wanting, our brain's reward system gets overwhelmed. This system, which normally helps us find pleasure in everyday experiences, becomes less responsive. It's as if the volume knob on joy gets turned down.

It's essential to recognize that greed isn't merely a moral failing or a personal weakness. It's a pattern of brain activity, a loop of craving and dissatisfaction that can quietly take over our lives. When we're stuck in this loop, it doesn't just make us unhappy; it clouds our judgment, strains our relationships, and keeps us chasing after satisfaction that never lasts.

However, there's good news: by shedding light on how this cycle operates, we can start to break free. When we become aware of our brain's tendency to adapt, we can learn to pause, savor, and appreciate the ordinary moments that truly enrich our lives. Recognizing these patterns is the first step toward change.

Mindfulness, reflection, and practice can help you think ahead and make choices that serve your long-term well-being rather than just your momentary desires. The next time you feel that familiar itch, whether it's envy, restlessness, or the urge to compare, pause for a moment. Take three slow, deep breaths. Notice what you're feeling, and name it: *"This is envy"* or *"This is wanting."* Simply acknowledging the emotion can loosen its grip.

Next, try shifting your focus to gratitude. Each evening, jot down three things you appreciated about your day, no matter how small. Maybe it's a warm cup of coffee, a smile from a stranger, or the comfort of your favorite sweater. Over time, you'll train your brain to notice abundance rather than lack.

Pay attention to how stress spreads in your environment. Notice if your mood shifts after scrolling through social media, watching the news, or talking with a stressed friend. When you sense stress catching, pause and ask: *"Is this mine, or am I absorbing someone else's tension?"* If it's not yours, imagine a gentle boundary, a soft light or shield around you, letting in warmth but keeping out unnecessary worry.

You can also set aside a few minutes each day to unplug from digital distractions. Step outside, listen to music, or simply take a moment to notice your surroundings. Observe how your mood and cravings shift, even in this short window. And when you catch yourself comparing, gently reframe the scoreboard. Ask, *"What is one thing I'm proud of today?"* Or *"How can I support someone else's success?"* Celebrating others can actually boost your sense of connection and satisfaction.

By incorporating these small practices into your daily life, you can begin to loosen the grip of greed. The brain's reward system is robust yet adaptable. With awareness, intention, and a little patience, you can step off the treadmill and rediscover the quiet joys that make life truly rich.

As we learn to interrupt the cycle of craving and find contentment in the present, something else becomes clear: the effects of greed reach far beyond our own inner world. Greed is not a solitary affliction. Like a slow, creeping fog, it seeps into the spaces between people, clouding trust and eroding the warmth that binds us together. When someone's focus narrows to the relentless pursuit of wealth, power, or constant validation, a subtle yet profound shift begins to occur in their relationships. Those closest—partners, friends, even children—start to feel less like cherished companions and more like rungs on a ladder, useful only for climbing higher.

The "greedy" person, consumed by their ambitions, becomes emotionally unavailable. They might be physically present at the dinner table or in a meeting. Still, their minds are always elsewhere, calculating, comparing, and planning the next move. As a result, conversations grow shallow; laughter fades, and the heart-to-heart moments that once defined the relationship become rare, replaced by a sense of distance and distraction.

This single-minded chase for *"more"* gradually creates a gulf. Friends and family, sensing their fading importance, may begin to pull away from them. They might stop sharing their joys and struggles, feeling unseen or undervalued. The connection built from shared memories, inside jokes, and mutual support starts to crumble, leaving behind something thin and fragile, a faint echo of what once was.

The corrosive effects of greed are not limited to personal relationships; they can be even more pronounced in the workplace. Here, greed breeds competition where collaboration is needed, allowing jealousy and suspicion to take root. The greedy individual might resort to manipulation, taking credit for others' work, or undermining colleagues to advance their own interests. These behaviors poison the atmosphere, making trust scarce and resentment common. Teams that once thrived on cooperation become divided, and the organization suffers as a whole.

Ultimately, unchecked greed isolates the individual and also damages the very fabric of the community. It turns allies into rivals, friends into strangers, and workplaces into battlegrounds. By recognizing how greed operates—not just within us, but between us—we can begin to choose a different path.

If you find yourself dealing with someone whose greed is straining your relationship, there are practical ways to protect your well-being and nurture healthier connections. Setting clear boundaries and communicating openly about how their actions affect you can help prevent resentment from building. Practicing compassion while refusing to enable harmful behavior allows you to support others without sacrificing your own needs.

In professional settings, focusing on collaboration and seeking out allies who value teamwork can counteract the divisive effects of greed. And sometimes, limiting your exposure to toxic dynamics or prioritizing your mental health is necessary. By modeling generosity and gratitude, you not only reinforce your own values but may also inspire those around you to shift their focus from relentless acquisition to genuine connection.

We can value people for who they are, not just for what they offer. We can nurture relationships, build trust, and rediscover the deep satisfaction that comes from genuine connection. Yet even when we make these conscious choices, life always has a way of testing us. The question is: *are we ready for it?*

PART TWO

A DECISIVE BRAIN

CHAPTER 4
THE DECISION DILEMMA: HOW STRESS, MEMORY, AND EMOTION SHAPE OUR CHOICES

CHOOSE A or B. No explanations. No justifications. Just choose.

Would you rather...

Say yes to a spontaneous adventure, or stick to your schedule?
Share a secret online, or keep it to yourself?
Confront a friend about an issue, or let it slide?

Every choice stirs something inside you: a flicker of impulse, a shadow of hesitation, a spark of curiosity, or a whisper of caution. The act of choosing is never just about the options before you. It's a quiet revolution, a moment when the world narrows to a single point, and your inner landscape comes alive. In these moments, you are both the observer and the actor, the storyteller and the story, standing at the intersection of desire and restraint.

With each decision, your mind becomes a stage for a well-known drama. Impulse leaps forward, eager and bright. It promises excitement or relief. Reason stands its ground, steady and measured, urging you to pause, to weigh the consequences, to remember what matters most. Curiosity beckons you to explore, to imagine what might be, while caution tugs at your sleeve, reminding you of the risks hidden just out of sight. These forces do not exist in isolation. They swirl together, shaping your path in ways both subtle and profound.

What drives your decisions?

The answer is as complex as you are. Your choices are shaped by the intricate wiring of your brain, by circuits honed through evolution, by memories etched through experience, by the chemistry of mood, and by the weight of your past. Sometimes, a single moment of adversity can tip the balance, making impulse louder or caution more insistent. Sometimes, the stories you tell yourself—about who you are, what you value, and what you fear—become the compass that guides you.

To choose is to reveal something of yourself, even when the decision seems small. Each choice is a mirror, reflecting not just your wants but your hopes, your regrets, your willingness to take risks, and your longing for safety. In this chapter, we'll journey into the heart of decision-making. We'll explore what drives your choices, how impulse and reason wrestle in your mind, and why you chose what you did. Along the way, you may discover that your choices are not just reactions to the world but moments when you shape your own story and perhaps see yourself in a new light.

~

Your fingers hover just above the glowing screen of your phone, the soft buzz of notifications humming like a distant chorus. It's another evening, the kind that slips quietly into routine, yet here you are. The endless scroll on TikTok, Facebook, or Instagram has you trapped in its web. The blue light washes over your face, calm and insistent, blending with the last golden threads of sunset spilling through the window.

In this suspended moment, there's a whisper of guilt, that quiet voice at the edge of your mind reminding you of the night's stillness waiting just beyond the screen. You hesitate, caught between the urge to keep scrolling and the pull to look away, to reclaim the night. Then the balance tips. Your thumb slides down again, and the screen flickers; the cycle continues. The choice is made—not once, but again and again.

This is a moment most of us know intimately: the pause before surrender. The electric charge of possibility is mixed with the weight of self-restraint. It's a small decision, yes, but inside your brain, a fierce tug of war unfolds. It's a clash of ancient impulses and deliberate thought, a seesaw of desire and reason that shapes not just this moment but the countless moments that follow. Our minds murmur questions both simple and profound: *Should I? Will I? What's the cost? What's the reward?*

Now, imagine that moment—but magnified a thousandfold. Picture yourself standing in a quiet room. The weight of a decision is pressing into your chest. Before you, an offer letter for a new job rests on the table, its crisp edges catching the light. Or perhaps you're walking through a house with sunlit rooms. Each breath is thick with the scent of fresh paint while you try to envision a life you haven't yet lived.

This choice will ripple through the years, shaping your identity, your relationships, and your future dreams. The stakes are higher, the unknowns more daunting. Beneath the surface, the same neural symphony plays. The spark of possibility ignites in your limbic system, lighting up your mind with visions of success, security, and a new beginning.

At the same time, your prefrontal cortex steps in, calm and deliberate, weighing the risks, whispering of sacrifice and what might be lost. Dopamine pulses through your veins, tempting you to leap, while circuits of caution remind you to pause, to think twice. The push and pull are electric, the tension almost palpable. It's like those moments spent scrolling, but now the screen is life itself, and every swipe feels like a leap into the unknown.

Whether it's the small, everyday choices or the rare, life-altering decisions that shape your path, the process is fundamentally the same. Our brains are wired to weigh desire against restraint, risk against reward, and impulse against reason. The mechanisms may be hidden, but the experience is universal. The glowing screen and the signed contract serve as metaphors for all the choices we face. Our brains may be complex, but the questions they ask are simple.

Will we swipe once more, or will we look up and step away?

Will we leap into the unknown or hold fast to what we know?

And what stories will we choose to tell ourselves in the quiet after the leap?

Desire, in all its forms, is a current running through the brain's reward circuits, a cascade of neurotransmitters. When we encounter a tempting stimulus, a lover's glance, a flash sale, or a tasty treat, the brain releases neurotransmitters and hormones. As you hover over choices, your brain is alive with a dynamic interplay of signals, emotions, and learned patterns. When we make a decision—whether it's as simple as what to eat for lunch or as complex as changing careers—chemical signals begin to flow through our brains. These neurotransmitters are the messengers that allow different regions of your brain to communicate, shaping your thoughts, feelings, and actions in real-time.

First is anticipation. It is primarily driven by a neurotransmitter we know well by this time: dopamine. Commonly referred to as the *"motivation molecule"* or the *"reward chemical,"* its release is triggered when you anticipate something desirable. This can start even before you make a choice, as soon as you notice a potential reward in your environment. Dopamine is released from neurons in a small region of the brain. It travels along pathways to the nucleus accumbens, a key part of the brain's reward system.

The surge heightens your focus, energizes your body, and makes the anticipated outcome feel more appealing. The more that is released, the stronger your urge to pursue the reward. This is why anticipation can feel so exciting and why it can sometimes override your rational plans. Dopamine is just one player in a much larger ensemble. Other chemicals also join in helping regulate mood and impulsivity.

Recall serotonin. It plays a key role in regulating mood, anxiety, and self-control and is produced in the brainstem and released throughout the brain, particularly in areas responsible for mood and decision-making. As a stabilizing neurotransmitter, it helps you feel calm and focused. When levels are low, you may experience restlessness, anxiety, or an increased tendency to act impulsively. This can make it more challenging to resist temptation or pursue long-term goals, especially when faced with immediate rewards.

Perhaps more interesting than the chemicals that power these feelings and desires is how and when exactly they do so. The release of neurotransmitters during decision-making is rapid and dynamic. As soon as you become aware of a potential reward or choice, dopamine levels begin to rise. This creates a sense of excitement and focus.

As you weigh your options, neurochemicals help regulate your mood and impulse control. This balance enables you to pause and consider the consequences before taking action. Once you make a decision and act, it surges again if the outcome is positive, reinforcing the behavior and making it more likely you'll repeat it in the future.

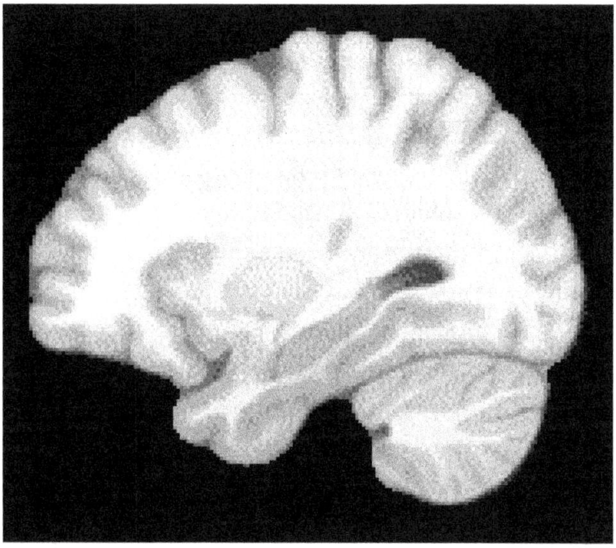

Figure 9. *Hippocampus highlighted in green on sagittal T1 MRI images.* Danielsabinasz on Wikimedia Commons

At this point, your brain's memory centers, especially the

hippocampus, spring into action. The hippocampus quickly retrieves relevant memories of past experiences, both good and bad. The hippocampus scans your mental library for similar situations, outcomes, and feelings. It recalls the satisfaction of past success or the regret of a poor choice. This allows us to anticipate what might happen if we choose a particular path. These memories shape expectations, guide reasoning, and can either encourage you to take a risk or hold you back.

Meanwhile, your amygdala acts like an emotional radar. As we've seen before, it scans for threats and opportunities, sending out signals of excitement, fear, or caution. If a choice feels risky, your amygdala may sound the alarm, prompting you to hesitate or reconsider the decision. If it seems safe and rewarding, the alarm quiets down, and you feel more confident to proceed.

At the same time, your prefrontal cortex weighs the pros and cons, thinks about consequences, and tries to keep your impulses in check. Sometimes, it's strong enough to help you resist temptation. At other times, especially when you're tired or stressed, you can feel overwhelmed, and your impulses take over.

Of course, every decision you make is not just a product of your brain's chemistry or anatomy. It is also profoundly influenced by the state of your body. The signals your body sends can tilt the scales of impulse and self-control, sometimes in ways that override even your best intentions. Your brain and body are in constant conversation. Hormones and physical sensations travel through your bloodstream and nervous system, sending real-time updates about your internal state. These signals can amplify or dampen the brain's response to temptation and risk, shaping your impulses in powerful ways.

When you're hungry, your body releases hormones like ghrelin, which travel to the brain and increase your desire for food. Ghrelin does more than make you crave snacks. It can heighten your sensitivity to all kinds of rewards, making you more likely to act impulsively, whether that means grabbing junk food or making rash decisions in other areas of life. Studies show that people are more likely to choose immediate gratification over long-term benefits when they are hungry.

When you're running on little sleep or feeling physically

exhausted, your brain's ability to manage self-control and decision-making takes a noticeable hit. The prefrontal cortex is especially vulnerable to fatigue. This area is responsible for planning, focusing attention, and resisting temptations. When it's well-rested, it acts like a wise coach, helping you stick to your goals and pause before acting on impulse. However, as exhaustion sets in, the prefrontal cortex becomes less effective. Its signals grow weaker, and it struggles to keep up with the demands of daily life. You may notice it's harder to concentrate, your patience wears thin, and your ability to weigh long-term consequences fades.

With the prefrontal cortex running on empty, your brakes on impulsive behavior are less powerful. A tired brain is a more impulsive brain. You're more likely to blurt out a secret, binge-watch another episode of a show, skip your workout, or snap at someone in frustration. Fatigue shifts your brain's priorities. Pleasurable distractions become more appealing because your brain is searching for quick bursts of energy or comfort. When you're tired, your brain is less able to plan or consider the long-term impact of your actions. This makes it easier to give in to whatever feels good at the moment, even if it contradicts your long-term goals.

The more you give in to these quick fixes, the more your brain learns to seek them out when you're tired. Over time, this can create a cycle: fatigue leads to impulsive choices, which can disrupt sleep, making you even more tired the next day. Speaking of stress, when you encounter it, your body's alarm system kicks into gear.

Hormones like cortisol and adrenaline surge through your bloodstream, priming your body to react quickly, an ancient response designed to help you survive threats like a predator's attack or a sudden danger on the road. In the short term, this fight or flight response sharpens your senses, increases your heart rate, and readies your muscles for action. In emergencies, it's a lifesaver.

However, when stress lingers, like when deadlines pile up, relationships strain, or worries never seem to end, your body stays in this heightened state far longer than nature intended. Chronic stress means cortisol and adrenaline remain elevated, keeping your nervous system on high alert. This constant state of readiness wears down your ability to pause and reflect. It makes you more reactive and less able to think things through.

Under stress, the brain's emotional centers, especially the amygdala, become more active. When stress is high, it takes charge, making you more sensitive to threats and quicker to react with strong emotions. When your emotional brain is in overdrive, and your rational brain takes a backseat, you may find yourself seeking comfort in familiar pleasures despite knowing these choices may not be the healthiest. This emotional state can also lead to impulsive actions, where you make snap decisions without fully considering the consequences. Furthermore, it's common to fall back on established patterns, whether good or bad, because your brain instinctively seeks the quickest and easiest ways to feel better or regain a sense of control.

The bodily sensations we just discussed—hunger, exhaustion, or the physical tension of stress—are not separate from the brain's chemical messengers; they are part of the same system. In moments of intense bodily need, instinctual drives can override the brain's more deliberate processes, causing you to act before thinking. We've all experienced the overwhelming drive from our bodies, so it's easy to imagine...

It's late afternoon, and you're sitting at your desk, the pale glow of your computer screen casting tired shadows across your face. Your stomach growls a low, insistent ache that seems to echo in the quiet room. You promised yourself you'd stick to your intermittent fasting plan. Still, now, the hunger gnaws at your resolve despite having at least another two hours in your "fasting window" before you can eat. The memory of last night's leftovers or the bakery around the corner grows vivid in your mind.

You try to focus, to reason with yourself. *"You'll feel better if you wait,"* you whisper, recalling your goals and the promises you made to yourself. Yet, the hunger is more than a suggestion; it's a wave, rising and relentless, washing away your careful plans. Your body feels heavy, your mind foggy. The world narrows to the idea of food, and suddenly, your feet are moving, almost of their own accord, toward the kitchen or out the door. Each step is a small surrender, a quiet rebellion against your own intentions.

Now, picture another day. You're not hungry, but stress presses in from every side. Emails pile up, and your phone buzzes with reminders. Your heart beats faster; your breath is shallow. In this storm, your brain's voice of reason grows faint. You scroll through your phone, searching for relief—a flash sale, a new gadget, a treat you don't need but suddenly want. Logic flickers in the background, warning you to pause, but the promise of comfort is louder. You click ***"buy now,"*** feeling a rush of satisfaction, followed quickly by a pang of regret.

Your impulses are not just *"in your head"*. The rhythms and needs of your entire body shape them. Understanding this connection can help you recognize why willpower sometimes falters and why self-compassion is essential. In the end, every decision is shaped by a delicate balance: anticipation, memory, emotion, reason, and even your physical state. It's not just about what you want—it's about what you remember, how you feel, and what you think might happen next. It's a learning machine, reinforcing behaviors that bring pleasure and weaving them into the fabric of habit. Sometimes, it reins us in. Sometimes, it's swept away by the thrill.

Think about the last time you faced a decision. Maybe you were lingering in the kitchen, eyeing a second slice of pizza. Or perhaps you were staring at your phone, debating hitting the send button on a risky text. We've all been there, caught in that familiar tug-of-war between *"Why not?"* and *"Maybe not."* It's a moment where time seems to slow, and you can almost feel the invisible gears of your brain turning, weighing desire against restraint, curiosity against caution.

Impulse and reason aren't enemies locked in battle; they're more like dance partners at a wedding, sometimes stepping on each other's toes, sometimes moving in perfect sync. One moment, impulse twirls you toward a spontaneous purchase or a midnight snack. Reason gently pulls you back, reminding you of your budget, your health, or your early morning meeting.

Every choice, no matter how small, is shaped by this intricate choreography. It's a dance that has been evolving for millions of years, yet it plays out in ways as unique as your favorite streaming playlist or the way you tell a joke. The real magic is how your brain navigates these choices, hesitates, dares, and sometimes surprises even you with its next move.

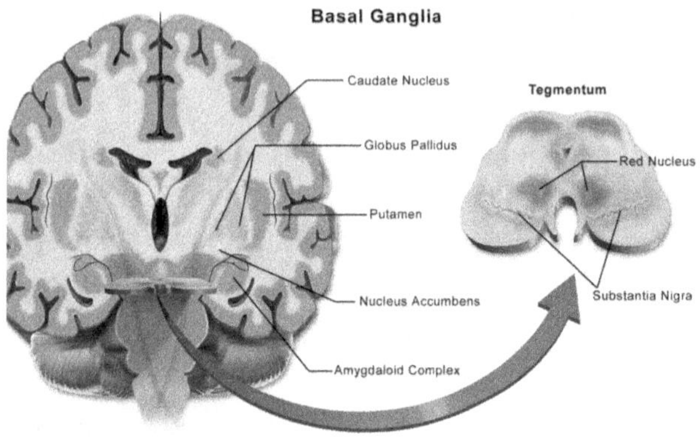

Figure 10. *Basal ganglia.* Blausen Medical

Beneath the chatter of conscious thought, the basal ganglia hum with activity. They sort through your possible actions in a split second. Every time you reach for a second cookie, the basal ganglia recall the pleasure from the last time and nudge you to repeat it. This region is the architect of making some choices feel almost automatic, as if your hand moves before your mind catches up.

When the stakes rise—say, a job interview or a first date—the amygdala takes center stage. This part of the brain colors your choices with urgency, flooding you with anticipation, anxiety, or even fear. Sometimes, these emotions push you to act on impulse; other times, they freeze you in place, urging caution when the unknown looms large. Meanwhile, the prefrontal cortex urges you to remember your long-term goals. When you resist temptation or take a moment to think before acting, your prefrontal cortex is working overtime, trying to keep your impulses in check and your actions aligned with your values.

We all share this machinery, but the way it works—how quickly we act, how long we hesitate, how strongly we feel desire—varies from person to person. Some people leap before they look, while others hold back, calculating every move. Science shows this variation comes from both biology and experience. Understanding this science doesn't just explain why you reach for that second cookie or hesitate before a big leap; it reminds us that every choice is shaped by a unique blend of nature, nurture, and the living, breathing reality of your own brain.

Genetics plays a starring role in shaping how we respond to temptation and regulate our impulses. Specific gene variants influence the activity of neurotransmitters. Some people inherit versions of genes that make their dopamine system more reactive. For example, individuals with particular gene variants that affect dopamine receptors tend to seek out new experiences and are more prone to impulsive behaviors. These individuals may feel rewards more intensely than others. A more reactive dopamine system means the "pull" of temptation is stronger, and resisting urges requires more effort.

Others may have less efficient serotonin systems, which can affect mood stability and impulse control. When signaling is weaker, it can lead to mood swings, increased impulsivity, and difficulty delaying gratification. Variations in the genes related to serotonin transport have been linked to greater impulsivity and emotional reactivity.

The architecture of the brain itself is also partly shaped by genetics. The prefrontal cortex can be more or less developed depending on your genetic makeup. Its connections to emotional centers, such as the amygdala, determine how effectively you can pause before acting or manage strong feelings. When these neural circuits are less robust, it becomes harder to resist temptations or think through the consequences of your actions. For example, people with ADHD often have differences in dopamine signaling and prefrontal cortex function, making it challenging to delay gratification or resist distractions.

While genetics play a role, they don't determine everything. The social and environmental world you grow up in leaves deep imprints on your brain's wiring. Early life experiences—such as nurturing or neglectful parenting, exposure to chronic stress, or living in environments filled with temptation—can shape how your brain develops its impulse and self-control systems.

Children raised in stable, supportive environments tend to develop stronger self-regulation skills as their brains are given the space and safety to practice restraint and decision-making. Cultural attitudes toward risk, reward, and self-control also play a role. In societies that value patience and long-term planning, children often learn to delay gratification more effectively than in cultures that reward immediate action.

In contrast, chaotic or unpredictable environments can heighten impulsivity, as the brain adapts to seek immediate rewards when the future feels uncertain. Ongoing traumatic experiences can wear down the brain's ability to pause and reflect. High levels of hormones can shrink the prefrontal cortex and strengthen the brain's impulse circuits, making it much harder to resist temptations or think through consequences.

~

To see this in action, we need to look no further than one of the most pervasive issues of our time: addiction. Most of us know addiction's shadow, whether through a loved one's struggle, a headline, or a quiet battle within ourselves. On the surface, it can look like a simple matter of willpower: *why not just stop?*

Beneath, addiction is a storm, a conflict between wanting and resisting, craving and control, that is shaped by the brain's deepest pathways and the scars of life's hardships. For those who have faced significant adversity like loss, neglect, or even the slow drip of everyday disappointment, the brain's wiring for impulse and desire can be changed at its core. Adversity comes in many shapes and sizes. It could be a childhood marked by chaos, a single traumatic event, or years of feeling unseen and unheard. What matters is not whether others would call it *"severe"* or *"traumatic"* but how the brain absorbs and responds to it. Even wounds that seem invisible to the outside world can leave deep marks inside.

When life delivers blow after blow, the brain adapts. The circuits that manage self-control and decision-making—the prefrontal cortex and its allies—can be worn thin, like a path trampled by too many storms. Hormones surge, shrinking the very regions that help us pause and reflect. Meanwhile, the brain's reward centers become hypersensitive, continually seeking relief and remaining vulnerable to temptation.

In this state, the drug or behavior of choice doesn't just offer pleasure. It provides escape, comfort, or the illusion of control. The more it's used, the more the brain learns to crave it. Every repetition strengthens the neural pathway, like a trail deepening in the woods. What starts as a choice becomes a habit, and what becomes a habit can harden into compulsion.

No two stories are the same, but the science is clear: adversity, in any form, can change the brain's impulse and restraint. It can make it easier to fall into patterns of risky behavior, harder to break free, and more challenging to make thoughtful decisions—even for those whose genes might otherwise offer resilience.

Today, our brains face temptations our ancestors could never have imagined. Scientists sometimes refer to this as a "Candyland world"—a landscape overflowing with instant gratification, from endless social media feeds to one-click shopping and ultra-processed foods engineered for maximum pleasure. Our neural wiring, however, remains tuned for scarcity, having been shaped by millennia of evolution to seek out rare rewards and act quickly when opportunities arise.

This mismatch between ancient circuitry and modern abundance creates a daily struggle. The same neural machinery that once helped us survive by seeking out sugar or fat now drives us to overindulge in a world where these rewards are everywhere. The impulse to accumulate, to click "buy now," to swipe right, is stoked by a world engineered to trigger our reward circuits at every turn.

Not all impulsivity is a pitfall. Sometimes, it's the very thing that sets life alight—a sudden spark that ignites creativity. This bold leap launches a new adventure, the courage to step beyond the familiar and try something untested. Impulse, in its purest form, is the force that nudges us out of our comfort zones and into moments that become stories worth telling.

Think of the artist who splashes color on a blank canvas before doubt can creep in or the writer who jots down a wild idea in the middle of the night. These moments of inspiration often arrive unannounced, catching us off guard. Impulse is the muse that whispers, *"Why not?"* before the inner critic has a chance to say, *"Don't."* It's the source of innovation. The quick decision to experiment, to combine old ideas in a new way, to take a risk on something no one has tried before.

Life's most meaningful changes rarely come from careful planning alone. Sometimes, it's the impulsive *"yes"* that leads to a new friendship, a career shift, or a move to a city you've never seen. These leaps of faith are fueled by a momentary surge of desire—a gut feeling that says, *"Go for it."* In these moments, the impulse isn't recklessness; it's trust in your instincts and a willingness to embrace the unknown.

Impulse can be the engine of passion, driving us to pursue what excites us, to speak up when silence feels safer, and to chase opportunities that logic alone might dismiss. It's the force that helps us seize the moment to act before hesitation builds a wall of regret. Without impulse, life can become predictable, even stagnant. With it, we find the energy to pursue dreams, to innovate, to connect deeply with others.

~

Not all choices carry the same weight. Some people are naturally drawn to risk and eager to leap into the unknown. Others instinctively seek safety, preferring the comfort of certainty. *What makes risk feel like an invitation to some and a warning to others?*

Recent neuroscience has uncovered a key part of the answer: a circuit in the brain, connecting the hypothalamus and the lateral habenula, that helps determine our risk appetite. For years, scientists believed that the lateral habenula—a small region located deep within the brain—primarily functioned as a warning system. It would light up when we experienced disappointment or made a mistake, steering us away from adverse outcomes. Think of it as the brain's internal "don't do that again" signal.

However, new research reveals that the lateral habenula does much more. Animal studies indicate that it doesn't just react after something goes wrong. Instead, it helps set our risk preferences before we even make a choice. This means the lateral habenula can influence whether you're likely to take a chance or play it safe, even before you realize you're making a decision. Some brains show more activity in this region when faced with a risky choice, almost as if preparing for a gamble. Others show less, signaling a preference for caution and certainty.

At the center of this process is a constant dialogue between the hypothalamus and the lateral habenula. The hypothalamus functions like the body's thermostat, monitoring basic needs to maintain balance. In contrast, the lateral habenula serves as a filter, helping to determine whether to pursue a reward or avoid a potential loss.

The hypothalamus sends two types of signals to the lateral habenula: excitatory signals and inhibitory signals. Excitatory signals encourage action, prompting us to take risks or seek uncertain rewards —such as trying a new food or applying for a new job—while inhibitory signals promote caution, making us more inclined to stick with what is safe and familiar. This ongoing neural conversation creates a unique balance within each individual, shaping how we respond to risk and reward in our daily lives.

The balance of signals between the hypothalamus and lateral habenula forms a subtle but lasting bias, a kind of neural fingerprint. For some, this system fosters excitement and exploration, making them more likely to take on risks. For others, it encourages caution, leading to more deliberate or cautious choices. This bias is often so ingrained that we're not even aware it exists. Yet, it quietly influences our decisions day after day. Understanding this science doesn't just demystify our quirks—it offers compassion for the subtle, persistent ways our brains color every leap, hesitation, and calculated risk. A biological conversation is happening in the background, shaping our unique approach to risk and reward.

Are our choices driven by impulse or by reason? The truth is more complex and more beautiful than a simple either-or. We are creatures of impulse. Our desires are sculpted by millions of years of evolution, our brains tuned to the ancient rhythms of hunger, longing, and survival.

Yet we are also storytellers endowed with the remarkable gift of reflection and restraint. We can pause, consider, and rewrite the narrative of our own lives, sometimes in defiance of our most primal urges.

The circuits of desire are ancient, yes—etched deep within the folds of our brains, whispering to us of risk and reward, of pleasure and pain. However, the stories we tell ourselves, about what matters, about who we are, about what we hope to become, can reshape the adventure in ways that biology alone cannot predict. Our myths, our memories, our dreams: these are the tools with which we chisel meaning from the raw stone of experience.

Every choice, no matter how small, is a leap into the unknown. The brain, ever vigilant, weighs the odds—calculating, remembering, yearning. And we, poised on the edge between caution and courage, must decide: *Will we leap, or will we wait for another day?*

In the end, perhaps the greatest adventure is not in the choices themselves but in the act of choosing—of embracing uncertainty, of daring to shape our own stories, of finding meaning in the delicate balance between impulse and reason. For it is here, in this perpetual dance, that we become truly human: not just the sum of our instincts but the authors of our fate.

CHAPTER 5
FROM INTENTION TO INSTINCT: THE SCIENCE BEHIND HABIT FORMATION AND CHANGE

YOU FIND it in the way your fingers reach for your phone before your eyes have opened, in the way your feet carry you to the coffee pot each morning, in the way your lips seek the familiar comfort of a cigarette when the day presses down. A habit is not merely an action repeated; it is a silent architect, shaping and steering you. It is the unseen hand that draws you back to the familiar, even as your conscious mind resists.

We often think of habits as choices gone stale. Choices made once, then repeated, until the will wears thin and the behavior carries itself forward. Yet beneath this lived experience is a story written not in ink but in neurons, not in memory but in circuits that etch themselves deeper each time you act.

Where do these habits come from, why do they stick so stubbornly, and how can they be transformed?

To answer these questions, we must descend into the brain itself, into the silent machinery that turns intention into instinct. Think of the first drag of a cigarette. The bitter smoke, the scratch of the throat, the light-headed buzz. It was no accident that it stuck with you. The brain registered that sequence—action and outcome, craving and release—

and began its work. It started to build a bridge, neuron by neuron, laying down a path that could be trodden again.

So it is with every habit. Brushing your teeth was once a nightly negotiation, your parents standing sentinel, reminding you again and again. Over time, the act slipped beneath the surface of awareness. Your hand finds the toothbrush before you have chosen to reach. Habit is the brain's way of economizing, conserving energy by tucking routines out of sight, below the threshold of conscious thought.

~

The brain's architect for this process is called the basal ganglia. More specifically, a region known as the dorsolateral striatum. This hidden machinery specializes in turning repetitive actions into automatic patterns. In these early stages of repetition, however, another brain region takes the lead: the prefrontal cortex. The prefrontal cortex says, *'Pick up the toothbrush. Put toothpaste on. Scrub the molars.'* Repetition here is a conscious effort—intention steering action.

With each repetition, the baton is quietly passed. The brain concludes: the lesson is learned, the teacher can step aside. The basal ganglia assume control, embedding the routine deep within neural circuits. The pattern no longer calls for your attention. Without realizing it, you are already brushing your teeth, driving familiar roads, and checking your phone. What began as conscious intention has become reflex.

Once installed, habits wear the armor of automation. They feel instinctive because, in a sense, they are. The commands no longer flow through the highway of the prefrontal cortex but through the side streets of the basal ganglia, bypassing conscious deliberation.

This explains the strange duality of trying to break a habit. The conscious self says: I will not check my phone again tonight. Yet the hand, almost without your permission, drifts to the screen. You catch yourself scrolling, and guilt follows. Outside, it looks like weakness. Inside, it is neurobiology.

Each repetition strengthens a neural pathway, much like feet trampling grass into a visible trail through a field. The first crossing barely registers. After days and weeks, the trail deepens; the path of least resistance reveals itself. Even if you decide to carve a new direction, your brain, like a wanderer seeking ease, inclines to return to the old groove.

Research in neuroscience affirms this. Magnetic resonance imaging reveals that once habits are encoded, they tend to resist decay. Even after years of abstaining, dormant circuits can reactivate in response to stress or fatigue. *Why?* Because the prefrontal cortex, especially under pressure, falters in control. Stress hormones impair its ability to "apply the brakes," allowing old circuits to flare back into action. It is not laziness but vulnerability in the system. This is why relapse is so common. The brain does not erase; it layers. Old pathways remain, hidden but intact, waiting for conditions to let them resurface. Habits, once etched, are never fully forgotten.

In the mid-1990s, experiments by psychologist Ann Graybiel, later popularized by Charles Duhigg, revealed that habits run on loops consisting of three elements: cue, routine, and reward. The cue is a trigger that tells the brain it's time to act. The routine is the behavior itself. The reward is the payoff, whether real or symbolic, that reinforces repetition.

Take the smoker again. Stress swells in the chest—*cue*. The hand finds the cigarette, lighting it with a practiced flick—*routine*. Nicotine soothes, releases dopamine, and brings a brief calm—*reward*. The brain remembers this chain and silently prepares to replay it the next time the cue appears.

Dopamine is the storyteller behind this loop. In this case, dopamine is the molecule of *anticipation*. It fires when rewards are predicted, not only when they arrive. The brain learns to expect, and in that expectation, desire grows. Thus, even looking at a cigarette pack can stir cravings before a puff is taken.

Every habit you carry follows this rhythm, whether you notice it or not. The coffee drinker hears the gurgle of the machine—*cue*, raises the steaming mug —*routine*, and enjoys the sharp clarity of caffeine—*reward*. The procrastinator sees the task ahead—*cue*, opens YouTube instead—*routine*, and feels the brief relief of avoidance—*reward*. Habits vary, but their architecture is universal.

Of course, as with all aspects of human behavior, numerous myths surround the nature of habits. You may have heard the phrase: *It takes 21 days to form a habit.* A neat, simple promise of transformation. However, neuroscience tells a murkier truth.

A study from University College London tracked participants as they attempted to build new habits, from drinking water with lunch to exercising daily. The results? On average, it took about 66 days for behaviors to become automatic. Some required only 18 days, while others took more than 250. The process was not linear. Progress came in fits and starts, with regressions, slow climbs, and plateaus.

The lesson here is humbling but freeing: habit formation is not ruled by a calendar. It is ruled by the brain's plasticity—its ability to remodel and strengthen connections. For some behaviors, the circuits form quickly. For others, especially those competing with old ingrained routines, the process is arduous. Timing depends on the complexity, environment, and persistence of the action.

~

Why, then, do bad habits seem to solidify faster than good ones?

The answer lies in reward. Many maladaptive behaviors supply immediate gratification: nicotine's rush, sugar's sweetness, the jolt of a notification. In contrast, healthier habits often bear delayed rewards—exercise today, but toned muscles months later. The human brain, designed for survival in a world of scarce resources, is wired to overvalue the present. We are creatures of *now*.

This architecture—immediate versus delayed gratification—tilts the playing field. Habits that comfort us swiftly are reinforced with ease. Those whose benefits lie in the future demand scaffolding, reminders, and patience before they become automatic. The ancient Stoics understood this long before neuroscience confirmed it. Epictetus observed that every habit and faculty 'acquires strength by being exercised.' What he sensed, neuroscientists now map: repetition and reward carve grooves in the brain, indifferent to virtue or vice.

Here is the hope: habits are not erased, but they can be reshaped. Neuroscientists call this neuroplasticity—the brain's enduring ability to forge new connections. Even when old grooves run deep, new paths can be carved with persistence. Researchers have uncovered several practical levers for changing habits.

Changing environmental cues can disrupt automatic behaviors; for example, removing cigarettes from easy reach, placing running shoes by the door, or silencing notifications all alter the signals that trigger habitual loops. Replacement routines are another powerful tool. Because old neural circuits persist, simply resisting an urge is often ineffective. However, substituting a new routine while maintaining the same cue and reward can be successful. Stress might still arise, but breathing exercises can replace a cigarette, offering calm in place of nicotine.

Mindfulness practices also play a crucial role. By cultivating awareness, you slow down the automation of habit. Observing cravings with detachment and naming them. Recognizing, for instance, that "t*his is anxiety pushing me to smoke"—inserts a* conscious choice into the cycle. Digital habit-tracking tools can further support individuals in making changes. These apps harness the brain's love of progress and small wins; watching a streak grow provides its own dopamine reward and reinforces new behaviors. Across all these approaches, the evidence converges on a central lesson: repetition, practiced in the right context, gradually rewires the brain, allowing a new pattern to acquire the same effortless automation as the old.

Let us not mistake the science for the whole story. Habit is not only about neurons. It is about identity.

~

When you say, *"I'm trying to quit smoking,"* you are still tethered to the smoker identity. Your words acknowledge a battle not only with cigarettes but with self-concept. Lasting change happens when behaviors align with *who you believe you are*. Instead of fighting to quit cigarettes, begin to whisper, *I am not a smoker.* Instead of striving to run, whisper, *I am a runner.* The brain loves consistency; identity becomes scaffolding for habit. This is why rituals matter. Ancient monks waking at dawn for prayer, athletes engaging in pre-game routines, writers lighting candles before work—these rituals reinforce not only the loop but the identity: *This is who I am. This is what I do.*

Interestingly, we can take this concept even further, as habits have shaped civilizations. Aristotle argued that virtue itself is habit made perfect—excellence, he said, is not an act but a habit. Confucian philosophy emphasized ritual as a means of repetition that molds character. The wisdom of ages converges on this: human destiny is, in no small part, the sum of our habits.

Modern consumer culture has learned to exploit this truth. Casinos, with their flashing lights and instant feedback, are engineered to foster habit formation. Social media platforms harness the dopamine system, turning every swipe into reinforcement. What was once a quiet loop of survival has become an industry of compulsion.

The journey of habit formation and change is not a test of brute willpower. Willpower wanes. The prefrontal cortex wearies. Real change demands a strategy: align cues, reshape rewards, enlist a new identity. Progress is not measured by perfection, but by gradually shifting the automatic in your favor.

Picture your future self: waking rested, saving more than spending, reaching for a glass of water instead of a cigarette. That self is not forged in grand resolutions, but in small, repeated grooves. Just as the bad habit once formed, so too does the good—step by step, day by day, until intention becomes instinct.

So consider your own habit—the nail biting, the overspending, the late-night scrolling. You may have believed it defined you. In truth, it is only the echo of neural repetition, not the core of who you are. Science now affirms what philosophers once proclaimed: you are not bound to the grooves you have walked. Through mindfulness, environment, identity, or repetition, you can strengthen new circuits. A habit is a path, not a prison. It is a trail you may choose to deepen or leave behind, depending on where you wish to go.

In the end, the story of habits is the story of freedom hidden within constraint. It is about how the brain automates and how it can relearn. It is about becoming not only a creature of habit, but a creator of them —so the roads you walk each day lead not in circles, but forward, *toward the life you choose.*

CHAPTER 6
LIFE ON AUTOPILOT: THE HIDDEN BRAIN NETWORKS GUIDING DAILY LIFE

IT IS LATE, you're exhausted, and your mind drifts while driving. Thoughts wander to work deadlines, to what you'll eat, to an offhand comment from a colleague that still lingers. And then, suddenly, you're home. The car has been steered, the lights obeyed, the turns made. Yet you remember almost none of it. As though another hand has been on the wheel, steering while your conscious mind wandered. This is life on autopilot—an invisible choreography of brain networks silently stitching your daily survival.

The brilliance of this machinery is stunning: it keeps you alive, moving, eating, avoiding danger, all while freeing your conscious self for other pursuits. It also raises unsettling questions. *If so much of what you do each day happens beneath your awareness, who is really steering your life?*

The silent partnership of procedural memory is housed in the basal ganglia. Driving, once effortful, has become a "chunked" habit routine. Each glance in the mirror, each press of the pedal runs within a circuit etched years ago. This is not magic but an economy. Conscious attention is expensive; evolution designed autopilot so the brain could multitask—one layer to maintain the body's trajectory, another to muse on life's dramas. This autopilot is not limited to driving. It stitches itself into countless acts: tying shoelaces, typing passwords, brushing teeth. Dozens of daily behaviors glide beneath awareness. The grace of this is efficiency. The danger is detachment: it allows one to sleepwalk through life.

For centuries, philosophers have debated the existence of free will and the extent of conscious control. The Greeks believed reason was sovereign, harnessing passions like a charioteer grasping wild horses. Modern neuroscience complicates this metaphor. Increasingly, evidence shows those "wild horses" do much of the steering.

Experiments conducted by neuroscientist Benjamin Libet in the 1980s challenged our understanding of deliberate choice. He asked participants to flex their wrist at a moment of their choosing while measuring brain activity. Astonishingly, neural preparations for movement—the so-called "readiness potential"—appeared several hundred milliseconds *before* participants reported consciously deciding. The unconscious brain had already initiated the action. Consciousness appeared more like it was arriving late to the party.

Though controversial, Libet's findings nudged science toward a sobering truth: much of human behavior is scaffolding erected beneath awareness. Choice feels deliberate, but it is often a surface ripple above deeper, underlying neural currents. This is not to say that free will is an illusion, but rather that it exists more in the editing process than in initiating. Consciousness selects, vetoes, redirects—but much machinery hums along without its command.

~

At the heart of automation is the basal ganglia, a collection of nuclei nestled deep in the brain, orchestrating the learning and execution of habits. Its role, once mysterious, is now illuminated by decades of neuroscience: it is the keeper of ritual, the engraver of repeated action.

By its side is the limbic system. It governs emotion, motivation, and primal drives. It also houses the amygdala, which responds to threats; the hippocampus, which shapes memory; and the nucleus accumbens, a dopamine-rich hub of reward. This duet—the habit engraver and the drive amplifier—creates much of life's autopilot.

When stress rises, you crave comfort food without thinking. When a sudden sound startles you, you jump before you reason. When boredom stretches too long, the hand drifts toward the phone. These acts are not deliberate but are orchestrated by circuits honed across evolution to preserve survival.

Neuroscientist Joseph LeDoux described the speed of limbic reflexes: the amygdala can trigger fear responses via a "low road" pathway—direct input from the thalamus—before the cortex has time to interpret the situation. That is why you leap from a coiled rope mistaken for a snake before realizing the error. Autopilot prioritizes speed over accuracy, a design that once saved lives.

However, autopilot is not all about physical reaction. There is also the autopilot of thought itself. Enter the default mode network—a constellation of brain regions spanning medial prefrontal areas, posterior cingulate cortex, and angular gyrus. This network awakens not when we pay attention outwardly, but when our minds drift inward. It spins daydreams, rehearses conversations, replays memories, and projects futures. When you find yourself rehearsing old arguments in the shower or scripting what you will say in tomorrow's meeting, it hums in the background.

It is often compared to an inner radio station, autoplaying even when you are not "tuned in." Some neuroscientists liken it to a browser with too many tabs, endlessly loading, shifting focus without command. Others compare it to Spotify shuffle, pulling up tracks of memory, fantasy, anxiety, or aspiration, depending on mood and past experiences.

The default mode network is central to what we refer to as the sense of self. It stitches together personal narrative, identity, and continuity across time. Yet it is also implicated in rumination and worry. Depression often reveals overactive default mode network activity, as though one is trapped on a playlist stuck in repetition. Here, autopilot becomes a prison of thought loops.

What is striking is the brain's ability to switch states fluidly. You may be driving on autopilot, immersed in the default mode network's inward play, and then suddenly a car swerves—the prefrontal cortex and attentional networks snap to control. Consciousness reclaims command instantly. The shift feels dramatic, like being wrenched from dream into wakefulness.

This dynamic between unconscious efficiency and conscious oversight is the rhythm of daily life. Neither is supreme. Unconscious systems supply speed, habit, and continuity. Conscious systems supply flexibility, intention, and correction. Too much autopilot, and life becomes passive drift. Too much conscious calculation, and life becomes exhausting, joyless, and micromanaged. Flourishing requires harmony between the two.

Beneath habit and thought lies another layer entirely—the brainstem, an ancient structure that bridges the spinal cord and the higher brain. It governs the body's autonomic functions, including heartbeat, respiration, and blood pressure. It also hosts reflex circuits that act without deliberation. When your hand touches a hot stove and jerks back before you "decide," that is the spinal withdrawal reflex. It's faster than cortical involvement. When your pupils shrink in bright light, it is the midbrain's reflex arc. These systems embody the primal autopilot: survival first, consciousness after. The brainstem also houses the reticular activating system, which regulates arousal and transitions between sleep and wake. In essence, it decides whether the theater of consciousness is lit at all. Without it, the show does not start.

Why would evolution shape such dense layers of unconscious control?

The answer is energy. The human brain, astonishingly, consumes about 20% of the body's energy despite comprising only 2% of body mass. Conscious attention is especially expensive. Autopilot conserves resources by offloading repeated or urgent tasks to streamlined circuits. This is why habits exist: to save the prefrontal cortex from micromanaging every move. It is why reflexes exist: to bypass costly deliberation in life-or-death moments. It is why the default mode network exists: to prepare scenarios and narratives in downtime, nurturing a sense of self. Efficiency is survival.

Yet the blessing is also a burden. Autopilot can trap us in loops—replaying worries, repeating addictions, reinforcing biases. Anxieties in the default mode network become self-perpetuating narrative webs. Bad habits in basal ganglia loops become ritualized prisons. Reflexive reactions, like anger outbursts or fear avoidance, can override rational goals.

Modern life magnifies these downsides. Social media exploits habit loops, slot machine-like reward designs, and embedding automatic checking behaviors. Advertising hijacks limbic rewards to nudge consumption. Even politics can exploit reflexive fear, bypassing deliberation to trigger automated tribalism. The autopilot that once protected survival can, in modern contexts, be manipulated against us.

The story is not so fatalistic as it may sound. Our autopilot can be influenced. Conscious systems, though often late to act, can redirect and even retrain these deeper networks. Neuroscience highlights several tools for this process. Functional imaging reveals that mindfulness practices can dampen default mode network overactivity, effectively shifting brain states. Simply put, this means that one strategy is to catch yourself when your mind wanders and gently refocus your attention on what you are doing. Practicing this skill, whether in meditation or everyday life, helps you snap out of autopilot and pay more attention to the present moment.

Environmental redesign is another option. The basal ganglia favor cues, allowing autopilot outcomes to adapt to environmental changes. Something as simple as placing fruit on the counter or hiding the chips can recode a routine by changing the cues.

Research in neuroplasticity reveals that while the basal ganglia encode rigid habits, the prefrontal cortex can override, especially when cued by conscious novelty. So, deliberate novelty also plays a role. Doing familiar routines differently recruits conscious attention and loosens rigid habit encoding. Switching the hand you use to brush your teeth or taking a new route to work jolts neural flexibility.

Finally, implementation intentions—a strategy shown to be effective by psychologist Peter Gollwitzer—involve forming if-then plans, such as *"If it is 7 am, I will run."* In this way, you piggyback conscious aims onto unconscious triggers, aligning autopilot with your goals.

These are not abstract ideas, but neural interventions; each practice reshapes circuitry through repetition and gradually adjusts what autopilot delivers.

To see this in real life, try an exercise. Once today, interrupt one routine. Switch the mug you use for coffee. Step outside barefoot. Brush with the opposite hand. It will feel strange, even irritating. That irritation is the prefrontal cortex being summoned. You wake from autopilot, if only for seconds, aware of life's texture, of the small sparks easily dulled by routine. Do this daily, and you train flexibility. You remind autopilot that it is a servant, not a master.

So, can we harness the scripts we didn't choose?

Yes—but not by abolishing them. Total control is impossible and undesirable. Autopilot exists for a reason. Instead, the goal is stewardship. To design your environment, to shape your habits, to cultivate thought practices, so that the automation aligns with who you wish to become.

Imagine life not as a Spotify shuffle stuck on morose tracks, but as playlists you curate, still occasionally surprised, yet steering overall mood. Imagine thought not as endless browser tabs overwhelming you, but as organized windows you close and reopen with intention. The idea is not to cling to control but to wield it wisely. Autopilot will carry you home, tie your shoes, and keep your heart beating at night. Consciousness can step in to redirect, to reshape, to infuse awareness into the script.

So, as you drive home next time, notice the moment you "arrive" without memory. Smile at the machinery that preserved you. Then, as the house rises into view, take the wheel consciously. Feel the road, touch the handle, step inside with awareness. Autopilot will always hum—*but you can decide when to awaken.*

PART THREE

AN EMOTIONAL BRAIN

CHAPTER 7
THE BIOLOGY OF DISAPPOINTMENT: COPING AND ADAPTING WITH REALITY

IT'S MIDNIGHT. You slip quietly to the pantry, careful not to disturb the hush of the house. You slowly crack the door, and then you see it. There in the moonlight glow sits the perfect blue package you were hunting for: *Oreos.*

You peel back the wrapper with delicate movements only to reveal...

It's empty.

The disappointment is so intense it practically squeezes your heart. It is not just about cookies. It is about expectation colliding with reality, the whispered promise of sweetness betrayed. Disappointment, whether over missing cookies or missed dreams, is far more than a fleeting emotional nuisance. It is a biological signal, wired into the brain's architecture. It shapes how we adapt, learn, and navigate the complex terrain between desire and reality.

Disappointment stems from unmet expectations. The empty Oreo package is a microcosm of the neural processes behind heartbreak, dashed ambitions, and rejection.

What happens in the brain when desire collides with denial?

The process begins with several interconnected regions. The amygdala, an almond-shaped cluster, constantly scans for threats, losses, or mismatches between what we expect and what actually happens. When our expectations collapse, the amygdala's circuitry lights up as if danger has arrived, flagging disappointment as a significant loss that demands attention. Meanwhile, the insula integrates bodily sensation and emotion, turning that abstract sense of letdown into a physical feeling. It's responsible for the pit in your stomach, the sting in your chest, the bodily ache of having your hopes thwarted. The insula ensures disappointment is not just a thought, but something you feel.

The prefrontal cortex steps in as moderator, working to calm the emotional storms stirred by the amygdala and insula. Through conscious reframing and interpretation, it can soften the blow, transforming loss into a valuable lesson and disappointment into a source of meaning. Disappointment, then, is not a solo note but a *symphony*: the amygdala's alarm, the insula's ache, the prefrontal cortex's search for understanding. Together, they compose the familiar sensation of a heart sinking or a hope dashed.

~

Knowing this, you may be thinking: *"Why should the absence of cookies, the rejection of an idea, or the denial of affection sting* ***so deeply****?"*

The reason lies in how the brain codes for prediction errors. Neuroscientist Wolfram Schultz's work showed that dopamine neurons fire not only when rewards arrive, but more critically, when rewards are greater than expected. Conversely, when rewards are *less* than expected—when the cookie pack is empty—dopamine activity plunges. This is the neurochemical signature of disappointment, a sudden neural silence where anticipation once sang. The sting is proportional to the gap between anticipation and reality: the greater the promise, the sharper the letdown. This measures not the object lost, but the expectation betrayed.

Evolution sculpted this disappointment system to optimize survival. Animals needed to register when reality fell short. They needed to recognize when a food source was exhausted, when safety failed. Disappointment's pain was the push to update strategies, to search anew. What was once adaptive for hunter-gatherers searching for fruit now manifests as heartbreak when love goes unreturned, or frustration when the internet buffer wheel spins endlessly on a Friday night.

It's important to note that occasional letdowns are tolerable, even instructive. However, repeated disappointment is another beast. The brain does not merely register each event in isolation—it adapts. With chronic letdown, two outcomes emerge: heightened sensitivity or strengthened resilience.

For some, repeated disappointment breeds hypervigilance. The amygdala grows reactive, the insula etches discomfort into the body, and the brain begins to expect disappointment. This forms the root of pessimism and depression: circuits rewired toward negativity, trapping the mind in a self-fulfilling cycle.

Others emerge stronger from setbacks. Research on resilience reveals that prefrontal circuits can be trained—like muscles—to recast disappointment as information, not failure. Over time, this practice builds emotional shock absorbers, dampening the amygdala's alarms. Resilience, like scar tissue, forms not by avoiding pain, but by healing well after the blow.

Given these diverging paths, a natural question arises: *Why does the brain end up on one path rather than another?*

Genetics, early experience, social context, and learned coping strategies all shape which path the brain takes. Culture, too, leaves its mark. The Stoics, for example, counseled lowering expectations as a kind of psychological armor, aiming to narrow the gap between desire and reality. Epictetus advised that expecting events to unfold as they do brings peace.

Meanwhile, Buddhism identified attachment and craving as the root of suffering, teaching that disappointment is inevitable when one clings to outcomes in an impermanent world, and that liberation comes through letting go.

Shakespeare captured the sting of disappointment in his plays: lovers undone, kings betrayed, ambitions thwarted. These dramas echo the same emotional currents that neuroscientists now map in the brain. Today, consumer culture amplifies expectation—advertising promises fulfillment with every product, setting the stage for disappointment when reality falls short of the glossy ideal. Across time and society, disappointment reveals not only truths about ourselves, but about the stories and values that shape our world.

Consider Sarah, who interviewed for her dream job. She rehearsed answers, visualized triumph, and allowed herself to imagine the celebration. When a polite rejection email arrives, her amygdala ignites. *Loss.* The insula brings nausea. Prefrontal cortex either sinks into self-blame or reframes: *This was practice, not finality. Next time, I'll be sharper.* Her trajectory forward depends on whether reappraisal takes hold.

Or Miguel, a teenager awaiting a text back from someone he likes. Each buzz of the phone spikes hope. Silence extends into hours. Anticipation collapses into disappointment. The gap between imagined connection and real-world void is felt viscerally. How Miguel interprets it—whether as confirmation of unworthiness or simply bad timing—will seed his resilience or deepen his insecurity.

These seemingly small scenarios reveal a profound truth: disappointment is the brain's way of managing life's steady stream of unmet expectations. How we respond—especially through cognitive reappraisal—determines whether disappointment becomes a source of growth or adversity. This ability to reinterpret events is one of our most powerful tools for strengthening resilience and adapting to reality.

Neuroscientist Kevin Ochsner's work shows that when individuals reinterpret an adverse event: *"This was a chance to learn"* instead of *"This proves I'm a failure"*, prefrontal cortex engagement increases and amygdala activation decreases. This is neuroplasticity at work. Each act of reframing forges new pathways that soften emotional reactions. With practice, the brain learns to blunt the sting of disappointment. Like a pianist repeating scales, the neural patterns of reinterpretation become second nature. In this, biology affirms what wisdom traditions have long taught: by choosing how we interpret events, we can shape the brain's response to adversity.

Physical activity is another effective approach. Exercise helps the body metabolize stress hormones, improves emotional regulation, and reduces the discomfort associated with disappointment. Practicing gratitude by redirecting attention to what remains rather than what has been lost can also build resilience against future letdowns.

Finally, novelty and creativity, such as starting a new project or engaging in artistic expression, are also options. They allow us to convert emotional energy from loss into growth and new possibilities. These approaches do not seek to numb pain, but rather to channel it into adaptive pathways, forging resilience and training the brain's capacity to recover and grow stronger.

Back in the pantry, the empty cookie package lingers—a small betrayal. Disappointment rises. You sigh, perhaps mutter a curse or two. Beneath the surface, your brain is recalibrating predictions and building resilience. This minor letdown echoes life's larger disappointments: the rejection letter, the failed venture, the love unreturned. Each empty Oreo tray is a lesson pressed into the brain's circuitry. With awareness, reframing, and practice, you can revise the narrative.

CHAPTER 8
EMOTIONAL LIFE AND BEHAVIOR: MAPPING JOY, ANGER, AND SADNESS IN THE BRAIN

IN THE DIM study of Down House, Charles Darwin sits over a notebook, the glow of a winter's lamp flickering across his ink-stained fingers. Outside, his infant son's laughter rings down the hall—a bright, irrepressible sound. Darwin pauses, listening, then returns to his notes. He is not recording the arc of a swallow's wing or the curl of a fern this evening but something far more elusive: the choreography of emotion itself.

He watched his children's faces flush with joy, crumple in grief, or twist in the throes of a tantrum. He also observed how animals, such as dogs, monkeys, and even birds, revealed their inner states through a universal language of movement and sound. *"The young and the old of widely different races, both with man and animals, express the same state of mind by the same movements,"* he would later write, marveling at the shared grammar of emotion that spanned continents and species.

This was the secret: that emotions, so often dismissed as fleeting or irrational, were, in fact, ancient, adaptive forces. They are biological currents running through every living thing. In *"The Expression of the Emotions in Man and Animals,"* published in 1872, Darwin sought to decipher this hidden language. He described, with almost cinematic detail, the trembling of muscles in fear, the baring of teeth in rage, the downward cast of the eyes in shame, and the convulsive joy of laughter.

"Fear is often expressed by the whole body trembling," he observed. "The lips being drawn back, the teeth being exposed, and the mouth opened wide, are signs of intense terror. The feeling of disgust is expressed by a slight protrusion of the lips, often accompanied by a slight raising of the upper lip. Shame is shown by a downward cast of the eyes, with a slight blush."

Darwin proposed three main ideas. The first is the *Principle of Serviceable Habits,* which states that certain emotional expressions originated as useful actions. For instance, widening the eyes in surprise allows a person to take in more information. Over time, these actions became ingrained and were passed down through generations as instincts.

The second principle is the *Principle of Antithesis,* which posits that some expressions exist simply as opposites. A clear example of this is the proud, upright posture of confidence contrasted with the slumped shoulders of defeat. Finally, there is the *Principle of Direct Action;* Darwin argued that many expressions arise directly from the nervous system and are beyond conscious control. Reactions such as a racing heart, blushing, or shivering are not learned behaviors but rather automatic responses to emotional stimuli.

For Darwin, these patterns were not mere quirks of human nature but evolutionary relics—evidence that our emotional lives are deeply rooted in our animal ancestry. He wrote, *"The far greater number of the movements of expression, and all the more important ones, are, as we have seen, innate or inherited; and such cannot be said to depend on the will of the individual."*

Before Darwin, emotions were often seen as mysterious, even spiritual. They were something that set humans apart from animals. But Darwin's biological lens revealed a different truth: the smile, the frown, the startled gasp, and the tears of grief are not just personal experiences. They are the echoes of millions of years of adaptation, survival, and connection.

His work was revolutionary, yet for many today, Darwin's name conjures memes about "survival of the fittest" or the infamous "*Darwin Awards*"—a tongue-in-cheek celebration of those who, through spectacular lapses in judgment, supposedly remove themselves from the gene pool. But the real Darwin was not a judge of folly; he was a chronicler of the heart's ancient wisdom. He saw that our emotions, far from being weaknesses, were the very tools that allowed our ancestors to thrive, bond, and endure.

Modern neuroscience now picks up where Darwin left off, tracing the neural circuitry of emotion from the amygdala's alarm bells to the dopamine-driven highs of joy and love. The foundation remains the same: to understand our feelings is to glimpse the deep, shared history written in every heartbeat, every tear, every laugh.

Anger is a sudden, unmistakable flash of heat that demands our attention. It's the pounding heart, the flushed cheeks, the tightness in the chest. In small, healthy doses, anger can be a gift, as it signals that something is wrong, a boundary has been crossed, or an injustice needs to be addressed. Anger, at its core, is the mind's way of saying, *"This matters. Pay attention."*

When channeled constructively, anger can be a powerful force for positive change. It fuels assertiveness, motivates us to stand up for ourselves, and can even spark movements for social justice. History is filled with moments where righteous anger—at unfair laws, broken promises, or abuses of power—became the driving force behind reform. When we learn to express anger clearly and respectfully, it can strengthen relationships, clarify values, and inspire action.

Anger is a force that demands respect. When it isn't allowed to move through us, when it's ignored, denied, or left to simmer beneath the surface, it doesn't simply fade away. Instead, it curdles into something more corrosive: aggression. Like a pot left boiling on the stove, anger that isn't acknowledged or expressed in healthy ways can eventually spill over, scalding everything in its path.

Neuroscience has begun to reveal just how deeply this process can affect us, especially in childhood. When aggression becomes chronic, whether from living in a home filled with shouting, experiencing repeated verbal abuse, or enduring early trauma, it can actually leave physical marks on the developing brain. The white matter pathways, the brain's internal highways that connect different regions, are especially vulnerable. These pathways are crucial for developing skills such as language, empathy, and emotional control. When they're damaged or altered, the effects can last a lifetime. This makes it harder to communicate, understand others' feelings, or manage one's own emotions.

Consider Jordan. In his childhood home, anger was a storm—sometimes crashing through the house in shouts and slammed doors, sometimes vanishing, leaving an eerie, suffocating calm. There was no safe middle ground. When anger erupted, it was volcanic and terrifying; when it was silenced, it hung in the air, heavy and unspoken. Jordan learned early to fear his own anger, to bury it deep in his chest where it simmered, unseen.

The brain doesn't forget what the heart tries to hide.

Each time Jordan swallowed his frustration, his amygdala's alarm bell flared, sending signals of threat and distress. The prefrontal cortex struggled to keep the lid on. The neural pathways connecting emotion and expression grew tangled, reinforcing a pattern: anger stuffed down, then boiling over in sudden uncontrollable outbursts.

As an adult, Jordan carried this legacy into the world. At work, a minor setback could ignite him—his voice sharp, his hands trembling, his mind flooded with adrenaline. Other times, he shut down completely, retreating behind a wall of silence. Relationships suffered. He felt misunderstood, ashamed, and alone with the intensity of his feelings.

It wasn't until Jordan began therapy that the cycle started to shift. In the safety of that space, he learned to recognize the early signals, such as tightness in his jaw, heat in his chest, and the quickening of his pulse. With practice, he named his anger out loud, engaging his prefrontal cortex and soothing the amygdala's alarm. Gradually, Jordan discovered that anger didn't have to be a threat; it could be a signal, a guide. He learned to express his frustration clearly and calmly and to advocate for his needs without resorting to aggression or withdrawal.

Over time, new neural pathways formed—connections that allowed him to pause, reflect, and choose his response. The old patterns softened. Jordan found himself building healthier relationships, no longer ruled by the ghosts of childhood rage. In his story, we see the brain's remarkable ability to heal, adapt, and transform, even after years of living in the shadow of unspoken anger.

Practices such as pausing, assertive communication, and seeking support can help us harness the energy of anger without letting it take over. By slowing and deepening each inhale and exhale, we activate the parasympathetic nervous system, which calms the body's stress response and reduces the intensity of anger. In a heated moment, a few slow, deliberate breaths can lower the heart rate and create space for a more thoughtful response.

Assertive communication is equally vital. Instead of suppressing anger or letting it explode, assertiveness means expressing feelings. It needs to be clearly and respectfully stated. This is often done using "I" statements, such as *"I feel frustrated when..."* These statements help maintain boundaries, foster mutual understanding, and reduce the likelihood of conflict escalation.

Seeking support from trusted friends, family, or mental health professionals can provide a safe outlet for processing anger. These supportive relationships offer validation, perspective, and guidance, helping to prevent anger from festering or becoming destructive. Therapy, in particular, can teach skills such as cognitive restructuring and emotional regulation tailored to individual needs. Cognitive techniques, like cognitive reappraisal, involve reframing the situation that triggered anger, allowing you to view it from a less threatening perspective. This shift helps reduce emotional intensity and encourages problem-solving rather than overreacting.

Physical activity is another powerful strategy. Exercise—whether it's a brisk walk, yoga, or martial arts—helps dissipate the physiological aspects of anger, releases endorphins, and improves mood. This makes it easier to return to a calm state. On the other side of this coin is relaxation as a strategy to calm anger.

Relaxation techniques, such as progressive muscle relaxation, guided imagery, or meditation, can help lower overall stress levels. This also makes it easier to manage anger when it arises. Sometimes, a simple timeout allows emotions to settle before responding, preventing impulsive reactions and promoting more thoughtful engagement.

By integrating these practices into daily life, anger can transform from a disruptive force into a valuable signal, highlighting what matters to us and guiding us toward healthier, more authentic connections with ourselves and others. Over time, these strategies strengthen the neural pathways involved in emotional regulation, enhancing resilience and overall well-being.

Yet, even when anger is managed skillfully, it often leaves a subtle imprint behind. As the heat of rage cools, another set of emotions can quietly emerge—shame and guilt.

Where anger demands action, shame and guilt draw us inward. They urge reflection and, sometimes, self-reproach. These feelings can cling like a shadow long after the outburst has faded. They are the echo in the empty room, the chill that lingers after the storm. Unprocessed anger leaves us not only isolated and misunderstood but also stuck in cycles of guilt and self-recrimination. It chips away at self-esteem, narrows the possibilities for healing, and can make the path back to connection feel impossibly steep—like climbing a mountain in the dark.

However, shame and guilt, though often lumped together, are not twins. They are related yet distinct. Guilt is action-focused: it arises when we recognize that we've done something wrong, and it nudges us gently—or sometimes not so gently—to make amends. Guilt says, *"I did a bad thing."* It is the internal compass that points us toward repair, the quiet voice that urges us to apologize, to fix what we have broken. In this way, guilt serves as a social glue by motivating us to restore trust, seek forgiveness, and mend the bonds that hold families, friendships, and communities together.

Neuroscientifically, guilt engages the prefrontal cortex—the brain's center for judgment, decision-making, and social reasoning. When we feel guilt, the anterior cingulate cortex is also activated, helping us process the conflict between our actions and our values. This neural circuitry enables us to reflect on our behavior, imagine its impact on others, and plan reparative actions.

Shame, by contrast, is self-focused. It whispers, *"I am a bad person."* Shame is a heavy cloak draped around the shoulders, convincing us that our flaws are not just in what we do but in who we are. While guilt can motivate growth and repair, shame can be paralyzing. It turns our gaze inward, shrinking our world and convincing us that we are unworthy of forgiveness or love. Shame is the fog that obscures the path forward, the weight that makes every step feel harder.

In the brain, shame activates not only the prefrontal cortex but also the insula and the amygdala—regions involved in processing emotional pain, bodily awareness, and threat detection. The insula, in particular, is associated with the visceral, gut-wrenching sensations of shame. At the same time, the amygdala registers the social threat and fear of rejection that often accompany it. This combination can trigger the body's stress response, flooding the system with cortisol and making it difficult to think clearly or reach out for support.

These emotions are not just personal burdens. They are social tools forged by evolution to help us navigate the complex world of human relationships. Guilt, in particular, is a force for social cohesion. Evolutionary neuroscientists suggest that the capacity for guilt is rooted in our need to maintain group harmony. This means our feelings of guilt evolved to help us recognize when we've harmed others, to motivate us to make amends, and to prevent the social fabric from unraveling. By activating brain regions involved in empathy and self-regulation, guilt helps us remain attuned to the feelings of others and motivates us to engage in prosocial behavior. In this way, guilt is a quiet architect of trust.

Shame, too, has deep roots in our social wiring. It evolved as a warning system, alerting us when we risk being cast out or rejected by the group. In small doses, shame can prompt humility and caution—reminding us to stay within the boundaries of what is acceptable and to learn from our mistakes. When shame becomes chronic and overwhelming or when it is fueled by harsh criticism, social exclusion, or unresolved trauma, it can spiral. The insula lights up with the sting of social pain: the flush of embarrassment, the ache of exclusion, the burn of humiliation. The brain can become overwhelmed, making it hard to see a way out.

Recent neuroimaging studies have revealed that the neural circuits underlying social pain, especially those involving the insula and the dorsal anterior cingulate cortex, overlap significantly with those activated by physical pain. This explains why shame and social rejection can feel physically excruciating and why these experiences can leave lasting marks on our emotional memory.

Consider Lena. In the house where she grew up, mistakes were never small things. A spilled glass of milk, a wrong answer in class, a forgotten chore—each was met not with a gentle correction but with sharp words or laughter that stung. Every error became a spotlight, every misstep a kind of public trial. Lena learned early to brace herself for the next wave of ridicule, to shrink a little smaller each time her imperfections were exposed.

Inside her, the pain of shame settled deep. Her brain became exquisitely tuned to the slightest hint of criticism. Repeated experiences of social pain can sensitize the amygdala and insula, making the brain hyper-vigilant to threat and rejection. Her prefrontal cortex was instead flooded with self-doubt and anxious rehearsals of what she might do wrong next. Over the years, Lena began to equate every error with unworthiness. The message was clear: to be flawed was to be unlovable.

As an adult, the echoes of that childhood followed her everywhere. A forgotten appointment, a misplaced word, a dish left unwashed—these minor slip-ups could trigger a flood of shame so intense it left her breathless. Instead of reaching out for reassurance or making amends, Lena would retreat. She canceled plans, let texts go unanswered, and built walls where bridges might have been. Her world grew smaller, her relationships more distant, her self-esteem eroded by the silent, relentless drumbeat of shame.

Lena's story is not unique. Many of us know what it is to be haunted by old voices, to feel our worth shrink in the shadow of a single mistake. Yet, in seeing Lena's struggle, we are reminded of the quiet courage it takes to face shame and the hope that, with compassion and understanding, even the deepest wounds can begin to heal. Shame, when met with kindness and self-awareness, can be transformed—its energy redirected toward healing, humility, and growth.

Guilt can lead us to repair and reconnect. The brain's remarkable plasticity means that, with support and practice, even the deepest grooves of shame can be softened. New paths of self-acceptance and connection can be forged. Therapies such as mindfulness and self-compassion training have been shown to strengthen neural pathways in the prefrontal cortex and reduce hyperactivity in the amygdala, gradually rewiring the brain's response to shame and guilt.

In the end, shame and guilt are not just scars; they are signposts. They point us toward what matters—belonging, integrity, and the hope of forgiveness. They remind us that, though we may stumble, we are never truly alone in our longing to be seen, to be understood, and to be whole. Yet even as we find the courage to face shame and guilt, another ancient companion often waits just beneath the surface. Sometimes, what holds us back from reaching out or daring to change is not only the memory of past mistakes but a deeper, older current—a pulse of fear that runs through the body and mind.

Sadness is not simply the absence of joy; it is a complex, deeply rooted emotion with a distinct biological signature. When we experience loss —whether it is the death of a loved one, the end of a relationship, or the collapse of a cherished dream—our brains respond with waves of sadness and grief. Neurotransmitters such as serotonin and dopamine, along with brain regions previously discussed, like the anterior cingulate cortex, insula, and amygdala, coordinate the complex interplay of sorrow and yearning.

Grief is a full-body experience. It is not just an ache in the heart. It's a storm that sweeps through the entire body and mind. When loss strikes, it can feel as if every part of you is on high alert. Emotions surge and crash, sometimes out of nowhere. The brain's fear center amplifies every pang of sadness, every flicker of anxiety. It's why memories can blur, why it's so hard to focus, why even small decisions suddenly feel overwhelming.

At the same time, another part of the brain—the anterior cingulate cortex—flares with the pain of emotional loss. It's the part that aches for connection. It makes you yearn for the sound of a loved one's voice or the comfort of their presence. The world feels emptier, and that emptiness is not just emotional; it's biological.

The prefrontal cortex, usually the brain's steady captain, can lose its grip. You might feel foggy, indecisive, or adrift as if you're moving through a thick mist. Even the brain's reward system, which usually lights up in response to pleasure and motivation, can become stuck on longing, replaying memories, and fueling a persistent sense of yearning. Letting go feels impossible because the mind keeps circling back to what—or who—has been lost.

Grief, in this way, is not just sadness. It's a full-body, full-mind experience, one that touches every corner of our being. And if you've ever felt lost in that storm, know that your brain is simply doing its best to make sense of the unimaginable, holding on until, little by little, the clouds begin to part.

Beneath the surface, mighty chemical messengers are at work. Neurotransmitters like serotonin and dopamine often fall out of balance during periods of deep sorrow. This chemical shift can leave you feeling drained, your energy sapped as if you're moving through molasses. Sleep becomes elusive or restless. Concentration slips away, making it hard to focus on even the simplest tasks. There's a heaviness, a sense of emptiness or hopelessness, that can settle in the chest and linger for weeks or months.

These symptoms can look and feel a lot like depression, and the line between grief and clinical depression is sometimes thin. Sadness, after all, is a normal and healthy response to loss—a sign that something or someone matters deeply. Yet, sometimes, the storm refuses to lift when the emptiness becomes all-consuming, and daily life feels hijacked by despair.

Chronic or "complicated" grief can reshape the brain. When loss is so profound or unresolved that it never quite recedes, the neural circuits responsible for reward and yearning remain on high alert. The brain's longing centers are unable to accept the absence. This persistent yearning can lead to depression. In this state, sadness no longer serves as a healthy adaptation but instead becomes a trap. The mind circles endlessly around what was lost, caught in cycles of rumination, withdrawal, and despair. The world grows smaller, pleasures fade, and hope seems to slip further away.

Understanding the difference between sadness and depression is crucial. Sadness, though painful, is usually tied to a clear object—a loved one, a dream, a chapter of life—and, even in its depths, often allows for moments of relief, connection, or meaning. It is a wave that rises and falls, sometimes bringing tears, sometimes bringing memories that warm the heart.

Depression, by contrast, is a fog that settles in and refuses to lift. It is pervasive and persistent. It cuts us off from life's pleasures, numbs relationships, and makes even simple joys feel unreachable. Beneath this emotional haze, the brain itself is caught in a complex interplay of disrupted circuits and chemical imbalances. In depression, the prefrontal cortex often grows quiet and dim, and its activity and even its size are reduced. This makes it harder to plan, to hope, or to see a way out.

The chemistry of depression is just as tangled. Serotonin often runs low or out of sync, opening the door to persistently feeling sad. Norepinephrine, which fuels alertness and energy, can dip. This leads to fatigue and trouble concentrating. Dopamine also dwindles, making pleasure and excitement feel out of reach—an experience known as anhedonia. Even the brain's networks get caught in the undertow.

The default mode network, which governs self-focused thought, can become overactive. This fuels endless rumination and negative thinking. The reward circuitry, once alive with anticipation, goes quiet, dulling the spark of curiosity and joy. To make matters worse, the body's stress response often shifts into overdrive. Inflammatory markers and cortisol rise. This further disrupts brain function and deepens the sense of despair.

Depression, then, is not simply a chemical imbalance or a fleeting feeling. It is a disorder of brain network dynamics, neuroplasticity, and the body's stress systems. It's a storm that can feel endless but one that science and compassion, together, are learning to calm. Treatments like antidepressants, psychotherapy, and lifestyle changes work to restore balance, rekindle hope, and help the brain find its way back to resilience and light.

Sadness is not a sign of weakness. It's a testament to our capacity for love and connection. Unlike depression, it serves a purpose in the landscape of healing. It draws us inward, prompting us to withdraw and rest, conserving energy for the slow work of repair. It is the emotion that allows us to let go of what cannot be reclaimed, to reimagine our place in a changed world, and to build new sources of meaning and connection. In this way, sadness is both a mourner and a builder—dismantling the old and preparing the ground for something new.

The journey through sorrow is rarely straightforward; it comes in waves, sometimes gentle, sometimes fierce, but always with the potential to move us, in time, toward adaptation and growth. Moments of laughter and connection can coexist with sorrow. Expressing positive emotions during grief is linked to better long-term adjustment. Sharing sadness with others can deepen bonds, invite empathy, and remind us that we are not alone. Over time, the brain's remarkable capacity for neuroplasticity allows us to integrate loss, restore balance, and rediscover hope.

After the ache of sadness and the fog of depression, another emotion rises: disgust. Fear alerts us, sadness prompts reflection, and disgust leads us to set clear boundaries between what is safe and what is forbidden. It is an emotion as old as life itself, etched into our biology as a first line of defense against the world's hidden threats.

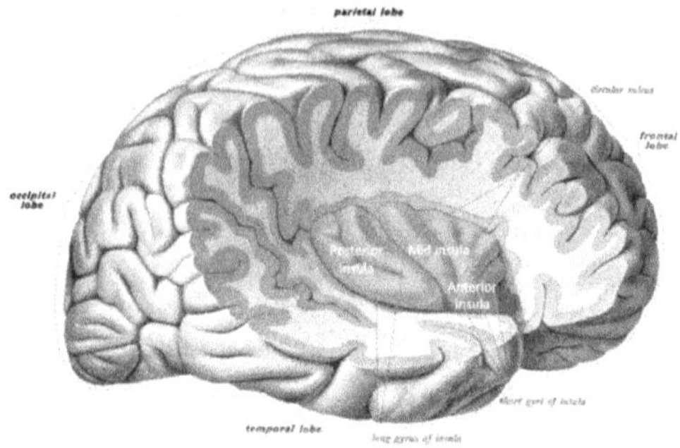

Figure 11. *The insula, divided into its anterior, mid, and posterior regions.* Schappelle on Wikimedia Commons

Disgust begins in the body. Its evolutionary roots run deep, protecting us from toxins, spoiled food, and disease. The insular cortex —tucked beneath the folds of the brain's outer shell—serves as the command center for this visceral reaction. When we encounter something rotten, foul, or infectious, the insula lights up. It triggers a cascade of sensations: a wrinkled nose, a curling lip, a wave of nausea. These responses are not learned; they are inherited, a universal language of survival.

Disgust is more than a biological reflex. As humans formed communities and cultures, this primal emotion was repurposed to guard not just the body but the group. Disgust began to shape our social and moral boundaries, drawing lines between what is pure and what is taboo and who belongs and who does not. The same insular cortex that recoils from spoiled meat also activates when we witness a betrayal, a violation of trust, or an act that offends our shared values.

Moral disgust is sometimes considered the glue that holds social groups together. It binds us together by defining what is acceptable and what must be cast out. When someone cheats, lies, or breaks a sacred rule, we feel a jolt of revulsion. It's as if the very fabric of our community has been soiled. This reaction is not just metaphorical; brain scans reveal that the insula responds to moral transgressions in much the same way as it does to physical contamination.

Disgust often works in concert with fear and anger. Fear alerts us to danger; anger rallies us to confront it; disgust draws the boundary, declaring, *"This must not enter."* In times of social upheaval, these emotions can reinforce one another. Sometimes fueling prejudice, exclusion, or even violence when boundaries are drawn too tightly or unjustly. Yet, at its core, disgust is a guardian. It protects us from harm, both physical and moral. It helps us maintain the integrity of our bodies and our communities, reminding us that survival is not just about what we take in but also about what we keep out.

In learning to recognize and understand disgust—its triggers, its wisdom, and its limits—we gain insight into the ways we protect ourselves and those we love. Yet, like all powerful emotions, disgust has a shadow side: it can be twisted, amplified, or misdirected, transforming from a tool of survival into a wedge that divides and isolates. Disgust, then, stands as both shield and signpost. Marking the boundaries of self, community, and the sacred, guiding us through a world where danger and belonging coexist. After the weight of such heavy emotions, the body and mind yearn for light.

~

Joy sometimes arrives as a sudden burst—a laugh shared with a friend, the first bite of a favorite meal, the quiet awe of a sunrise. At other times, happiness is a gentle, steady warmth. It can be a sense of contentment that lingers beneath the surface, even on ordinary days.

Beneath these feelings lies a dazzling orchestra of brain chemistry. Joy and happiness are the result of intricate neural choreography. The brain's reward circuitry becomes activated in response to pleasurable experiences, releasing a surge of dopamine throughout the system. Endorphins, the body's natural opiates, add another layer of euphoria. They soothe pain and amplify pleasure. Serotonin, too, plays a role. As we've discussed before, it stabilizes mood and promotes a sense of well-being.

These neurochemical surges are not just fleeting fireworks; they have a purpose. Joy motivates us to seek out rewarding activities such as play, learning, and social connection, and to repeat them. This is why happiness is so tightly linked to motivation and resilience. When we feel good, we are more likely to take risks, solve problems, and bounce back from setbacks. Joy expands our mental horizons, encouraging creativity, flexibility, and growth.

Yet, joy is more than a personal reward. It is a powerful force for social bonding. Happy people are more likely to form strong relationships. Those relationships, in turn, reinforce happiness in a virtuous cycle. Laughter, play, and shared celebration knit communities together, building trust and resilience that buffer against life's inevitable stresses. Yet, happiness, like all emotions, is fleeting.

As discussed in an earlier chapter, the brain is designed for adaptation. This is a phenomenon known as hedonic adaptation. It explains why the excitement of a new success or possession quickly fades, returning us to our emotional baseline. This impermanence is not a flaw. Rather, it is a beneficial feature of our biology. Hedonic adaptation encourages us to keep striving, learning, and growing rather than settling into complacency, ensuring that we remain engaged with life's unfolding possibilities.

The pursuit of lasting contentment isn't a frantic chase after endless highs. It's more like tending a garden, nurturing the habits and mindsets that allow joy to take root and flourish. Imagine starting each day with a few lines in a gratitude journal—pausing to notice the sunlight on your pillow, the laughter of a friend, the taste of your morning coffee. With every entry, you're quietly rewiring your brain, teaching it to spot and savor the good, however small.

Joy also lives in movement. It might be a brisk walk beneath swaying trees or a spontaneous dance in the kitchen as your favorite song spills from the speakers. These moments flood the body with endorphins and dopamine, brightening mood and sharpening focus. Small acts of kindness, like a handwritten note, a helping hand, or a genuine compliment, also send ripples of happiness through your mind and the minds of others. Then there are the moments of awe. Standing beneath a vast sky, watching a child discover something new, losing yourself in the beauty of a painting or a piece of music. Each of these experiences feeds the brain's happiness circuits, inviting joy to visit more often and linger a little longer.

Joy is a powerful buffer against adversity. Positive emotions help regulate stress by lowering cortisol levels, broadening our perspective, and opening us up to support and fresh solutions. In classrooms, workplaces, and homes, a joyful atmosphere is fertile ground for learning, creativity, and resilience. It turns even the toughest challenges into opportunities for growth. In this way, joy becomes a wellspring we can return to again and again as we move through life.

Happiness is not a permanent state, nor is it meant to be. Like morning dew, it sparkles and fades, but in its wake, it leaves a landscape more vibrant for its passing. The secret is not to cling to joy but to cultivate the conditions—connection, gratitude, movement, meaning—where it can return again and again. Of course, just as we settle into the gentle cadence of contentment, life has a way of shifting the tempo.

The next emotion we will cover arrives unannounced—sometimes with a crash, sometimes with a whisper. One moment, you are sipping coffee in the hush of morning; the next, the mug slips from your hand and shatters, shards skittering across the tile like startled insects. Or a siren wails outside, slicing through the silence. Or a message blinks onto your screen: news that flips your world on its head. Even the ordinary can tilt suddenly; an unexpected laugh bursting from a stranger's lips, a forgotten song flooding your memory, the sharp tang of lemon where you expected honey.

Surprise is a lightning strike in the middle of the routine, a jolt that ricochets through your body. Your heart leaps. Your breath halts. The edges of the world sharpen, and for a moment, everything is possible.

Surprise doesn't whisper or wait its turn. It crashes in, upending the ordinary and scattering your expectations like leaves in a gust of wind. This is the power of surprise: it interrupts, it awakens, it reminds us that beneath the surface of every predictable day, the unexpected is always lurking, ready to rewrite the script.

The startle response is automatic. When something unexpected happens, sensory receptors in the eyes or ears send signals racing through the brain. The information is routed to the amygdala, which activates the sympathetic nervous system. This is the classic *"fight or flight"* reflex, but it is also the brain's way of asking, *"What just happened?"*

Surprise is more than a reflex; it is a gateway to learning. When our expectations are violated, the brain releases a surge of noradrenaline, also known as norepinephrine. It floods neural circuits and heightens alertness. This chemical burst primes us to pay extra attention, amplifies curiosity, and marks the moment as important. In these startling moments, the brain's prediction machinery—rooted in the hippocampus and dopaminergic pathways—springs into action, updating our internal models of the world.

The orienting reflex, first described by Ivan Pavlov, is the body's way of pausing and turning toward novelty. Eyes and ears shift, breath catches, and the mind suspends its usual routines to take in new information. This reflex is not just about survival; it is about exploration. Each surprise is an invitation to learn, adapt, and grow.

Surprise is a master engraver of memory. Studies show that unexpected events are more likely to be encoded and recalled than predictable ones. The emotional jolt of surprise etches details into the hippocampus. This is why we remember where we were during a shocking news event or the exact words of an unexpected compliment.

Not all surprises are created equal. Positive surprises, such as an unexpected gift or a sudden burst of laughter, can spark joy and reinforce social bonds. In contrast, negative surprises, like a sudden loss or a frightening encounter, may be remembered even more vividly. Both types, however, serve the same purpose: they force the brain to update its expectations. They strengthen synaptic connections and fuel neuroplasticity.

With repeated exposure, the brain learns to distinguish between true threats and harmless novelties. This process, known as startle response habituation, enables us to tune out background noise and focus on what truly matters. Over time, the startle fades, anxiety diminishes, and the world feels a little safer. This ability to adapt is crucial for emotional regulation and resilience.

Surprise is not just about disruption; it is about possibility. In the classroom, a well-timed surprise can ignite curiosity and deepen learning. In everyday life, surprise keeps us flexible, open to new experiences, and ready to rewrite our stories. It is the emotion that bridges the gap between what we know and what we have yet to discover. In the grand symphony of emotion, surprise is the cymbal crash—a sharp, bright note that commands attention and leaves a lasting echo in the mind. It is the spark that keeps us learning, adapting, and alive to the wonders of an unpredictable world.

Modern neuroscience bridges the gap between ancient wisdom and contemporary understanding, revealing how emotions are not just fleeting experiences but deeply rooted in the brain's architecture. Stress, for example, floods the body with chemical messengers, while unprocessed anger can leave lasting marks on neural circuits. Chronic craving dulls our capacity for everyday joy. Yet, these discoveries do not doom us to a life dictated by our biology; instead, they offer a pathway to change.

For centuries, efforts to control desires and subdue emotions were often framed as battles of willpower or fate. Neuroscience, however, reframes this struggle as an opportunity. The brain is not a static machine but a dynamic, living system—capable of growth, adaptation, and renewal. This is the promise of neuroplasticity: the brain's remarkable ability to reorganize itself by forming new neural connections throughout life.

To thrive, our brains must master emotion regulation. This is a skill as vital as any other for well-being. Think of emotions as a symphony: sometimes the music swells, sometimes it quiets. Emotional regulation is the conductor's baton, ensuring no single feeling overwhelms the rest. The goal is not to silence emotions but to adjust their intensity, allowing us to experience the full spectrum without being overpowered.

Techniques like labeling emotions—simply naming what we feel—activate the prefrontal cortex and calm the amygdala's reactivity. Cognitive reappraisal, or reframing a situation to change its emotional impact, also strengthens neural pathways in the prefrontal cortex, enhancing our capacity for emotional control.

Emotion regulation is not fixed at birth. Children develop these skills through social learning and brain maturation, while adults can continue to refine them throughout their lives. Older adults often exhibit improved emotional regulation, likely due to the accumulation of experience and shifts in brain function that prioritize well-being. This adaptability is a testament to neuroplasticity.

Neuroplasticity is the brain's ability to rewire itself in response to experience, reflection, and deliberate practice. Even if we have spent years reacting with anxiety or falling into destructive emotional patterns, we are not bound to repeat those cycles forever. Each time we pause before responding, practice mindfulness, or seek therapeutic support, we lay down new neural pathways. Old, automatic responses can be softened; healthier patterns can be established and strengthened.

The process is not always linear. Setbacks are natural, just as a new path in the woods can become overgrown if not used. Persistence and self-compassion are crucial—every effort to notice, pause, and choose a new response reinforces the connections that support emotional resilience. Over time, these new neural pathways can become the brain's preferred routes, making positive change sustainable.

Our emotional tendencies are shaped by both genetics and environment. Twin studies reveal that while our DNA provides a starting script, life experiences continually rewrite the story. Some people may inherit a heightened sensitivity to stress, while others are born with greater resilience. However, thanks to neuroplasticity, everyone can adapt and grow, regardless of their starting point.

Understanding the neuroscience of emotion regulation and neuroplasticity empowers us to respond rather than react—to pause, reflect, and choose new paths even when old habits feel entrenched.

Emotional resilience is not about suppressing feelings but about navigating setbacks, managing stress, and staying motivated through life's ups and downs. With self-awareness, support, and persistent effort, we can soften the grip of destructive patterns and cultivate greater freedom, connection, and joy. Each moment offers a new opportunity to rewrite our emotional stories, strengthen new neural pathways, and grow into wiser, more compassionate versions of ourselves.

CHAPTER 9
FROM ANCIENT SURVIVAL TO MODERN ANXIETY: GROWING IN THE FACE OF STRESS AND FEAR

MOVING EVEN FURTHER into the neurobiology of emotion, we continue to follow in Darwin's footsteps—part scientist, part story-teller—seeking not just to map the brain's hidden pathways but to honor the ancient, universal language of feeling that connects us all. It's within this intricate web of shared emotion that we encounter one of the most powerful forces shaping our daily lives: stress.

Stress is rarely a private affair. It's like a pebble dropped into a pond. Its ripples extend outward, touching everyone nearby. This phenomenon, known as "stress contagion," is more than just a metaphor. When one person in a family, classroom, or workplace is anxious or overwhelmed, others often pick up on those signals, sometimes without even realizing it.

A sigh, a tense jaw, a clipped tone of voice: these small cues can transmit stress like a subtle virus. In groups, stress can synchronize, amplifying collective anxiety and eroding everyone's confidence. Even children and pets can sense and react to the emotional climate, mirroring the tension around them.

Consider a workplace where a team faces a looming deadline. The atmosphere in the office tenses as the deadline approaches. The manager, usually a steady presence, now moves through the room with clipped footsteps and averted eyes, her voice losing its warmth, each word sharpened by urgency. This tension is contagious. It seeps into the posture of her team: shoulders draw inward, and conversations dwindle to terse exchanges. The room, once alive with collaboration, now feels constricted, as if the very oxygen has thinned.

This is not merely a poetic observation; neuroscience tells us that emotions are, in fact, social contagions. Through subtle cues like tone, gesture, and even the micro-expressions that flicker across a face, stress transmits itself from one nervous system to another. Cortisol levels rise, cognitive flexibility narrows, and the collective intelligence of the group falters. Mistakes proliferate, creativity withers, and even after the project is delivered, a residue of unease lingers, echoing in the silence that follows.

A similar choreography unfolds in the home. Picture a parent returning from work, shoulders heavy with invisible burdens. The front door closes, and with it, a subtle shift in the household weather. Children, attuned to the smallest changes, grow quieter, their laughter subdued. A partner, sensing the undercurrent, grows irritable, words edged with impatience. Even the family dog, ever the emotional barometer, paces restlessly from room to room. Here, too, stress moves like smoke—tangible yet elusive, curling into every corner.

Yet, this phenomenon is not a failure but a feature of our biology. Human beings are exquisitely sensitive to the emotional states of those around us, a legacy of our evolutionary past when attunement to the group meant survival. Mirror neurons fire, hormones shift, and the boundaries between self and others blur. The science is clear: our moods are not entirely our own.

They are shared, shaped, and amplified by the collective pulse of those with whom we live and work. In this way, the narrative of stress, whether in the boardroom or the living room, reminds us of our profound interconnectedness. The emotional climate we create is both a private weather and a public atmosphere.

Not all stress is harmful. Acute stress, the kind that flares up in response to a sudden challenge or threat, can be life-saving. Imagine a cyclist swerving to avoid a car or a babysitter catching a falling child.

In these moments, the body's alarm system kicks in: the heart races, senses sharpen, and muscles tense. The "fight or flight" response, driven by a burst of adrenaline and a surge of cortisol, prepares us to act quickly and decisively.

When the danger passes, the body's natural brakes engage, and we return to baseline—a state of calm and recovery. However, when stress becomes chronic, the body never quite shuts off. Cortisol lingers in the bloodstream, and the stress response becomes a background hum, wearing us down day after day.

Biologically, stress is a chain reaction set off by the brain. When we sense a threat or experience frustration, the hypothalamus springs into action. It sends a signal to the adrenal glands, perched atop the kidneys. These respond by flooding the bloodstream with adrenaline and cortisol.

The hippocampus, the brain's primary memory center, is particularly vulnerable during these periods of stress. Chronic stress can damage its delicate cells, making it harder for the brain to form new memories or recall old ones. At the same time, the prefrontal cortex grows weaker under the constant barrage of stress hormones. This is why, under stress, we might snap at loved ones, forget important details, or make impulsive choices we later regret. Meanwhile, the amygdala also becomes more reactive, primed to detect threats everywhere. It's a vicious cycle that makes us ever more sensitive to stress.

If left unchecked, stress can take a toll on nearly every system in the body. It can suppress the immune system, raise blood pressure, and disrupt sleep. It can also increase the risk of anxiety, depression, and even heart disease. Emotionally, it can erode our patience, strain relationships, and sap the joy from everyday life.

Stress, though powerful, is not destiny. The brain is plastic—capable of change and adaptation, even in adulthood. Evidence-based coping strategies can buffer the effects of stress. They can quite literally reshape the neural pathways that govern our emotional responses.

Exercise, for instance, acts as a natural stress reliever, burning off excess adrenaline and flooding the body with mood-enhancing neurochemicals. Alternatively, social support, whether it's leaning on friends, family, or colleagues, can provide comfort and calm us. It reminds us that we are not alone in our struggles.

There is also something called cognitive reframing. This involves viewing challenges from a new perspective. It helps us break free from cycles of worry and see setbacks as opportunities for growth rather than defeat. Additionally, mindfulness and breathing practices anchor us in the present moment, lowering cortisol and restoring a sense of balance. Each of these tools, practiced regularly, can help transform stress from an overwhelming force into a manageable and even motivating part of life.

To see these strategies in action, consider Maya—a teacher whose classroom hums with the energy of thirty restless children. During exam season, Maya feels the stress in her jaw. It's tight as a drum. Her patience is stretched thin by the relentless demands of the day. In the past, she might have tried to simply push through, letting stress pile up like ungraded papers on her desk. Now, however, Maya chooses a different path.

Between classes, she pauses for a few slow breaths, letting the swirl of anxiety settle. She shares a quick laugh with a fellow teacher in the hallway. The sound is a small lifeline in the chaos. At home, she opens her notebook and writes down three small things she's grateful for—a student's smile, a moment of quiet, and the taste of her morning coffee. These simple rituals become her anchor. Over time, Maya finds herself more resilient. She's not immune to stress but can ride its waves with steadier hands and a softer heart.

Recognizing the signs of stress—both in ourselves and those around us—is the first step toward breaking the cycle. Creating moments of calm, even in small ways, can help buffer the effects of stress and restore a sense of balance. Ultimately, stress is not just a personal burden; it is a shared human experience. When we acknowledge its presence, respond with compassion, and reach for evidence-based tools, we transform stress from an invisible epidemic into a challenge that we can meet— together.

If shame is the shadow that dims our sense of worth, fear is the chill that tightens our chest and sharpens our senses, ever alert to what might go wrong. To truly understand the emotional landscape, we must journey further down into the oldest chambers of the brain, where it has been quietly shaping our instincts and choices since the dawn of humanity.

Beneath the polished surface of our thoughts and intentions, the lower regions of the brain are always at work with ancient, instinctive patterns. Think of these areas—the cerebellum, amygdala, and brainstem—as the foundation stones of a castle built over millions of years of evolution. Long before we learned to reason or reflect, these structures sustained our ancestors, keeping them alive in a world of lurking predators and sudden storms.

Here, in the shadowy depths, fear is born. The amygdala, in particular, acts like a smoke detector for danger. It scans the world for threats, often reacting before we're even aware of what's happening. You might jump at a sudden noise or tense up when you sense someone's anger, even before your conscious mind catches up. This is fear working below the surface faster than thought.

Interestingly, fear is not just about snakes in the grass or shadows in the night. In the modern world, it often wears subtler masks: the fear of rejection, the fear of failure, the fear of being exposed or left behind. These social and existential fears are just as real—sometimes more so—than the primal terrors our ancestors faced. Neuroscientists have found that these activate many of the same brain regions as physical threats. They also recruit the prefrontal cortex, which, sometimes in vain, tries to reason with our worries and anticipate social consequences.

Our lower brain is not just a sentinel for the present—it is a meticulous archivist, quietly recording every brush with danger. Conditioned responses are like deep grooves worn into a forest trail, guiding our steps long after the storm has passed. Imagine a child bitten by a dog: years later, even the jingle of a collar or the sight of a wagging tail can send a jolt of anxiety through their chest, the brain taking action before reason can intervene.

Or picture someone who once stood before a crowd and felt laughter turn sharp and cold. Now, decades on, the mere thought of public speaking can make their palms sweat and their hearts pound as if the audience were still waiting to pounce. These learned fears do not fade with the threat. They linger, quietly tinting the lens through which we see the world, fueling anxieties that seem to come from nowhere. It's as if the lower brain keeps a secret ledger, tallying every peril we've ever faced, just in case we need to run—or hide—again.

What of anxiety, that quieter, more persistent cousin of fear?

The feeling that creeps in not with the roar of a lion but with the whisper of unseen dangers. Anxiety is a low, electrical hum beneath the surface of daily life. This current flickers through the body and mind, sharpening senses, tightening muscles, and coloring the world in shades of anticipation.

Inside the brain, anxiety is both an ancient and modern puzzle. Signals race along neural highways, activating the body to flood with noradrenaline. Heartbeats quicken. Palms grow damp. The world narrows to a pinpoint of worry. Anxiety is not simply a matter of sirens blaring in the dark. In those prone to anxiety, the dialogue between the emotional brain and the rational mind can become a tug-of-war: the urgent warnings overwhelm our attempts at reassurance.

Neuroscientists have traced these patterns in living color, watching as the amygdala glows with activity during moments of apprehension, especially when faces turn angry, or the future feels uncertain. In some, this response is so pronounced that even minor social slights or ambiguous cues can trigger a cascade of anxiety. This leads to a cycle of hypervigilance and avoidance. The brain is perpetually scanning for what might go wrong.

Evolution shaped anxiety as a survival tool, a way to prepare us for threats that might never materialize. In moderation, it sharpens attention and readies the body for action. When the system misfires—when the amygdala's alarms ring too loudly, or the prefrontal cortex cannot quiet the storm—anxiety becomes a cage rather than a shield, confining rather than protecting us.

We are, all of us, the inheritors of these ancient circuits. They are powerful and persistent. They aren't easily silenced by logic or willpower alone. You can't simply "think your way" out of a panic attack or snap your fingers to erase a lifelong phobia. Instead, these patterns must be understood and respected. They need to be brought into the light of awareness, integrated into our broader sense of self, and, where possible, gently rewired.

Here, the science of neuroplasticity offers hope. The brain, even in adulthood, can learn new responses to old fears. Exposure therapy, a cornerstone of modern psychology, works by gradually and safely introducing a person to the source of their fear. Over time, the brain signals quiet; new, calmer pathways are forged.

Sam's story begins in a moment of childhood panic. One afternoon, the elevator he was riding in shuddered to a halt between floors. The walls seemed to press inward, the air thick and unmoving. The hum of the machinery grew into a roar in Sam's ears, his heart pounding like a drum in a silent room. Minutes stretched into what felt like hours. From that day on, elevators became more than metal boxes—they were tombs. For years, Sam chose the stairs, even when it meant climbing ten flights, each step a silent echo of that trapped feeling.

However, fear, as ancient as the brain itself, is not set in stone. In Sam's case, he had learned to associate elevators with threat, triggering anxiety even when no real danger was present. This learned fear was etched into the neural pathways of his brain. It shaped his choices and reactions.

With the help of a compassionate therapist, Sam began a journey of exposure therapy—a gradual, step-by-step process to retrain his brain. At first, he simply stood near an elevator, feeling the pulse of fear but choosing to stay. Then came a short ride to a single floor. Then two. Each small victory was a rewiring of the brain, a lesson: elevators are safe, not prisons. What once felt impossible became routine. The elevator transformed from a tomb into a vehicle, carrying Sam upward with ease.

Sam's story is not unique. Many of us carry fears—some rational, some less so—that quietly shape the contours of our lives, sometimes in ways we barely notice until they hold us back. Think about the fear of spiders, a common phobia that affects roughly 3.5 to 6.1% of people worldwide. Maybe you know someone who freezes at the sight of a tiny spider, or perhaps you feel a shiver yourself when one scuttles across the floor. It's a fear rooted deep in our ancient brain circuits. This survival mechanism once helped our ancestors avoid venomous bites.

Then there's the fear of heights—acrophobia—which grips millions. Standing at the edge of a balcony or looking down from a tall building can send the heart racing and the stomach flipping. It's a visceral reminder of our vulnerability. This primal warning keeps us safe but can also limit our experiences. Flying, too, is a source of anxiety for many. The thought of being thousands of feet above the ground, enclosed in a metal tube, triggers a cascade of fear responses. It's a modern fear, born not from evolutionary necessity but from the unfamiliar and uncontrollable.

Who hasn't felt the knot of dread before speaking in public? Glossophobia—the fear of public speaking—touches nearly three out of four people at some point in their lives. Interestingly, it's more common than fears of heights, spiders, or even death itself. You might remember your own hands trembling before a classroom presentation or the way your mind raced before a wedding toast or a big meeting. Maybe you've watched a friend's voice quiver at a podium or seen a colleague's face flush as they stumbled over their words. This fear is so universal because it strikes at something ancient and fundamental: our need for acceptance, our fear of judgment, and our deep-rooted instinct to avoid social rejection.

These fears, whether born from real danger or old memories, live in the same ancient circuits of the brain. They can feel overwhelming, isolating, and sometimes even embarrassing. However, like Sam, we have the power to face them, to understand their roots, and to change our relationship with fear. Recognizing that fear is a shared human experience can be the first step toward reclaiming freedom and peace.

Take a moment. Consider your own fears—those shadows that linger in the corners of your mind. *What holds you back? What might you gently approach, step by step, to reclaim your freedom and peace?*

Not every mind flinches at the same shadows. For some, fear arrives like a sudden chill—unexpected, visceral, impossible to ignore. For others, it is a faint draft, barely noticed, passing quickly through. The difference is etched in the subtle interplay of memory, biology, and temperament.

Some of us are born with nervous systems tuned to a higher pitch, and our brains are more sensitive to the possibility of social scrutiny. The amygdala flares at the hint of judgment. At the same time, the rest of the brain sometimes struggles to calm the tide. Genetics, early experience, and even culture shape the volume and texture of our fears, making some of us more vulnerable to the sting of embarrassment, the threat of rejection, or the memory of a single, searing mistake.

Others seem to thrive on fear—roller coaster lovers, horror movie buffs, the friend who volunteers to give every group presentation. For them, fear can trigger a rush of endorphins, turning anxiety into excitement. Brain structure and chemistry play a role here, too. People with a more active prefrontal cortex or a different balance of neurotransmitters may find fear exhilarating rather than paralyzing.

So the next time you feel your heart pounding before you speak or see someone else hesitate at the microphone, remember: this is not just nerves or weakness. It's the echo of our evolutionary past, the legacy of old memories, and the unique wiring of each brain. It's a reminder that fear, in all its forms—whether of spiders, heights, flying, or speaking up—is both deeply human and, with understanding and practice, something we can learn to face and even reshape.

By acknowledging the ancient wisdom of our lower brain, we can begin to work with, rather than against, these deep-seated patterns. We reclaim a sense of safety and freedom, not by erasing fear but by learning to navigate it with compassion and skill. Fear, after all, is not our enemy; it is a guardian that sometimes needs gentle retraining.

PART FOUR
A MOTIVATED BRAIN

CHAPTER 10
THE SCIENCE OF ICK: HOW ESCAPING DISCOMFORT BECOMES HABIT

ON A RAINY MONDAY MORNING, you sit at your desk, staring at a blank screen. The cursor blinks, steady and indifferent. Your coffee cools beside you. You know you need to start that report for work—the deadline is looming. Your manager's reminders echo in your mind. Yet, your fingers hover, unmoving, above the keyboard. You scroll through messages, check the weather, and wipe a crumb from the table. The urge to begin is there, but so is something else: a restless discomfort, a prickling unease that makes starting feel strangely impossible.

Most of us have been here, in some form or another. Sometimes it's the gym shoes by the door, untouched for days. Sometimes it's a difficult conversation we keep postponing, or a creative project that stays locked in our imagination. Discomfort is not just pain or fear. It's that invisible resistance that tugs at us when we try to move forward. It's a shadow that stretches across our intentions.

Discomfort is not a single note, but a spectrum—a gentle itch, a whisper at the edge of awareness, or a sudden stab that commands immediate retreat. Our brains are exquisitely tuned to these signals. For many of us, the simple act of beginning, of pushing through inertia, can feel like scaling a mountain. The question is: *why do some of us struggle more than others to get started, to stay motivated, to persevere?*

Imagine the body as a grand concert hall. The nerves are musicians, each section tuned to a particular instrument. Some play the high, insistent notes of itch, others the deep, resonant chords of pain. The spinal cord is the stage where these signals first gather and mingle. Specialized groups of nerve cells, each with its own unique shape and sensitivity, wait for their cue. Some are awakened by the feather-light brush of an itch, others by the sharp clang of pain.

As these signals ascend, they are carried upward like melodies rising through the air, reaching the thalamus, the brain's relay station where sensory information is sorted and directed. From here, the signals are sent to the anterior cingulate cortex. This region acts like an emotional conductor, orchestrating the brain's response to discomfort. Some nerve cells are versatile, responding to both itch and pain.

In contrast, others are specialists, firing only in response to one or the other. The anterior cingulate cortex does not merely register discomfort; it interprets, assigns meaning, and guides our actions with remarkable precision. Pain sounds the alarm, prompting immediate withdrawal and protection. Itch, in contrast, is subtler. It is a crescendo that demands resolution, urging us to scratch, rub, or shift, often before we even realize it.

Discomfort is not only about sensation. It is also about meaning. Our brains are not passive receivers of signals; they are storytellers, writing narratives from every flicker of sensation. A mild ache in the muscles after exercise can be interpreted as a sign of progress, indicating growth. The same ache, in the context of illness, becomes a warning.

The prefrontal cortex shapes this interpretation. It's where experience and future goals collide. It's also where the cost of discomfort is weighed against the promise of reward, and sometimes, the scales tip toward avoidance. We hesitate, procrastinate, and tell ourselves stories of danger, incompetence, or failure until the discomfort of beginning outweighs the pain of staying still. It is a delicate balance, shaped by both biology and history.

Speaking of discomfort and aversion, sometimes, a single bite is all it takes. One taste can turn infatuation into aversion, flipping yesterday's obsession into today's "ick." One day, you're filming TikToks about your daily matcha latte, or a pot of that viral pasta recipe. The next moment, however, just the idea of those once-enjoyed delights sends a wave of unease through you. It twists your stomach and prompts memories of a past enjoyment now overshadowed by discomfort. In a moment, a food that once lit up your reward pathways—your so-called *"dopamine food"*—becomes unappealing, even repulsive.

Surprisingly, this isn't just a fleeting or fickle change in taste; it's an ancient survival mechanism that has been honed over millennia to keep us safe from harm. The insula acts as a translator between the raw data of bodily sensation and the emotional responses that guide our choices. When we eat something that makes us sick, whether from genuine contamination or a single overwhelming experience, the insula erupts in a burst of neural activity. This region, along with the amygdala and parts of the hippocampus, forges a powerful memory that links the taste, smell, and even the sight of that food with a sense of danger or disgust.

Neuroscientists call this phenomenon *"conditioned taste aversion,"* and it is one of the most robust forms of learning in all of biology. A single episode of food poisoning can override years of positive associations, rewriting your cravings in an instant and ensuring you steer clear in the future. This rapid, almost primal learning is a marvel of evolutionary engineering.

In animal studies, rats and monkeys develop lifelong aversions to flavors paired with illness after just one exposure, a testament to the crucial role this mechanism plays in survival. For humans, the effect is just as powerful. The insula's neural signature of disgust can be detected on brain scans within seconds of tasting something spoiled or toxic. The memory can persist for decades. It's a system designed to protect us from acute threats—like spoiled meat or poisonous berries—by making the cost of a second mistake unthinkably high.

In today's digital era, this ancient biology collides with the relentless novelty of modern technology. Social media doesn't just reflect our cravings; it amplifies them, transforming *"dopamine foods"* into viral obsessions. Rainbow bagels, molten chocolate lava cakes, the latest TikTok coffee trend—these treats are engineered for visual spectacle and maximum pleasure, their images flooding our feeds and our kitchens.

The brain's reward pathways, especially those involving dopamine, light up at the mere anticipation of these foods. It fuels desire and drives trends. Yet, as quickly as these foods rise to fame, they can fall from grace. Sometimes, all it takes is a single bout of food poisoning, a stomachache, or even the slow, creeping fatigue of overindulgence for the insula to flip the switch from craving to aversion. What was once irresistible can become intolerable overnight.

Our brains are far less adept at warning us about the dangers that unfold slowly over time—the excess sugar, the hidden trans fats, the chronic harms that never trigger a dramatic *"ick"* response. The circuits that govern aversion are designed for acute peril, not for the gradual, cumulative risks of modern eating. This is a vulnerability that food marketers and manufacturers exploit by crafting products that encourage repeat consumption.

In this way, the "one bad bite" effect is both a blessing and a blind spot: a vivid reminder that our appetites are sculpted by forces both ancient and modern, by the chemistry of survival and the culture of the moment, by the primal wiring of our brains and the algorithms that shape our feeds. It is a testament to the enduring power of our biology—and a cautionary tale about the new frontiers of appetite in an age of abundance and algorithmic influence.

~

When discomfort arrives, we each stand at a familiar crossroads. Maybe you recognize it in your own life: the moment you hesitate before sending an important email, the way you put off a doctor's appointment, or the urge to distract yourself when a difficult feeling surfaces. Sometimes, you take action—making a plan, seeking support, or facing the problem head-on. This is active avoidance, a process powered by the brain's planning centers and fueled by the sense that you have some control over the outcome. When you believe you can shape what happens next, discomfort becomes a challenge to meet rather than a wall to hide behind.

Other times, you might freeze or withdraw, caught in the grip of passive avoidance. Perhaps you scroll endlessly on your phone, zone out in front of the television, or simply hope the problem will resolve itself if you wait long enough. Here, the amygdala takes the lead, urging stillness and retreat. In the wild, this instinct can save lives. In modern life, it can leave us stuck, cycling through inaction and regret, feeling our bodies tense and our minds racing, yet unable to move forward.

Imagine yourself at the edge of a dark forest. Somewhere within lies a challenge: a task, a conversation, a risk you must take. You feel the thrum of discomfort in your chest, the flutter of uncertainty in your stomach. At this moment, the mind stands at a fork, choosing between two paths: to step forward or to retreat. Neuroscience reveals that these choices—active and passive avoidance—are not just matters of will, but of wiring. They are the work of overlapping yet distinct neural circuits, each shaped by the hand of evolution.

Active avoidance is the path of the strategist, the problem-solver. It is the decision to act: to make a plan, to take a step, to shape fate rather than be shaped by it. When we choose this route, the prefrontal cortex lights up. As we know, this region, nestled behind the forehead, is responsible for planning, decision-making, and weighing consequences. Alongside it, the striatum, a deep cluster of cells, helps us evaluate risks and rewards. It motivates us to move.

There is another ingredient as well: control. When we believe, even faintly, that our actions can influence the outcome, the brain's circuits for active avoidance hum with energy. This sense of agency transforms discomfort from a wall into a doorway. We push through, not because the path is easy, but because we sense our own power to shape what lies ahead.

Passive avoidance is the path of the sentinel, or the watcher. It is the instinct to freeze, to withdraw, to hope that danger will pass us by. Here, the amygdala takes the lead. This almond-shaped cluster is finely tuned to detect threats. When fear or overwhelm rise, the amygdala sounds the retreat, shutting down action and urging stillness. In the wild, this response can be lifesaving. Picture a rabbit frozen in the grass, invisible to the circling hawk. In our modern world, when passive avoidance becomes our default, it can trap us in cycles of inaction and regret.

Our experience is not shaped solely by biology. We are social creatures, born into a blend of customs, expectations, and unwritten rules. The way we interpret and respond to discomfort is choreographed by the culture and community that surround us. In some societies, stoicism is regarded as the highest virtue, characterized by the stiff upper lip and the silent endurance of pain.

In others, emotion is a river to be shared, its currents navigated together. Family attitudes and peer influences write early scripts in our minds: *"Be brave,"* "Don't *complain,"* or *"It's okay to cry."* Over time, these messages become part of our neural choreography, shaping the very circuits that govern avoidance and resilience.

Consider the child who scrapes a knee. In one home, tears are met with gentle comfort; in another, with a brisk *"You're fine, walk it off."* These moments, repeated over the years, become the foundation for how we approach discomfort as adults. The brain, ever plastic, ties these social lessons into its fabric, tuning its responses to match the expectations of the world around us.

The difference between active and passive paths is not just psychological, but biological. Both paths have their place. Sometimes, the wisest move is to wait, to gather strength, to let danger pass. Other times, action is the only way forward. The key lies in balance, knowing when to step up and when to step back. Too much passive avoidance, and we become prisoners of our own fear. Too much action, and we risk leaping without looking.

~

As we mature, the connections between the regions of our brains become stronger, enabling adults to manage discomfort and motivation with greater flexibility and resilience. Yet even in adulthood, the chemistry of motivation is not uniform. Each of us carries a unique blend of sensitivity, learning, and neurochemical balance, shaped by our genes, experiences, and circumstances.

Throughout history and across cultures, humans have sought to understand the invisible forces that propel us—or hold us back. Ancient philosophers spoke of willpower as an inner fire. This flame could be kindled or extinguished by discipline and desire. Poets painted desire as a wild river, rushing and swirling, sometimes calm, sometimes tempestuous. Today, we peer beneath these metaphors to find the currents themselves. They are chemical rivers flowing through channels carved by evolution and experience. The story of wanting, focus, and action is not just poetic; it is biological, delicate, and dynamic, written in the circuitry of every brain.

Dopamine, often misunderstood, is the wind that fans the flames of wanting. It is the spark that ignites anticipation. When we imagine a reward—a sweet taste, a word of praise, the satisfaction of a task completed—dopamine surges. We now distinguish between three intertwined experiences: *"liking,"* the quiet contentment of reward; *"wanting,"* the restless urge to pursue; and *"learning,"* the gradual building of memory and expectation. Dopamine is the architect of wanting, its pathways stretching from the ancient midbrain through the nucleus accumbens and onward to the prefrontal cortex.

As we've seen before, dopamine does not work alone. In the orchestra of attention, another player stands ready: noradrenaline. This chemical is a close cousin of adrenaline that surges in moments of danger. Imagine you're walking through a quiet forest, when suddenly, a twig snaps nearby. Instantly, your senses sharpen: your ears tune in, your eyes scan the shadows, your heart beats a little faster. This surge of alertness is the work of noradrenaline, which is always on guard for what's new, important, or potentially threatening.

Noradrenaline, also known as norepinephrine, triggers our "fight or flight" response. While adrenaline prepares the body for immediate action, noradrenaline plays a subtler yet equally vital role in the brain. It is released when we encounter something novel, challenging, or stressful, anything that demands our attention. When noradrenaline is released, it acts like a spotlight operator in the theater of your mind. It brightens the stage, making essential details stand out and helping you react quickly to what matters most. It also enables you to tune out background noise—both literally and figuratively.

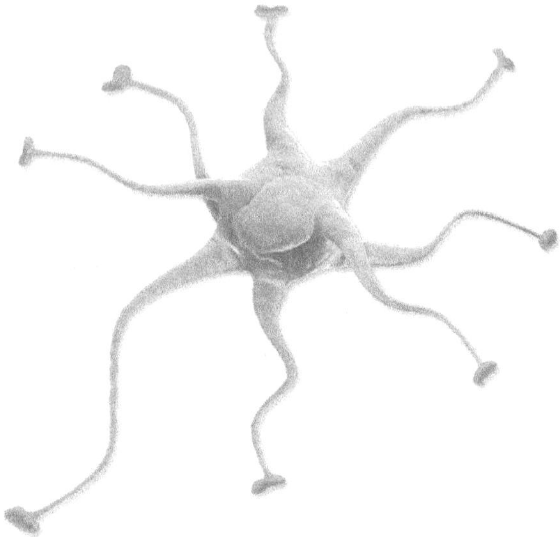

Figure 12. *Astrocyte.* Blausen Medical

Noradrenaline communicates with astrocytes, star-shaped support cells that help manage the brain's environment. When noradrenaline signals these cells, they help quiet down excessive brain activity, much like gently applying the brakes on a car. This calms the mental "chatter" that can make it hard to concentrate, especially when you're feeling overwhelmed. By working with astrocytes, noradrenaline helps you regain control when distractions accumulate or stress becomes overwhelming. It's as if your brain has an internal mechanism to pull you back from the brink of overload and help you zero in on what's truly important.

In essence, noradrenaline is the mind's watchful gatekeeper. It helps us attend to what matters most, filtering the urgent from the unimportant with a steady, vigilant eye. This intricate system ensures that, even in a world full of distractions, our brains can find clarity and focus when it counts. Just as noradrenaline sharpens our focus and helps us filter the world's noise, there is another essential player in the brain—one that determines not only what we notice, but what we actually do.

While noradrenaline acts as the vigilant gatekeeper, ensuring our attention is directed where it matters most, our brains also need a way to decide whether to move forward or hold back. This is where glutamate comes into play. If dopamine is the spark that ignites our desire and noradrenaline is the watchman who keeps us alert, then glutamate is the crucial switch, flipping us between action and restraint, pursuit and avoidance. Glutamate is the brain's primary excitatory neurotransmitter. This main chemical messenger increases the activity of neurons and gets circuits firing. Think of it as the accelerator pedal in the brain's engine, ready to rev up our motivation and drive when the situation calls for it.

Glutamate is released when we are gearing up to pursue a goal, solve a problem, or respond to something meaningful. It energizes neural pathways, making us ready for action. Some neurons are exceptionally versatile—they can release both dopamine and glutamate. This means the brain can rapidly switch between states, from eager pursuit to careful restraint, depending on what is needed. Glutamate also helps the brain determine when to pursue rewards and when to hold back from doing so. When glutamate is active, we are more likely to seek out new experiences, take risks, or work toward a goal.

If glutamate is blocked, animals lose the urge to seek rewards—they become passive, even if they still avoid harm. Conversely, if dopamine is blocked, the drive to escape discomfort fades, but the desire to pursue rewards can persist. This interplay serves as a kind of neural crossroads, enabling the brain to weigh risks and rewards and choose the most adaptive path. In this way, glutamate completes the trio of the brain's motivational chemistry. It is the switch that toggles us between movement and stillness, pursuit and pause, helping us navigate the complex landscape of choices, risks, and rewards that make up our daily lives.

To bring this to life, let's consider a scenario many people have witnessed or experienced: the difference between depression and anxiety in daily motivation. Picture someone who once loved playing music, meeting friends, or pursuing hobbies. Over time, they begin to withdraw. Not because they no longer recognize danger, but because the spark to seek out pleasure or rewards has faded. They still get out of bed to avoid the discomfort of hunger or the risk of losing their job, but the drive to chase after what once brought joy is gone.

This is often seen in major depression: people may avoid "harm" like paying bills, eating enough to survive, but lose motivation for anything beyond basic survival. This mirrors what scientists observe when glutamate is blocked in animal studies. The urge to seek rewards —such as exploring, playing, or working for treats—disappears. Still, the basic instinct to avoid pain or danger remains intact. The animal becomes passive, not out of fear, but because the neural drive for reward-seeking has been switched off.

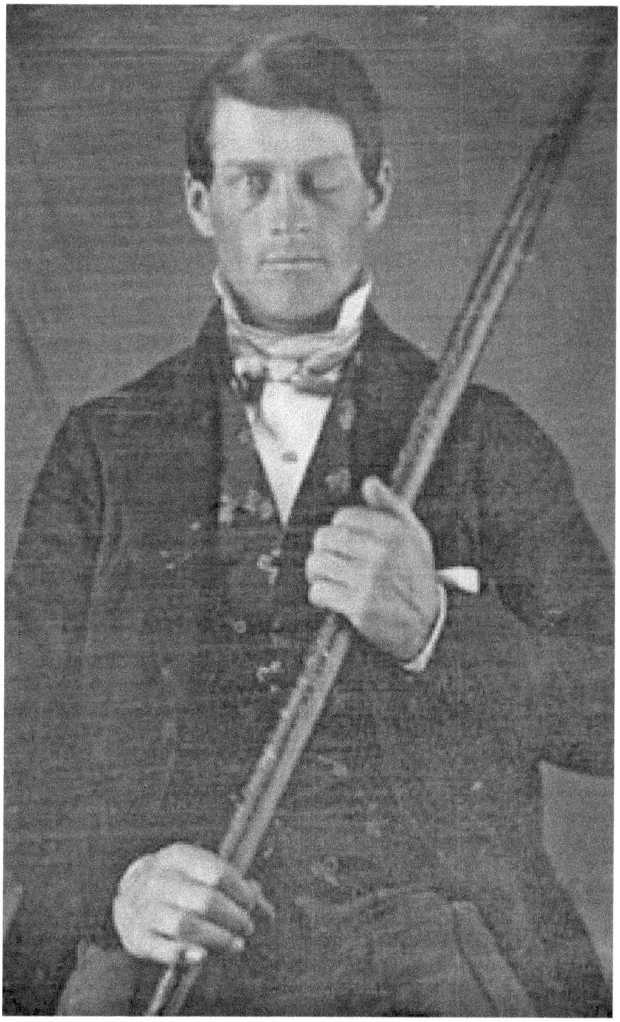

Figure 13. *Phineas Gage.* Based on a photograph by Jack and Beverly Wilgus of a daguerreotype originally from their collection, and now in the Warren Anatomical Museum, Center for the History of Medicine, Francis A. Countway Library of Medicine, Harvard Medical School

Now, imagine someone with a different imbalance—where the drive to avoid discomfort is blunted. However, the desire to pursue rewards is still present. Specifically, let's consider the famous case of Phineas Gage, a railroad foreman in 19th-century America whose life changed in a flash of iron and fire. In 1848, Phineas Gage was using a tamping iron to pack explosive powder into a rock. A sudden spark ignited the powder, and the iron rod shot upward, passing through Gage's cheek and out the top of his skull. Remarkably, he survived, but the rod destroyed much of his prefrontal cortex.

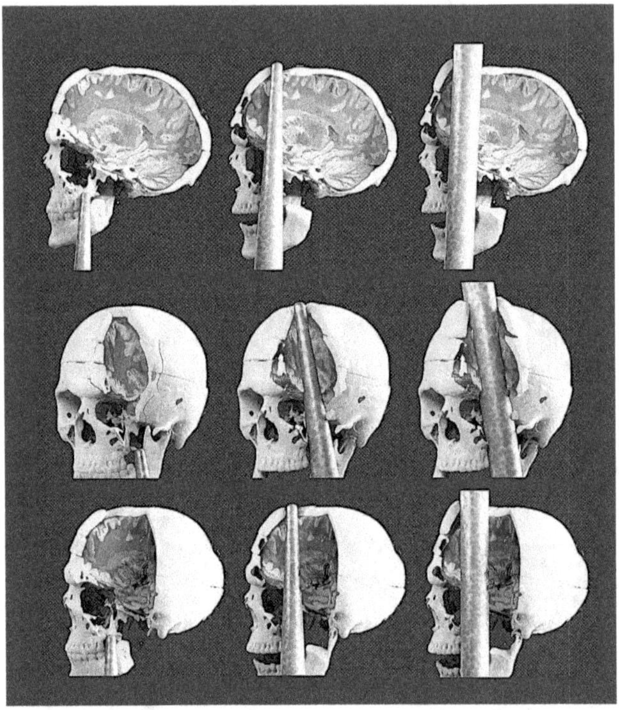

Figure 14. *Phineas Gage accident, Side view of the trajectory.* Cicero Moraes on Wikimedia Commons

Before the accident, Gage was known as a responsible, hardworking, and dependable employee and friend. After the accident, Gage's personality and behavior changed dramatically. He became impulsive, unreliable, and prone to risky decisions. He chased after things he wanted—pleasure, excitement, immediate rewards—without regard for future consequences or potential harm. He seemed to lose his ability to avoid discomfort or negative outcomes. He ignored social norms, took dangerous risks, and failed to plan for the future, even when it led to trouble or pain. Gage's friends said he was "no longer Gage"—he would make choices that brought immediate satisfaction but ignored the discomfort or harm those choices would cause down the line.

Like Gage, people with similar brain injuries may pursue what feels good in the moment, but struggle to avoid situations that could cause harm or discomfort. This uncoupling explains why someone might repeatedly make risky choices, neglect their responsibilities, or fail to protect themselves, even when the desire for pleasure or excitement remains strong.

Thankfully, most of us experience a balance—sometimes we push forward for rewards, sometimes we pull back to avoid pain. Understanding this balance helps explain why, in conditions like depression, people can still avoid harm but lose the drive for joy, and why, in other conditions, someone might pursue rewards without proper caution. Yet, even as we marvel at the brain's power to tip the scales between risk and restraint, it is essential to remember: our experience of discomfort is not confined to the mind alone.

~

For discomfort is not merely a whisper in the corridors of the mind. It is played out in the flesh and bone of our existence. Long before the mind crafts a story about suffering, the body is already speaking in its own ancient language: a language of racing hearts, fluttering stomachs, and lungs that seem to shrink with every breath.

The signals that shape our decisions—whether to chase a reward or retreat from pain—do not begin and end in the brain's circuitry. They ripple outward, stirring muscles, tightening skin, sending a cascade of sensations through every organ and nerve. Sometimes, it is the body that first alerts us to unease: a clenched jaw before a difficult conversation, a restless leg before a leap into the unknown, a stomach that knots with anticipation or dread. Our biology is not just a backdrop to the drama of motivation and avoidance; it is an active participant, amplifying or softening the messages that the brain sends and receives.

Our nervous system is a vast and intricate network that extends far beyond the brain to every corner of the body. Sensory receptors embedded in the skin, muscles, joints, and internal organs constantly monitor the body's state and the environment. Receptors in our body detect different types of signals, like temperature changes, pressure, chemical imbalances, and muscle tension. These signals can indicate possible harm or discomfort.

The process of interoception enables our body's internal sensing system, which uses specialized nerve fibers, to transmit information about our physical state directly to the brain. Interoceptive signals provide a continuous stream of feedback, informing the brain about states like hunger, thirst, pain, or anxiety. Alongside this, proprioception monitors the position and movement of our limbs and body in space, often alerting us to tension or imbalance before we become consciously aware of it.

These bodily signals travel through the spinal cord and cranial nerves, converging in several key regions of the brain that process and integrate sensory information. The brainstem, thalamus, insular cortex, and anterior cingulate cortex all play a role in this symphony of sensation. The insula, in particular, acts as a hub for interoceptive awareness, translating raw bodily sensations into feelings that influence our emotional and motivational states.

The relationship between body and brain is not a one-way street, but a dynamic, bidirectional dialogue. Sensory information from the body ascends to the brain, alerting it to states of discomfort or threat—a tightening in the chest or a fluttering stomach can signal anxiety or impending stress. The brain, in turn, sends signals back down to the body through the autonomic nervous system, modulating heart rate, muscle tone, and hormonal release. This feedback can amplify or dampen sensations of discomfort. It is this loop that explains why bodily states can intensify or soothe our experience of discomfort: a racing heart can escalate anxiety, while slow, deep breathing activates the parasympathetic nervous system, promoting calm and reducing the brain's alarm signals.

Central to this process is the autonomic nervous system, which regulates involuntary bodily functions and plays a pivotal role in how discomfort is experienced and managed. The sympathetic branch, often called the "fight or flight" system, prepares the body to respond to perceived threats by increasing heart rate, dilating airways, releasing adrenaline, and redirecting blood flow to muscles. These changes heighten alertness and readiness. They also create sensations we recognize as discomfort.

The parasympathetic branch, known as the "rest and digest" system, counterbalances this by slowing the heart rate, promoting digestion, and encouraging relaxation. Activation of the parasympathetic system can soothe the body's alarm signals. This reduces the intensity of discomfort.

The vagus nerve, a significant conduit between the body and brain, is a vital link in this ongoing conversation. It carries sensory information from the heart, lungs, and digestive tract to the brainstem, influencing emotional regulation and stress responses. Higher vagal tone—a measure of the vagus nerve's activity—is associated with better emotional regulation and resilience to stress. Techniques that stimulate the vagus nerve, such as slow breathing and meditation, can help calm bodily sensations of discomfort and reduce avoidance behaviors.

Discomfort often manifests physically before it is consciously recognized. Chronic or acute stress can cause muscles to tighten, creating aches or a sense of restlessness. This tension sends signals back to the brain, reinforcing feelings of unease and sometimes triggering avoidance. The skin, rich with sensory receptors, is often the first site where discomfort is felt—a prickling itch, a burning sensation, or a cold shiver—all of which can prompt reflexive or conscious responses.

Even the gut can play a starring role in this drama. Sometimes referred to as the "second brain," the gut contains an extensive network of neurons that communicates bidirectionally with the brain via the vagus nerve and hormonal pathways. The enteric nervous system governs digestion and is intimately linked to our emotional states. Stomach discomfort—such as "butterflies" or nausea—is a common physical manifestation of anxiety or anticipation. These sensations feed into the brain's interpretation of discomfort and can either heighten avoidance or motivate action.

Together, these systems create a rich spectrum of signals that inform our experience and guide our behavior. Bodily signals can amplify brain signals of discomfort, making avoidance more urgent and compelling. Think of those moments when your heart pounds before a difficult conversation, your palms sweat before a test, or your stomach twists as you contemplate a big change. These are not random quirks; they are the body's way of alerting you to challenge or uncertainty. Sometimes, the body's messages make avoidance feel urgent and compelling, like the impulse to put off an awkward phone call, or the sudden need to tidy your desk instead of tackling a daunting task. Other times, a surge of energy or a calming breath can motivate you to act, to step forward despite the discomfort.

Interestingly, discomfort, for all its shadows, can also be a catalyst. It's a spark that ignites change. When we learn to listen, to interpret the signals, to understand their source, we can transform discomfort from a barrier into a guide.

Consider the story of Hippocrates. He was a Greek physician often referred to as the father of medicine. Picture him in the past, moving through the sun-dappled courtyards of Kos, his white robe stirring in the Mediterranean breeze. In his world, illness was not a matter of flesh and bone. It was a conversation with the gods. When a patient arrived, clutching a wounded arm or doubled over with abdominal pain, Hippocrates saw a message.

To him, pain was not a meaningless torment. It was a divine messenger, dispatched by the gods to warn, to instruct, to demand attention. He listened closely to the cries and groans of his patients, believing that each pang and ache was a clue, a sacred signal pointing toward imbalance or injury. Pain, in this ancient view, was both a warning bell and a teacher. It urges rest, caution, and sometimes, a change in the patient's way of living.

Centuries later, we have traded the language of gods for the language of science. We now know that pain and itch are not supernatural punishments, but the result of intricate neural circuits that have been refined over years of evolution. Tiny receptors in our skin and tissues detect injury or irritation and send urgent signals up the spinal cord. Then they move through the thalamus and into the brain's emotional and sensory centers. The message is the same: *pay attention, protect, adapt.*

Modern neuroscience reveals that the brain's response to discomfort is not fixed. It can be shaped by attention, expectation, and belief. Mindfulness practices, for example, teach us to observe discomfort without judgment, to notice its ebb and flow. This simple act of awareness can quiet the brain's alarm bells, reducing the urge to escape and increasing our capacity to endure.

All of us, at one time or another, stand at the edge, feeling the pull of retreat and the urge to act. Our beliefs, our stories, and our sense of control shape the neural circuits that govern our approach and avoidance behaviors. When we choose to act, we strengthen the pathways of agency. When we reframe our struggles with metaphor, we give ourselves new reasons to try.

CHAPTER 11
THE FIRE WITHIN: REWIRING HABITS FOR A LIFETIME OF MOTIVATION AND PURPOSE

IF AVOIDANCE IS the shadow that dims our resolve, motivation is the fire that propels us forward. At its best, motivation is a living flame. When it burns bright, the smallest spark can ignite sweeping action. When it wanes, even simple tasks feel cold and insurmountable. Like any fire, motivation requires the right conditions: fuel, oxygen, and a spark. These elements, pulled together by the brain's intricate circuitry, determine whether our inner fire blazes or burns out.

At the heart of this lies a fundamental question: *what compels us to move? What transforms inertia into purposeful action?*

The ventral tegmental area, a cluster of neurons in the midbrain, provides an elegant answer. From here, a river of dopamine surges into downstream regions. These regions, including the nucleus accumbens, serve as a hub for reward anticipation. This pathway, often referred to as the mesolimbic dopamine system, is the spark plug of motivation

Contrary to common belief, dopamine does not merely produce pleasure. It encodes *incentive salience*—the *"wanting"* rather than the *"liking."* When you imagine the taste of morning coffee, dopamine rises not only when you sip but when you anticipate. Neuroscience refers to this phenomenon as the reward-prediction error: sudden bursts occur when outcomes exceed expectations, while dips occur when hopes aren't met. In this ebb and flow lies the fire of pursuit.

Motivation is not confined to the brain. It courses through the body, carried by noradrenaline—a chemical also known as norepinephrine. If dopamine sparks the flame, noradrenaline gives it momentum. Released by the locus coeruleus, a tiny structure in the brainstem, noradrenaline heightens alertness and sharpens focus. It is the oxygen that sustains our drive.

Think of those moments of flow where you lose yourself in writing code, playing an instrument, or lifting weights. Here, noradrenaline balances in a sweet spot—not too high, which causes anxiety, not too low, which causes lethargy. The body hums in synchrony with brain networks, a well-tuned engine firing on all cylinders.

The body shapes motivation in subtler ways as well. For example, hormones such as cortisol can inject a sense of urgency, but in excess, they cloud concentration. Testosterone modulates drive. It fuels the pursuit of mastery or competition. Even the gut microbiome, sending chemical messages to the brain, can energize or sap our motivation.

While the initial spark of motivation emerges from the brainstem and limbic circuits, it requires direction to become purposeful. Without guidance, desire disperses like sparks carried by the wind. The prefrontal cortex serves as the heart by aligning long-term goals with immediate actions. Alongside it, the anterior cingulate cortex monitors effort, detects errors, and allocates resources for persistence. Together, these regions transform raw desire into sustained pursuit.

Consider a college student staring down their research proposal. The limbic system, fueled by dopamine, signals, *'Achievement ahead—reward awaits.'* The prefrontal cortex translates this promise into concrete steps, such as deadlines, page targets, and research outlines. Without this translation, motivation fizzles. With structure, the flame channels into productive flow. The motivational engine comes together: spark, fuel, and direction.

Yet motivation, like fire, is fickle. The brain's motivational circuits are sensitive and easily disrupted. For example, stress floods the brain with cortisol, impairing the prefrontal cortex and making it difficult to plan. Meanwhile, fatigue reduces dopamine. This drains pleasure from once-enjoyable tasks.

In our digital age, constant distractions trap us in endless cycles of seeking novelty. Every ping, buzz, or pop-up offers the promise of something new—a text message, a headline, a like. Each delivers a tiny surge of dopamine, briefly lighting up the brain's reward circuits. However, as we chase these micro-rewards throughout the day, the cost accumulates: our ability to sustain focus, sit with discomfort or boredom, and make deep progress on meaningful tasks is gradually eroded. The mind becomes conditioned to expect continual stimulation, making it harder to resist temptation and easier to avoid the challenging work that leads to lasting fulfillment.

Self-doubt, too, can cast a long shadow across motivation's flame. Even when dopamine sparks the initial desire to act, fragile confidence can be quickly extinguished by the persistent murmur of inner critics. These voices whisper, *'Why try? Why bother? Failure is inevitable.'* Over time, this internal narrative not only dampens enthusiasm but can also short-circuit the brain's reward pathways, making it more difficult to ignite and sustain the fire of motivation.

Yet, there is hope: just as embers can reignite, motivation too can be rekindled—even in seasons that feel dormant. Neuroscience offers insight into this process. Motivation rises and falls not just with the value of a goal, but with how attainable and immediate it feels. Tasks that are close in time activate motivational circuits more powerfully. This is why we respond quickly to emails but procrastinate on long-term projects. By breaking large ambitions into smaller, proximal steps, we reduce psychological distance and create a steady 'dopamine drip' that sustains momentum. The unfinished novel or business plan often stalls not because of a lack of desire, but because the reward seems too distant.

All of this underlines one of the most transformative revelations of neuroscience: *motivation is not fixed*. Circuits can be reshaped. Habits can be trained to feed the fire daily. Like a muscle, motivational systems strengthen with specific practices.

Every time you break a daunting challenge into smaller, manageable actions, you trigger a series of dopamine surges. These micro-wins build momentum. Marathon training does not begin with 42 kilometers; it starts with a single lap around the block. Each step reignites the motivational circuit.

Humans are wired to discount delayed rewards, but strategies like temptation bundling—pairing exercise with a favorite podcast—link long-term effort to immediate pleasure. This bridges the gap between present-focused circuits and future goals. Research on growth mindset, pioneered by psychologist Carol Dweck, reveals that viewing challenges as opportunities transforms avoidance into pursuit. When setbacks become lessons rather than sources of shame, dopamine continues to be released, even in the face of adversity.

Motivation, however, is not always beneficial. When taken to excess, it can also consume. Mania offers a stark example of motivation gone awry—relentless drive without restraint. In these states, the prefrontal cortex loses its moderating influence, and the fire of motivation burns unchecked. Balance is essential. Motivation must be cultivated as a disciplined flame, not allowed to burn out of control.

~

The architecture of motivation is not fixed at birth. It is built, brick by brick, as we grow. This is why motivation changes across age. In childhood, novelty sparks dopamine freely; curiosity is a natural blaze. Adolescence exaggerates this, with surging dopamine making risk and reward hypersalient. This developmental gap explains why young people may leap before they look or freeze in the face of perceived discomfort.

In adulthood, the motivational flame stabilizes, anchored by a mature prefrontal cortex and the routines of daily life. As we age, dopamine levels wane, but motivation endures—now fueled by meaning, relationships, and legacy rather than novelty. The fire changes form but does not go out. What was once a wildfire of curiosity in youth becomes a steady hearthfire of purpose in later years. Each stage of life calls for its own kindling.

At its deepest, motivation transcends productivity hacks. It roots in purpose, the story that gives life coherence. Neuroscience alone cannot define purpose, but it shows how narratives ignite durable motivation. Dopamine surges sustain when tethered not to fleeting rewards but to identities and values: *I am a writer; I am someone who helps others; I am building a legacy.*

Motivation is not a static trait. It is fire—living, flickering, shaped by the interplay of biology and environment. Some mornings it blazes forth; other days, it smolders beneath the surface. Science shows that through habits, environment, mindset, and meaning, we can reshape the brain's motivational pathways.

Cultivate motivation through small victories. Protect it from distraction. Anchor it in a meaningful purpose. When nurtured, motivation—sparked by dopamine, fueled by noradrenaline, and guided by the prefrontal cortex—becomes a steady force, supporting lasting progress toward what matters most.

PART FIVE
MY BRAIN VS YOUR BRAIN

CHAPTER 12
GENES AND JOURNEYS: NATURE, NURTURE, AND THE BRAIN

IN THE GRAND gallery of existence, an intricate mosaic stretches endlessly across the walls—a living portrait made of countless glimmering tiles. No one tile gleams in isolation. A shard of a father's laughter catches the light at breakfast; hands, shaped by a grandmother's steady rituals, move with inherited echoes. Freckles scatter across skin like pressed memory: stories carried through genes, years beneath open skies, and the soothing touch of those who came before.

Perhaps this mosaic is *you*.

It is tempting to want simplicity. To blame everything on inheritance—*"I'm just like my father," "It runs in the family."* Or to credit experience—*"the streets taught me," "my childhood shaped me."* The truth, as neuroscience reveals, does not play in binaries. It unravels as a dynamic duet, a braided rope of *both* nature and nurture, wound tightly around one another, inseparable and alive. This means the real story is not *nature versus nurture.* It is *nature through nurture.*

Before you could walk or breathe air, instructions had been etched into your DNA. Inside each of your cells are 3 billion base pairs—the letters A, T, C, and G composing your genetic script. This code forms genes, each of which codes for proteins that build your physical body and, indirectly, your brain's architecture.

Twin studies, which compare identical twins who share the same DNA and fraternal twins who share only partial DNA, indicate that intelligence, temperament, and many personality dimensions are heritable to a significant degree. This means that genes load the dice: your likelihood of being extroverted, anxious, or musical is partly determined by your unique genetic sequence.

Yet it is important to recognize the metaphor: genes load the dice, but they do not determine the outcome. A gene is not a command, but a predisposition—a first note in a symphony that changes as environment and experience join the performance. One twin may inherit a tendency toward introversion, but whether that becomes quiet reserve or creative reflection depends on the world that shapes them.

The brain's construction follows genetic scaffolding. Early in fetal development, billions of neurons migrate, guided by molecular signals encoded by genes. Like architects sending out blueprints, genes shape the cortex's six layers, the hippocampus's horseshoe curve, and the cerebellum's dense folds.

What sets the human brain apart is its unfinished state at birth. We arrive incomplete, our neural wiring deliberately left open to possibility. This plasticity enables the environment to complete what genes have initiated. In early childhood, synapses—the connections between neurons—proliferate in astonishing numbers. Experience then acts as a sculptor, strengthening the pathways we use and trimming away those we do not.

So, to be born with certain genetic tendencies is not to be bound by fate. Life after birth continues to shape the brain's circuitry. A child with a gift for music must hear melodies and explore instruments for those neural pathways to flourish. A child inclined toward anxiety may thrive in a nurturing environment, yet struggle if neglected. Genes provide the script, but experience writes the performance.

Picture the brain as a vast forest. Genes plant the trees, set the soil, and influence the rainfall. Nurture is the weather, the footpaths, the fires, and storms that determine which trails deepen and which trees reach for the sky.

Attachment bonds in infancy play a profound role. Secure, consistent caregiving strengthens prefrontal–limbic regulation. These circuits enable children to calm down after experiencing distress. Neglect, in contrast, disrupts development. As studies in Romanian orphanages revealed, deprivation in the earliest years left measurable marks—smaller hippocampal volume, altered stress responses—even into adulthood.

Adversity in adolescence sculpts differently. Chronic stress, poverty, and maltreatment increase cortisol, impairing the hippocampus's ability to form resilient memory networks, while over-activating the amygdala, priming fear responses. Yet alongside these risks lies remarkable adaptability. Supportive mentors, safe schools, and opportunities enrich neural growth. They thicken the prefrontal cortex, strengthen executive function, and enhance cognitive abilities.

Opportunity matters too. The lives of the Beatles remind us: four Liverpool youths played in Hamburg dive bars for hundreds of hours, unwittingly engaging in what neuroscience calls deep practice. Their eventual brilliance was not due to DNA alone—it was due to DNA plus environment. Nature and nurture struck chords in harmony.

To believe genes are static would be like believing books never open. In reality, genes are scripts whose pages can be folded, highlighted, or silenced depending on context. Epigenetics is the science of these modifications.

Chemical tags, known as methyl groups, can attach to DNA, silencing genes without altering the underlying genetic code. Proteins known as histones can tighten or loosen, making DNA more or less accessible for reading. These changes act like bookmarks, guiding which passages are read and when.

Why does this matter for the brain and for us?

Epigenetic modifications are shaped by experience. Childhood trauma can add methyl groups to genes linked to stress reactivity, leaving an adult more anxious. Joyful enrichment, in contrast, reduces chromatin tightness around genes, promoting neuroplasticity and boosting cognitive flexibility. These are not mere theories; studies in rodents show pups groomed more frequently by their mothers develop calmer stress responses, mediated by epigenetic marks on specific genes. Humans reflect this process. Holocaust survivors and their children show altered methylation on stress-related genes. Conversely, adults who practice mindfulness, gratitude, or exercise exhibit beneficial epigenetic changes, which enhance their resilience. Genes do not sit idly. They remember. They encode our encounters with adversity and love alike.

Genes also forecast vulnerabilities. Variants in the serotonin transporter gene have been linked to heightened risk of depression under stress. Here's the nuance: risk manifests only under adversity. With nurturing environments, such individuals perform as well as, or even better than, others. Some researchers refer to this as the orchid–dandelion hypothesis: dandelion children, those with robust genes, survive anywhere, while orchid children, those with sensitive genes, wilt under neglect but bloom magnificently under care. Thus, what appears to be genetic risk can be recast as a potential for extraordinary growth, given the right nurturing environment.

Interestingly, the human brain remains plastic throughout life, meaning our choices etch themselves onto circuits. Habits—whether procrastination, exercise, or mindfulness—reinforce synaptic patterns until they become automatic, housed in the basal ganglia. Stress, likewise, leaves molecular imprints. Chronic stress shrinks the hippocampus while overactivating the amygdala; calming practices, on the other hand, literally regrow dendritic branches. Your daily rituals, therefore, are not trivial. They are microscripts inscribed in biology. Reading nightly sculpts memory circuits. Gratitude reshapes regulation circuits. Doomscrolling at midnight strengthens pathways of compulsion and comparison. Nurture is every choice repeated.

Genes and journeys do not stop with you. Epigenetic changes can pass across generations. Studies in mice demonstrate trauma echoes in offspring's stress reactivity. In humans, the grandchildren of famine survivors from the Dutch Hunger Winter exhibit metabolic changes decades later. Some epigenetic shifts echo like whispers across bloodlines.

Yet inheritance is not a curse alone—healing passes too. Work on intergenerational resilience suggests nurturing environments not only buffer children, but can *reverse* imprinting of parental trauma. A mother facing adversity yet practicing sensitive caregiving offers her child an altered, healthier epigenetic legacy. Nature and nurture ripple forward like two entwined rivers shaping future landscapes.

Beyond the immediate family, culture is also an architect. Cultural scripts teach languages, values, taboos, and aspirations. Neuroscience reveals that bilingual individuals exhibit denser gray matter in language areas; cultural norms of collectivism or individualism are correlated with brain activity patterns in social cognition networks. Even concepts of self differ: Western brains activate differently when thinking of "self" versus "mother." Chinese brains show overlapping regions for both, highlighting cultural shaping of neural identity. Culture, in this sense, is a massive environmental funnel pouring meaning into the brain. Genes prepare the clay, but culture molds forms no gene could predict.

~

Understanding the interplay between nature and nurture is not just academic trivia. It has tangible, everyday implications for how we live, raise others, and organize our society. The realization that both biology and experience shape us gives each of us a measure of agency in crafting our futures and the futures of those around us.

For parents, this knowledge means your care and attention do more than guide behavior—they reach into biology itself, shaping how genes are expressed in your child's developing brain. Building secure attachments is not just about comfort. It sculpts the neural circuits of the prefrontal cortex and limbic system, laying the groundwork for emotional regulation and resilience.

For adults, the process does not end. Habits, routines, and our responses to stress continue to shape our brains and gene expression throughout life. Practicing resilience, pursuing growth, and nurturing healthy routines are not mere slogans. There are ways to reinforce and rebuild the brain's architecture, keeping us adaptable and resilient.

For societies, policy is a tool for shaping biology on a large scale. Decisions about poverty, education, and nutrition are not only political or economic—they are biological interventions. Unaddressed inequity can leave lasting marks on DNA expression and health for generations. By expanding opportunity and support, we can rewrite the possibilities encoded in our bodies and minds.

Recognizing the entwined roles of nature and nurture brings a sense of responsibility. While we cannot alter our genetic inheritance, we can shape the environments—our own and those of others—that foster growth. In doing so, we create the conditions for human flourishing, building worlds where even the most sensitive among us can thrive.

Who, then, made you who you are?

It was your mother's lullaby and your father's absence. It was the city you walked in and the books you read. It was dopamine's flickers and cortisol's floods. It was the methyl groups glued atop strands of DNA responding to traumas known and unknown. It was joy, loss, risk, and care.

You are not simply the sum of your bloodlines, nor merely a product of circumstance. You are a mosaic. Some pieces gleam with ancestry, others with experience, and some cracks await the healing of resilience. Together, they form a portrait that is unique, unpredictable, and always evolving.

The truth resists simplification. Genes and journeys merge ceaselessly, like waves blending into shore. To ask which matters more is to ask whether light or warmth makes the fire glow. The answer is both. Always both.

Within that union lies freedom. You inherit, and you are shaped.

But more than that, *you can still sculpt*. You can choose your environments, your habits, your relationships. You can kindle fires where genes provide fuel, and calm storms where ancestry left its mark. Nature offers possibilities. Nurture offers paths. *The self is a journey, and the journey is yours.*

CHAPTER 13
THE STORY OF YOU: HOW MEMORY AND EXPERIENCE SHAPE THE SELF

WHO ARE YOU? *What makes you "you"? Are you more than your name, your address, your hobbies, your personality? What sets each of us apart, and why does this uniqueness exist at all?*

These questions resonate through philosophy and poetry, through the hush of temples and the hum of MRI machines. Perhaps it's human nature to wonder these things, *but has anything ever come of these wonderings?*

If you ask the philosopher, the answer is both a lantern and a labyrinth. *"Knowing yourself is the beginning of all wisdom,"* Aristotle reminds us—simple, luminous, yet endlessly deep. Or perhaps, as Nietzsche muses, *"One's own self is well hidden from one's own self; of all mines of treasure, one's own is the last to be dug up."* The self, it seems, is both the map and the mystery.

Turn to the poet, and the reply is a gentle urging: *"Your real self may be hiding somewhere, look for it within, when you find yourself, you can freely be what you want to be,"* writes Michael Bassey Johnson. Here, the self is a secret garden, waiting to be discovered.

Ask the artist, and the answer is painted in bold strokes. *"Painting is self-discovery. Every good artist paints what he is,"* says Jackson Pollock. The canvas is a mirror; every color, a confession.

In the hush of the sanctuary, the priest counsels acceptance: *"Do not desire to be other than you are, but desire to be very well what you are,"* offers St. Francis de Sales. The self, in this light, is a calling to be answered, not a mask to be worn.

What if you ask a machine, such as an MRI?

The answer is neither riddle nor rhyme, but a constellation of flickering lights. The self, it tells us, is a pattern of activity, a choreography of neurons. It is both more mysterious and more tangible than we ever imagined. So we begin: with questions as old as breath, with answers that shimmer and shift, with a journey inward—toward the mirror in the mind.

Within your brain, tucked away in the middle of the parietal lobe, lies a region called the precuneus. If you placed a finger on the very top of your head and imagined going straight down toward the middle, you'd be pointing right at it. For much of scientific history, this area was overlooked, dismissed as just another patch of neural landscape. But as brain imaging technology advanced, the precuneus quietly stepped into the spotlight, revealing itself as one of the brain's most important architects of who we are.

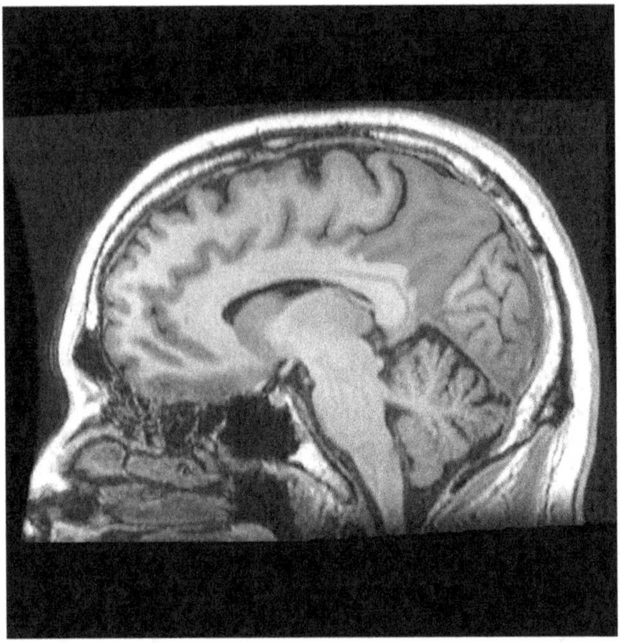

Figure 15. *Sagittal MRI slice with the precuneus shown in red.* Geoff B Hall

Far from being a passive bystander, the precuneus acts as a kind of internal guide or compass, integrating memory, imagination, and self-reflection to help shape our sense of identity. It orchestrates the seamless flow between our inner world and outward experience, quietly directing how we process, relive, and even rehearse the story of ourselves.

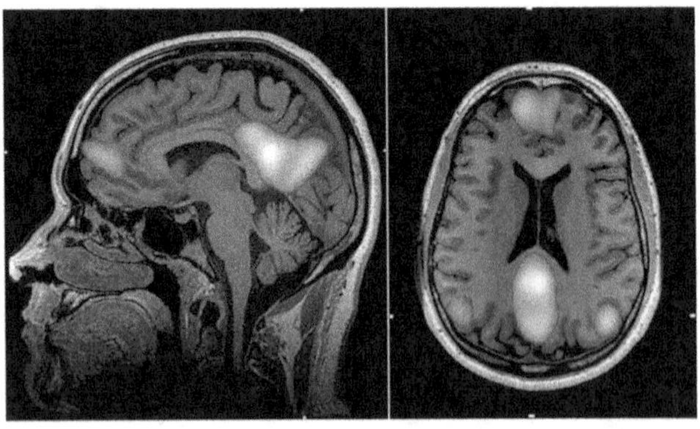

Figure 16. *Magnetic resonance imaging of areas of the brain in the default mode network.* John Graner

The precuneus is also a central player in what we now call the "default mode network"—a group of brain regions that become active when we're not focused on the outside world. Think of it as your brain's background app, switching on when you're daydreaming, remembering, or letting your mind wander. If you've ever arrived home and realized you barely remember the drive, you've experienced your brain's remarkable ability to operate on autopilot.

When you "zone out" behind the wheel, your brain is running two programs at once: the habit system stored in regions like the basal ganglia keeps you on the road. At the same time, the precuneus opens the door to your inner world. It's the silent conductor that lets you slip seamlessly from the present moment into the real-life movie of your memories. You don't just remember the facts; you experience the scene: the taste of gooey cookie dough, the warmth of a blanket, the smell of your favorite candle.

This inner cinema doesn't just replay the past—it allows you to leap forward, rehearsing future plans or imagining yourself in someone else's shoes. The boundaries between now and then, between real and imagined, blur and dissolve. Nothing embodies this more relatably than that shower time pep talk we give ourselves before a big confrontation.

Imagine you're standing in the shower, hot water streaming down, and your mind starts to wander. You know you have a difficult conversation coming up. Instinctively, you begin to play out the scenario in your head, picturing the other person's face, imagining what they might say, and crafting the perfect, witty responses.

Maybe you even replay the scene a few times, tweaking your words, trying out different tones, or imagining how you'll feel when it's over. In these moments, the precuneus is not focused on remembering the past; it's leaping forward into the future, running simulations of what might happen, and preparing you for what's to come. Your mind can jump back to similar conflicts you've had before, borrowing lines or emotions, and then fast-forward to possible outcomes, letting you practice and refine your approach—all without ever leaving the shower.

Just like a film director editing together scenes from different times and places, your brain stitches together memories, hopes, and imagined conversations. This inner movie keeps your identity whole, helping you learn from the past, navigate the present, and step bravely into the future. The precuneus acts as the cutting room floor, arranging these moments into a continuous reel, so that who you were, who you are, and who you might become all play out as one unfolding story.

~

What makes the precuneus so fascinating isn't just what it does on its own, but how it acts as a crossroads for some of the brain's busiest highways. Picture the precuneus as a central train station. It has tracks running in every direction, connecting neighborhoods. Each of those has its own specialties.

One of its main connections is with the prefrontal cortex, which sits just behind your forehead. As we've explored in earlier chapters, the prefrontal cortex is often called the brain's "executive," because it helps you make decisions, weigh options, and plan for the future. When you're deciding whether to speak up in a meeting or what to cook for dinner, your prefrontal cortex is hard at work. By staying in close contact with this region, the precuneus helps blend your memories and sense of self into your decision-making. This means your choices reflect not just logic, but who you are and what you've experienced.

Another important partner is the hippocampus, a small, curved structure in the brain. It is essential for forming and recalling memories. It's the brain's archivist, helping you remember your first day of school, your favorite vacation, or even where you parked your car. The precuneus works with the hippocampus to bring these memories to life, adding detail and emotion so they feel real and personal.

The precuneus also connects with the sensorimotor regions, which are responsible for sensing your body's position and controlling movement. These areas allow you to sense where your arms and legs are, even with your eyes closed. They help you move smoothly through the world. By linking up with these regions, the precuneus grounds your sense of self in your physical body, so you don't just know who you are—you know where you are, and how you fit into the space around you.

All of these connections make the precuneus perfectly positioned to tie together the many threads of your identity: your memories, your decisions, your sense of presence in the world. It's this teamwork that allows you to feel like a single, continuous person, even as you change and grow over time.

Sometimes, these relationships are also responsible for that feeling when you walk into a room and forget why you're there. That's your brain "buffering," like Spotify pausing to load the next song. When you're deciding what to do next, it's like your brain is shuffling through tracks, picking the one that fits your mood and history.

So, whether your mind feels like a Spotify playlist shuffling through moods, or a browser with too many tabs open, remember: the precuneus is the behind-the-scenes multitasker, editing together the highlight reel of your life—one memory, one plan, one mental track at a time.

How do we know all this?

For centuries, the brain's inner workings were hidden, its secrets locked away behind bone and mystery. The arrival of magnetic resonance imaging, or MRI, changed everything. MRI scans let scientists peer inside the living brain, watching different regions light up as people remember, imagine, or reflect on themselves.

When you are asked to think about your personality: *Am I generous? Am I brave?*—the precuneus lights up, a lighthouse in the neural fog. When you call to mind a cherished memory or gaze at your own face in a photograph, this same region pulses with activity. It is as if, in these moments of self-reflection, the brain draws a bright circle around the idea of *"me."*

In a sweeping meta-analysis, dozens of imaging studies found a consistent pattern: the precuneus, along with the medial prefrontal cortex, forms the beating heart of self-referential thought. When you ponder your own story, the precuneus is the narrator, the editor, the archivist, and the location. When you turn your thoughts to someone else—imagining their feelings, recalling their face—the glow shifts. The precuneus dims, ceding the spotlight to other regions. The distinction is clear: the brain keeps a separate chamber for the self, a neural sanctum where your own identity is assembled and maintained.

Yet the MRI reveals more than just the mechanics of memory or imagination. It shows us the architecture of the self. It shows the way the brain constructs a continuous, evolving identity from the raw materials of experience. When you ask, *"Who am I?"* it is the precuneus that assembles your answer, drawing on a lifetime of stored scenes and future rehearsals. It is here, in this quiet fold of cortex, that the philosophical and biological meet: the self as both story and structure, both question and answer.

This is not just a scientific curiosity. It is a universal inheritance. Most of us, at some point, have gazed into a mirror and wondered about the person staring back. Thanks to the marriage of technology and curiosity, we now know that this act of self-recognition is measurable, visible, and alive within our brains.

When the precuneus is damaged by injury, stroke, or disease, individuals may experience a loss of self. The vividness of personal memories can fade, leaving only pale outlines where once there were rich, sensory details. Some people find themselves struggling to recognize their own face in the mirror, or to recall the emotional texture of their most cherished experiences.

In the most profound cases, the line between self and others blurs entirely. This is seen in certain psychiatric conditions like depersonalization disorder and some forms of schizophrenia. The boundaries that usually keep *"me"* separate from *"not-me"* begin to dissolve, leading to confusion, anxiety, and a haunting sense of unreality.

The story of Phineas Gage, recounted in a previous chapter, stands as a foundational example of how brain injury can profoundly alter a person's sense of self. Gage's traumatic accident—an iron rod passing through his frontal lobes—transformed him from a responsible, sociable foreman into someone impulsive and unpredictable. His case was among the first to show that our identity and personality are deeply rooted in the physical structure of the brain.

Not all wounds are visible on a scan. We are taught to look for scars on the skin, to measure harm by the blood that stains a bandage. Yet some injuries are etched into the soul, as indelible as smoke after fire. These are moral injuries. They are wounds that do not bleed. They occur when we cross the boundaries of our own morals, or are forced to witness acts that violate the very code by which we live. The result is a fracture, not of bone, but of self. A shattering of trust in the goodness of the world, and in the person we believed ourselves to be.

The language of medicine is ill-equipped for this kind of pain. No scan can reveal a soul torn by guilt or shame; no bandage can heal a conscience in crisis. Yet the symptoms are unmistakable: guilt that clings like a second skin, shame that seeps into every waking thought, a loss of faith—not just in others, but in oneself. Some retreat from the world, withdrawing into a shell of silence. Others are haunted by memories that replay in the mind's theater, each scene more vivid than the last. It is a wound that festers in the absence of acknowledgment, growing deeper with every attempt to ignore it.

Science, ever the cartographer of the unseen, has begun to chart this territory. Moral injury is not classified as a mental disorder. It is a dimensional wound, one that can hollow out the emotional, psychological, social, and spiritual core of a person. Unlike post-traumatic stress disorder, which is rooted in fear and the body's primal response to threat, moral injury is the aftermath of ethical conflict. This wound gnaws at the very narrative of who we are.

This fragility of self is built into the very biology of our brains. The precuneus is particularly active during moments of self-reflection, when we think about our own traits, recall autobiographical events, or envision ourselves in the future. When this region falters, the internal narrative that stitches together our identity can unravel, leaving us feeling fragmented or adrift. It's like waking up one morning and finding yourself watching your life from a distance, a spectator rather than the main character. For some, this unsettling detachment is not just a fleeting sensation but a persistent reality. A world grown hazy, the self slipping out of focus.

Yet, this vulnerability also hints at something deeper: the self is not built in a day. In fact, the precuneus is not fully formed at birth. It develops slowly, unfolding throughout childhood and adolescence, paralleling the gradual process by which we all come to understand ourselves as unique individuals. Young children are often blissfully unaware of how they appear to others. Only later do they develop the capacity for self-consciousness, introspection, and the nuanced sense of *"me"* that marks adult identity. The slow maturation of the precuneus reminds us that selfhood is not fixed, but grows and changes over time.

It is also important to mention that not everyone's precuneus operates in the same way. Some people are naturally introspective, with rich inner worlds and a tendency toward self-reflection. Others are more outwardly focused, living in the moment. We believe these differences may be linked to the degree of activity or connectivity within the brain's default mode network. Age, mental health, and even lifestyle habits, such as meditation, can influence its function.

For instance, studies suggest that regular mindfulness or contemplative practices can enhance activity in the precuneus. This potentially strengthens our sense of self and emotional resilience. While you can't "work out" your precuneus at the gym, you can nurture it through habits that encourage self-awareness and reflection. Mindfulness meditation, journaling, or simply taking time to pause and notice your thoughts can all help keep this neural lighthouse burning bright. These practices may not only sharpen your sense of self but also buffer against the mental fog that sometimes creeps in with stress, aging, or illness.

As we turn from the intricate wiring of the brain to the broader stage of existence, we find that the story of identity does not begin in the sterile glow of a laboratory, nor in the flicker of a brain scan. It starts in the wild, in the raw theater of survival. Long before humans puzzled over the meaning of *"me"* or *"I,"* evolution was already shaping the foundations of selfhood. In the animal kingdom, a sense of self is not a philosophical luxury—it is a matter of life and death.

To survive, a creature must know where its body ends and the world begins, must distinguish kin from predator, must remember friend from foe. Even in the silent depths of the ocean, the octopus that solves a puzzle, or the dog that recognizes its scent—these are the first glimmers of identity. Across species, the brain has evolved clever ways to maintain the individual's integrity amid the chaos of the world.

For a jellyfish, the self is a membrane, a thin veil separating saltwater from the soft machinery of life. For a bird, it is the knowledge of wings and feathers, the ability to sense the air's pressure, and the ability to adjust in flight. For a wolf, it is the memory of pack and territory, the recognition of kin by scent and sound. These are not abstractions; they are the architecture of survival itself.

Even the simplest creatures possess mechanisms for distinguishing themselves from their environment. The sea slug withdraws from touch; the crab repairs its own limb but ignores a foreign object. Social animals, from elephants to magpies, remember individuals and relationships, forming social maps that guide behavior. A handful of species—great apes, dolphins, elephants, magpies—can recognize themselves in mirrors, a sign of higher-order self-awareness, a flicker of the *"me"* or *"I"* that burns so brightly in our minds.

Charles Darwin, in his work *The Descent of Man*, argued that the differences between human and animal minds are *"one of degree and not of kind."* He observed that animals exhibit emotions, form social bonds, and even display rudimentary forms of self-awareness. Darwin described dogs showing pride and shame, elephants displaying grief, and primates using tools—behaviors that hint at a complex inner life.

"The lower animals, like man, manifestly feel pleasure and pain, happiness and misery," Darwin wrote, noting that animals can recognize themselves and others, remember past experiences, and anticipate future events—the very foundations of what we call the *"self."* For Darwin, it was clear the seeds of selfhood were sown deep in our evolutionary past, blossoming in myriad forms across the tree of life. Today, we can see that more clearly with discoveries that have shed light on our collective past.

Fossil endocasts, natural molds of the braincase, reveal that the precuneus began to expand dramatically only in the last half-million years. This is after our lineage split from Neanderthals and Denisovans. While Neanderthals possessed large brains, their parietal lobes, particularly the precuneus, were less developed compared to those of modern humans. Without a fully developed precuneus, as in Neanderthals, the capacity for nuanced self-reflection and sophisticated social networks may have been limited. The Neanderthal mind lacked the intricate web of self-other distinctions and future-oriented thinking that propels human culture.

If the early animal self was a campfire, flickering alone in the wilderness, the human self—illuminated by the precuneus—is a bonfire, drawing others near, casting long shadows of memory and hope. It is the hidden architect of empathy, the silent conductor of the social symphony. It's clear the precuneus did not appear overnight. It was sculpted by the slow chisel of natural selection, each groove and fold a testament to the growing complexity of our inner worlds. In its emergence, humanity found the neural soil in which society could take root and flourish.

For us, the self has become something richer and more intricate. It is the lens through which we experience pride, shame, ambition, and love. It is the quiet voice that colors our choices, sometimes nudging us toward greatness, at other times tripping us up with old fears or stubborn habits. Pride, especially, is a double-edged sword. It can fuel our boldest dreams or blind us to our own shortcomings. In the intricate circuitry of the brain, pride is not just a fleeting feeling—it is a compass. It points us toward belonging, achievement, and recognition, guiding us through the complex undercurrents of social life.

Pride is the ego's constant companion, a force that can sharpen our focus or cloud our judgment. It whispers in our ear, urging us to take risks, to stand out, to defend our choices even when doubt creeps in. It helps us seek recognition, avoid shame, and find our place in the world. Pride can also blind us, making us stubborn or defensive, trapping us in patterns that no longer serve us.

Every choice we make is a negotiation—a subtle dance between memory and desire, between the lessons of the past and the hopes for what might come next. Here, the ego acts as both judge and advocate, weighing options, calculating risks, and nudging us toward decisions that feel true to who we are. Neuroscientists have found that this process is a measurable activity in the brain. Within the folds of the cortex, networks known as "egocentric value maps" light up as we evaluate our choices, constantly updating our internal sense of what matters most to us.

It's like standing in front of a bakery case, torn between a decadent chocolate cake and a fruit tart. Your imagination might conjure the taste, the texture, the memory of birthdays past. Your ego steps in to weigh pride against prudence: *"Will I regret this later? Will I feel better if I choose the tart?"*

This inner debate is not just about calories or cravings; it's about much more. It's about reinforcing the story you tell yourself about who you are. *Are you disciplined? Are you indulgent? Are you spontaneous or careful?*

The ego is the quiet voice that frames these questions and pushes you toward an answer. Modern brain imaging reveals that the regions involved in ego-driven decision-making overlap with those that support self-reflection and imagination. In these moments, the prefrontal cortex works in concert with the precuneus and other areas to weigh the value of different actions. They predict outcomes and monitor how our choices align with our self-image. These "egocentric value maps" are dynamic—they shift with context, mood, and memory, ensuring that the self we present to the world is always a work in progress.

Ultimately, ego is a silent partner in every decision, a backstage manager keeping the show running smoothly. It draws on the raw materials of imagination and memory, shaping them into action, guiding us through the infinite crossroads of daily life. Whether we are choosing dessert, defending our beliefs, or chasing a dream, the ego is there. Sometimes it is bold, sometimes cautious, always shaping the story of who we are becoming.

Here, the neurobiology and philosophy of self intertwine. Identity is not a static label or a single moment of self-awareness; it is a dynamic and evolving concept. It is a living, evolving toolkit—shaped by ancient instincts, refined by memory and imagination.

Across continents and centuries, beneath painted ceilings and flickering screens, humans have always circled the same questions: *Who am I? Why do I remember? What does it mean to change?*

From the ancient fireside tales of gods and shapeshifters to the silent hum of MRI machines mapping the brain's hidden folds, our search for self is relentless, universal, and endlessly inventive. We have peered into mirrors—bronze, glass, digital—hoping to catch a glimpse of the soul behind the eyes. We have written epics and memoirs, built temples and laboratories, all in pursuit of the elusive *"me"* or *"I."* Some have sought answers in the stars, while others have looked to the intricacies of the brain's circuitry. Still, the questions remain, refracted through culture, language, and time.

The self is not a static monument but a living, breathing story. One told by the brain to itself, scene by scene, day by day. The precuneus, tucked deep within the parietal lobe, acts as the silent editor, stitching together memories, sensations, and dreams. The hippocampus archives our past; the prefrontal cortex weighs our choices; the sensorimotor regions anchor us in the present moment. Together, these regions form the neural orchestra that scores our private epic.

Yet, for all our searching, the self remains partly veiled, a mystery and a mirror. It reflects our past, refracts our hopes, and is always, always becoming. We are the sum of our memories, the echo of our choices, the silent witness to our unfolding.

To know the self is to step into the stream of time, to feel the current of change, and to recognize, if only for a moment, the face in the water as our own. We are, all of us, unfinished stories, blueprints in motion, forever shaped by the interplay of biology, memory, imagination, and choice. And so the search continues: in science and story, in the quiet of reflection and the noise of daily life. The self is not a destination, but a journey—a question we live, an answer we become.

CHAPTER 14
THE BRAIN'S PLAYGROUND: THE NEURAL BASIS OF CREATIVITY AND IMAGINATION

A RUSH of wind presses against your face as a dragon's wings thunder overhead, the air shimmering with heat from its breath. Scales catch the light, flashing iridescent colors that shift with every movement. In a blink, the scene transforms: neon rain streaks down the glass of a future city, chrome-lined alleys pulse with energy, hovercars rumble overhead, and a chorus of voices filters through the static of mechanized speakers. The mind's eye is a restless traveler, conjuring worlds both ancient and yet to be.

Nothing of this exists outside you. And yet—for you—it *does exist*. Your brain has become an architect of experiences, conjuring whole universes, reshaping fragments of memory into impossible worlds. This is imagination. It is the playground of the self, the canvas of creativity, the hidden theater where inner worlds come alive.

Think of the fantasy author mapping out entire continents, languages, and histories in their head before a single word hits the page. Or the musician who hears a melody in a dream and wakes to bring it to life. Even the everyday act of scrolling through a feed, imagining yourself in someone else's shoes, is a quiet act of invention.

Imagination lets us step outside the boundaries of the present to visit worlds that never were and return changed. It is the crucible of possibility. Every story, every invention, every decision about who we might become begins here. And creativity itself—whether in poetry, engineering, or problem-solving—is the practical outgrowth of this capacity. Imagination builds scaffolds where none exist, carving *"what ifs"* and *"why nots"* into the bedrock of reality.

Imagination is not a fixed trait, nor is it evenly distributed across time or cultures. It is shaped and colored by our social environment and the stage of life we inhabit. Societies encourage different forms of creativity. Collectivist cultures often emphasize incremental improvement, collaboration, and harmony within the group. Individualist cultures, by contrast, celebrate radical novelty and unique self-expression. The landscape of imagination is as varied as the societies that nurture it.

Throughout a lifetime, creativity takes many forms. In childhood, imagination is abundant and uninhibited. Children invent imaginary friends and fantastical worlds with ease, fueled by a period of synaptic exuberance. As they grow into adolescence, imagination becomes more self-reflective. Teenagers use creative powers to envision various selves, explore identities, and imagine complex social scenarios, experimenting with who they might become.

In adulthood, creativity becomes more focused and applied. Many adults channel imaginative energy into problem-solving at work or honing a personal craft. Later in life, memory deepens. Imagination often turns toward reflection and meaning-making as novelty fades. Creativity focuses on storytelling and legacy. While imagination evolves, it remains essential throughout life.

When you imagine, the brain is not idle. Neurons fire in precise symphonies, meshing memory, perception, and emotion. Think of it as a forge: molten fragments of past experience are poured into molds of possibility, hammered into visions, fears, and dreams.

The hippocampus, a structure located in the temporal lobe, plays a central role here. Known famously for its role in memory, the hippocampus allows you to relive the feel of your grandmother's kitchen—the smell of simmering soup, the cool linoleum beneath your toes. The line between memory and imagination is faint, sometimes vanishing altogether. When you recall a childhood birthday, your mind fills in the gaps. Taking it further, the hippocampus also allows you to recombine those memories into novel imaginings: perhaps the kitchen stretches into a palace hall, or perhaps dinner is served by robots.

The hippocampus works in conjunction with the visual cortex. This region is located at the back of the brain and is responsible for processing what the eyes see. When you recall or imagine a dragon, your visual cortex reactivates in patterns overlapping with those of real sight. Imagination piggybacks on sensory systems, summoning mental imagery almost as though you were looking through your own eyes. This explains why mental rehearsal of movement—such as a pianist imagining scales or an athlete simulating swings—activates the motor cortex in ways parallel to actual practice. Imagination is not the ghost of action but its rehearsal.

The work of the imagination is also further distributed across several interconnected networks. Recall our default mode network from earlier chapters. This network comes alive when the mind wanders. Our thoughts drift inward, and we find ourselves daydreaming. It links areas such as the medial prefrontal cortex, posterior cingulate, angular gyrus, and hippocampal formation. It's the brain's movie projector. It ties together scenarios, self-reflections, and autobiographical memories that form the fabric of our inner worlds.

Working alongside is the executive control network, found in the lateral prefrontal and parietal regions. This network organizes, critiques, and selects among the many visions generated by the default mode network. While the default mode network offers unfettered freedom to generate wild associations, the executive network steps in to ask: *How feasible is this idea? Which vision is worth pursuing?* Creativity depends on the interplay between the freedom of the default mode network and the disciplined guidance of executive control.

The salience network, anchored in the insula and anterior cingulate cortex, acts as a conductor for the other two networks. It helps the brain shift attention between the external world and internal thought, deciding whether we tune in to inner imagery or respond to outer signals. Without the salience network's direction, imagination might never surface to consciousness, or could drift untethered from reality.

Altogether, creativity emerges from a dynamic conversation between these networks. The default mode network proposes ideas, the executive network evaluates them, and the salience network shifts the spotlight of attention. This triadic dance is evident in brain imaging studies of improvising jazz musicians, writers immersed in a state of flow, and problem solvers experiencing moments of "aha!".

One of the most intriguing discoveries of modern neuroscience is the profound differences in inner worlds. Not all minds imagine alike. Some people live with aphantasia, a condition where the mind's eye is blind—they cannot summon mental images at will. For them, memory is a list of facts, not a movie played in Technicolor. When asked to picture a beach, those with aphantasia report seeing *"nothing at all—just darkness."* This condition also highlights that vivid imagery is not required for imagination. Such individuals rely more on conceptual or semantic representations. Their creativity emerges in abstraction rather than visual replay.

At the other end are those whose mental imagery is stunningly intense and immersive. This condition is known as hyperphantasia. For these individuals, simply closing their eyes and summoning a thought can set off a vivid, multisensory experience. A single idea, like imagining a dragon or recalling a childhood home, can conjure scenes with the sharpness and color of a movie projected on the mind's inner screen. Some hyperphantasic people report being able to *"see"* details. Some can visualize sunlight glinting on water, the shifting patterns of shadow among trees, or the precise layout of a room from decades ago.

Yet their imagination is not limited to visuals. Mental images may be accompanied by imagined sounds, smells, or even tactile sensations, blurring the line between thought and perception. This vividness can inspire creativity, allowing stories, inventions, or artistic visions to unfold with cinematic clarity. But it can also be overwhelming: intense images may intrude unbidden, making daydreams deeply absorbing or difficult to ignore. For the hyperphantasic, the theater of the mind is not a dim, abstract space, but a living landscape—sometimes a gift, sometimes a challenge, always astonishingly real.

Why do these differences exist?

The answer lies in the intricate wiring of the brain. Mental imagery, the ability to "see" with the mind's eye, relies on a specific combination of the networks we discussed before. It also includes the visual cortex, which processes actual sight, the parietal and frontal lobes, which help us manipulate and control images, as well as the connections between them.

In people with aphantasia, this network functions differently. Brain scans reveal less activation in visual areas when they try to imagine. Suggesting that the neural pathways responsible for conjuring images are less active or less connected. For those on the opposite end—sometimes referred to as hyperphantasia—the brain's visual centers light up almost as if the person were actually seeing the imagined scene, making their inner world strikingly vivid.

This diversity in mental imagery is just one facet of how our inner experiences can differ. A few years ago, a viral social media trend swept the internet, with people astonished to discover that not everyone has an "internal monologue"—that running commentary of words and thoughts in the mind. Some people "hear" their own voice narrating their day, arguing with themselves, or rehearsing conversations. Others think in pictures, emotions, or abstract concepts, with little or no verbal narration. The revelation that these differences exist sparked widespread fascination and debate, as people realized that their own experience of their minds is not universal.

At its core, creativity in the brain is often the recombination of existing parts. The hippocampus blends fragments—a dragon wing here, a subway tunnel there—stitched into new visions. Studies show that creative individuals exhibit heightened semantic distance, the ability to connect unrelated concepts: sunset and typewriter, sorrow and weather. This capacity depends on flexible network interconnectivity, not on any single creativity center.

Famous creative breakthroughs illustrate this process of recombination. When August Kekulé famously dreamed of a snake swallowing its tail, he wasn't just seeing an idle image—he was unconsciously providing the key to the structure of the benzene ring. Similarly, Einstein's iconic thought experiment, imagining what it would be like to ride alongside a beam of light, drew on the sensations and memories of his childhood bike rides. It fused the memories with the deep questions of physics that preoccupied his mind. In both cases, imagination did not simply replay the past but metabolized fragments of memory into something entirely new and transformative.

This alchemy of imagination and memory often leads to dramatic moments of sudden insight. This is often what we call the "aha!" moment, or an epiphany. The story of Archimedes is perhaps the most famous of these. As he stepped into his bath and watched the water rise, the solution to a perplexing problem suddenly came to mind. He reportedly leapt from the tub, shouting *"Eureka!" or "I have found it!"*

Such moments are not random; they are the culmination of the brain's creative networks working behind the scenes, testing combinations and searching for patterns until the pieces lock into place. In fact, sudden insight carries its own neural profile. Brain scans show that just before an "aha!" moment, the brain's right side suddenly becomes very active. Other brain areas register the surprise and release dopamine, producing a feeling of well-being. This dopamine rush makes the insight feel rewarding, motivating continued exploration for new solutions. This explains creativity's addictive quality: the joy of writing, inventing, or solving a puzzle comes with a neurochemical reward.

~

Beyond art and survival, imagination is the crucible of self. The brain generates model scenarios. Computational neuroscientists call this mental simulation, akin to running algorithms in a virtual environment before acting in the real world. This sandbox creativity is why humans outpace rigid artificial intelligence in novel contexts. A brain can recombine half-forgotten fragments, draw inspiration from metaphor, and leap from linear logic to sudden insight. Imagination is not a luxury; it is a survival advantage.

When you picture a future self delivering a speech, when you replay a past error at night, when you construct moral scenarios to decide what you'd do *"if"*—you are sculpting identity through inner rehearsal. Functional MRI reveals that imagining oneself activates the same regions as remembering oneself. The hippocampus and medial prefrontal cortex collaborate not just to recall who we were but to simulate who we could be. Psychologists propose the *constructive episodic simulation hypothesis*: the brain's ability to imagine futures derives from its ability to reconstruct past events. Imagination is memory repurposed forward.

Try it now. Set aside two minutes.

Imagine something that awaits you—perhaps tomorrow's conversation with a friend, or delivery of a presentation, or even shopping for groceries. Picture not only the events but alternate versions: *What if it goes well? What if it doesn't?*

Notice what arises. *Do you see images? Hear voices? Feel the event in your body? After* the event, pause. Did *mental simulation change your confidence? Did the outcome feel easier or strangely familiar?*

This is imagination's practical gift. By rehearsing possible futures, you prepare without risk. You inoculate yourself with familiarity. Yet this has its downside. The capacity to simulate futures also lets us ruminate, worry, and catastrophize. Anxiety disorders involve overactive simulation of possible threats. PTSD replays traumatic scenes, reactivating the hippocampus and amygdala until the imagined becomes felt once again.

In depression, imagination shrinks. Individuals report difficulty seeing positive futures. The playground grows desolate. Imagination directly shapes well-being. Too much catastrophic simulation fractures resilience; too little future vision erodes hope.

Therapies often target imagination. Cognitive-behavioral interventions train clients to visualize coping scenarios and situations. Exposure therapies reimagine trauma within a safe context. Mindfulness dampens default mode overactivation, allowing prediction error to quiet. Imagination wounds, but also heals.

~

If imagination has the power to both wound and strengthen us, a natural question follows: *can it be trained?*

Scientific research suggests that the answer is yes. Imagination is not a fixed trait; it is a faculty that can be cultivated and expanded through deliberate practice and the right environment. One way to train imagination is through deliberate daydreaming. Setting aside a few minutes each day to let your mind wander can boost creative output by activating the brain's default mode network. Rather than seeing daydreaming as a waste of time, it can be reframed as mental exercise, a rehearsal space for new ideas.

Cross-domain learning is another powerful tool. By exposing your brain to different fields, such as music, art, science, or literature, you provide more raw material for your imagination to recombine. Polymaths and creative thinkers often draw inspiration from a variety of sources, allowing connections to form across seemingly unrelated domains.

Sleep and dreaming, especially during REM sleep, also play a vital role in nurturing imagination. During dreams, the brain makes associative leaps. It combines fragments of memory and experience in ways that can spark creative insight. In this sense, dreams may be the nocturnal workshop of imagination, strengthening creativity while we rest. Meditative practices, particularly those that encourage open monitoring of thoughts and sensations, have also been shown to enhance the generation of creative ideas. By altering attentional networks and allowing the mind to observe without judgment, meditation can lead to more flexible and original thinking.

Play is not just for children. Adults who regularly engage in playful activities—games, improvisation, unstructured exploration—maintain more flexible communication between the default mode and executive control networks. This flexibility supports creative thinking and keeps the mind nimble.

Ultimately, training imagination is less about forcing creative output and more about nourishing the right conditions. It's about creating space for association, encouraging recombination, and giving yourself permission for free mental play. In this way, imagination can be strengthened. The key takeaway is that imagination thrives through practice, exposure to new domains, rest, meditation, and play. Nurturing these elements can expand your creative capacity at any stage of life.

The landscape of inner life is far more varied than we might assume. Some of us navigate by images, others by words, some by feelings, or even by silence. The brain, in its complexity, offers many paths to self-awareness and creativity. Whether your mind is a silent stage, a crowded theater, or a blank canvas, these differences are variations on the theme of being human.

In our digital age, imagination is both amplified and challenged. We binge-watch epic sagas, lose ourselves in video games, and curate online personas. Our brains are constantly remixing the stories we consume, knitting them into the fabric of our own identity. The memes we share, the avatars we build, the fan theories we debate—these are all acts of collective imagination, shaping not just how we see the world, but how we see ourselves.

Ultimately, imagination is an engine of the self. It allows us to rewrite our past, envision our future, and create meaning where none existed before. It is the reason we can fall in love with fictional heroes, mourn the end of a series, or dream up new worlds on the bus ride home. The self is not a static character, but a storyteller. It is forever editing, embellishing, and expanding the narrative of who we are and who we might become.

The dragon's wingbeats fade. Rain-streaked neon dims. Slowly, your inner cinema dissolves into quiet. Yet the brain's playground remains open, ready. It is always there, conjuring scenes of desire, fear, ambition, and art. In this playground, we invent futures, rehearse ourselves, and sculpt our identities. Here, every story is written, every tool forged, every choice rehearsed.

Imagination is not escapism. It is a rehearsal for existence, a blueprint for invention, therapy for wounds, fuel for art. It makes us human in ways no other species fully rivals. So visit often. Wander through imagined landscapes. Converse with futures. Reshape memories. Picture your life not only as it is but as it could be. In that act of daring to imagine, you are already molding neural circuits toward possibility. *Your playground awaits.*

CHAPTER 15
THE LIVING GARDEN: HOW MEMORY AND SLEEP PRUNE AND RESTORE THE MIND

WHERE WERE *you when the world shut down in March 2020?*

Many of us can still recall with vivid clarity: the moment schools announced closures, the eerie quiet of empty streets, the endless Zoom calls. And then, of course, the Great Toilet Paper Shortage—when a single mega-pack felt like gold, and neighbors whispered tips about which store might still have a few rolls left.

Now ask yourself something more ordinary: *where is your phone charger right now?* You might pause, scan your mental map—*bedroom outlet? Living room? Did you leave it in your bag? And your earbuds—where have they wandered off to?*

You retrace your steps, flipping through mental snapshots. Perhaps the nightstand, a coat pocket, or some nameless place just out of reach. Then comes the familiar frustration: w*hat was the name of that show on Netflix, the one with that actor whose face you can picture but whose name escapes you?*

The answer hovers on the tip of your tongue. You can sense it, almost grasp it, yet it slips away, just out of reach. Memory speaks in fragments, offering echoes but rarely the whole. It is both loyal and elusive—a trickster that plays by its own rules. Some memories anchor themselves, immovable in time. Others drift, vanishing the moment you try to seize them.

Memory is not a static vault, but a living garden. It is constantly pruned and reshaped by time, sleep, and emotion. It's not a warehouse with fixed shelves, but a fertile soil bed where recollections sprout, wither, and regrow. Some memories bloom in vivid color decades later; others become tangled in confusion or fade away entirely. Memory is not simply stored, but cultivated. It grows wild across the years, shaped by sleep, trauma, joy, and repetition.

Every memory begins as experience—a sound, a sight, a taste, an emotion. Yet only some experiences are granted the privilege of planting a seed in the brain. At the heart of this process lies the hippocampus, tucked deep in the medial temporal lobe. This small, seahorse-shaped structure is astonishingly powerful. It stitches together time and space, recording where things happen and when. Think of it as a gardener sowing seeds into rich soil beds, tagging experiences with coordinates so they can be retrieved later. A birthday party from childhood lingers because the hippocampus bundled the cake, the candles, the song, and the faces at the table into one coherent "episode."

The brain organizes memory into distinct types. Episodic memories are the stories of our lives—birthdays, adventures, moments of joy or sorrow—relying heavily on the hippocampus. Semantic memories are facts and knowledge, like the capital of a country or the rules of a game, distributed more broadly across the brain. Procedural memories are the skills we master, such as riding a bike or playing an instrument, governed by deeper structures like the basal ganglia and cerebellum.

Yet not every seed of memory survives. Many wither before they can take hold. You might pass a hundred strangers on the street, but unless something remarkable happens, their faces will fade by tomorrow. The hippocampus cannot nurture every seed; it must choose with care. Each new experience floods the brain with information, but only a select few are cultivated into lasting memories.

The hippocampus gathers and organizes this flood of information, deciding what to retain and what to discard. Memories are not stored in a single place. Instead, they are distributed across the brain in networks of cells called engrams. The sound of laughter may reside in one region, the image of a friend's face in another, and the feeling of joy in yet another. When we recall a memory, the brain reactivates this network, piecing together fragments to reconstruct the original experience.

Emotional memories burn especially bright. They are colored by fear or happiness and are shaped by the amygdala. These flashbulb memories remain seared across decades. The amygdala tags events based on their emotional intensity. Fear sharpens memory consolidation; joy, too, can elevate recollection. In evolutionary terms, this makes sense: remembering danger kept us alive, remembering bonds kept us connected.

Neuroscientists have found that when the amygdala activates strongly during an experience, hippocampal encoding becomes stronger. The neurotransmitter norepinephrine floods circuits, heightening attention, locking in detail. That is why trauma can feel unforgettable. It's seared sensory fragments return unbidden. The same mechanism explains why you remember a first kiss in sensory detail: the warmth of lips, faint scent of perfume, trembling heartbeat. Emotion is biological fertilizer. It grows vivid flowers, though sometimes thorned.

~

Once these seeds of memory are sown, another gardener steps in: the prefrontal cortex. This frontal lobe region, the brain's decision-making center, helps sift through memory content. It asks: *Which recollections matter? Which are trivial weeds?* When you cram for an exam, it directs attention to relevant details. When you try to forget a painful night, your mind attempts to suppress recall.

The brain's garden also thrives on a careful balance of chemical caretakers—neurotransmitters and neuromodulators that nurture, prune, and shape our memories. Among these, dopamine plays a central role by rewarding learning and signaling which experiences are most important. When dopamine spikes, it marks pleasant or significant moments, making them more likely to be stored in long-term memory.

Acetylcholine is crucial for encoding new information, especially in the hippocampus; without enough of it, forming new memories becomes difficult. Norepinephrine heightens attention and arousal, especially during emotionally charged events, helping to encode those moments with extra vividness. Serotonin acts subtly, shaping the overall mood context in which memories are formed and coloring them with positive or negative tones. Glutamate, the brain's primary excitatory neurotransmitter, is essential for synaptic plasticity. The process that strengthens the connections underlying memory storage is known as long-term potentiation.

Together, these chemical messengers act as caretakers. They determine which memory sprouts receive nourishment and which remain stunted. However, the system is delicate. Stress hormones like cortisol can overwhelm the garden, stunting growth and even damaging the hippocampal neurons responsible for planting new memories. Too much cortisol—often released during chronic stress—can make it difficult to form or retain new memories. Just like a real garden, a healthy memory system depends on balance: the right mix of nourishment, pruning, and protection from stress.

Interestingly, the brain does not simply record memories and file them away. Each time we remember something, we are not just retrieving it. We are also rewriting it. This process, known as reconsolidation, means that our memories are continually updated and reshaped by new experiences, emotions, and even the act of remembering itself. The prefrontal cortex helps us decide what is important enough to remember and what can be forgotten.

Here's the twist: just as plucking a flower to admire it risks bruising its petals, each memory retrieval opens a period where it can be altered, subtly rewritten, before being stored again. Over time, stories shift. We add details that never were; we lose those that were present. In this way, memory is a living thing, trimmed every retelling. It explains family arguments over "who said what" years ago. It explains nostalgia that paints the past with soft hues.

This living nature is what makes memory vulnerable. It can even be intentionally distorted. Psychologist Elizabeth Loftus famously demonstrated how easily people can be led to believe in events that never occurred. In one foundational study, Loftus presented volunteers with slides of a car crash and then asked questions with subtly misleading wording. For example, asking *"How fast were the cars going when they smashed into each other?"* versus *"...when they hit each other?"* elicited different responses. The word "smashed" was enough to prompt higher speed estimates and even false recall of broken glass at the scene, when none existed.

Another experiment, called the "Lost in the Mall" study, had family members tell participants stories from their childhood—three true events, and one invented tale of being lost in a mall. Astonishingly, after repeated interviews, nearly a third of subjects developed a partial or full memory of the false event, describing vivid details and emotions about a childhood experience that had never occurred. Loftus and colleagues demonstrated that external suggestion, especially from trusted sources, can implant not only altered memories but also wholly fabricated episodes.

All of these findings explain why eyewitnesses in court may mistakenly identify familiar faces, recall events in distorted ways, or even "remember" seeing things they only heard about in conversation or on the news. In therapy, intense imagination exercises or suggestive questions can lead clients to recall scenes from childhood—sometimes true, sometimes crafted anew from the fragments of fantasy, hearsay, or cultural stories. "Imagination inflation" refers to the phenomenon where repeatedly imagining an event can make people more likely to believe it actually happened.

Perhaps most interestingly, memory distortion is not limited to individuals. On a collective scale, it shapes communities and cultures. Just as families rework stories for reunions or holidays, entire nations revise history, omitting inconvenient details and amplifying myths to craft a shared narrative. These rewritten memories can take on lives of their own, blurring the line between truth and fiction in ways that feel startlingly familiar to most of us.

A striking example of this phenomenon is known as the Mandela Effect. Coined by researcher Fiona Broome, the term describes incidents where large groups recall the same event or fact incorrectly—often with remarkable confidence. Broome and many others vividly "remembered" South African president Nelson Mandela dying in prison during the 1980s. These memories come complete with imagined news coverage and social reactions. In reality, Mandela was released in 1990 and lived until 2013.

The Mandela Effect extends far beyond this one historical event. People collectively misremember the Monopoly Man as wearing a monocle, or the Fruit of the Loom logo as having a cornucopia, when neither detail was ever true. Movie quotes are also famously distorted. Many remember Darth Vader saying, *"Luke, I am your father,"* instead of the real line, *"No, I am your father."* Some even insist on recalling a 1990s genie movie called "Shazaam" starring Sinbad, which never existed. The Mandela Effect and false memories are a clear demonstration of how memory, both individual and shared, is an active, living process. It's subject to trimming, fertilizing, and sometimes wild mutation.

It's essential to recognize that forgetting is not a failure. It's a vital part of healthy memory. Like a garden overwhelmed by unchecked growth, our minds would be in chaos without regular pruning. The hippocampus is highly selective. It chooses what to nurture and what to let go, but even after memories have sprouted, pruning continues. Synaptic connections weaken over time if we don't revisit or rehearse them. This is a process known as "synaptic downscaling," which helps keep our brains energy-efficient and focused on what matters most.

Imagine if you remembered every face in every crowd, your mind would be swamped with unbearable clutter. Forgetting allows for balance. It acts as a compost heap where unused memories decay and nourish the ecosystem as a whole. Sherlock Holmes, the famous and ever precise, fictional detective, put it like this in A Study in Scarlet: *"I consider that a man's brain originally is like a little empty attic, and you have to stock it with such furniture as you choose... It is a mistake to think that the little room has elastic walls and can distend to any extent. Depend upon it, there comes a time when for every addition of knowledge you forget something that you knew before. It is of the highest importance, therefore, not to have useless facts elbowing out the useful ones."*

In Holmes's attic, only the most useful tools are kept, meticulously arranged. The rest—astronomical trivia, idle gossip—are tossed out with deliberate indifference. For him, forgetting is not an accident, but a necessary part of housekeeping. Neuroscience has come to echo Holmes's insight: the brain is no limitless warehouse, but a living thing that curates and prunes its inventory. This clears tangled paths so that vital memories, such as the faces of loved ones, critical facts, and moments of insight, can occupy the foreground and remain accessible when truly needed. Indeed, forgetting allows flexibility. If you cannot let go of outdated knowledge, learning new patterns would be hindered. Thus, pruning is not a loss, but rather a preparation for growth.

German philosopher Friedrich Nietzsche, one of history's boldest critics of convention and inherited wisdom, argued that the art of forgetting is essential for genuine health and vitality. Nietzsche wrote in *On the Genealogy of Morals*: *"Forgetfulness is not just a vis inertiae, as superficial people believe, but is rather an active ability to suppress, positive in the strongest sense of the word... active forgetfulness, like a doorkeeper or guardian of mental order, rest and etiquette."*

This suggests that forgetting is about temporarily shutting the doors and windows of consciousness. It's about inviting a little peace and making room for new growth and nobler pursuits. Therefore, above all, forgetfulness makes space for rest. Just as the mind needs periods of silence and reset to remain clear and flexible, so too does the body: sleep is our nightly invitation to close the attic, to sweep out old dust, and let the garden of memory renew itself. Only in those quiet hours do our brains perform essential housecleaning—consolidating, sorting, and discarding—so we can rise restored, ready to learn anew.

~

During deep, slow-wave sleep, the brain doesn't simply switch off. Instead, it replays the day's experiences, strengthening important memories and pruning away those deemed superfluous. The brain carefully refines and integrates key experiences with existing knowledge networks, chiefly within the hippocampus and neocortex. This is like a gardener pruning a rose bush, ensuring that only the healthiest branches thrive. The process, known as memory consolidation, transforms fragile new memories into robust, long-term recollections.

During these slow-wave stages, encoded memories are reactivated. In animal studies, scientists have observed neurons firing in patterns similar to those observed when the animals were awake and exploring —literally replaying the experience in miniature. In this way, the brain brings together emotional and skill-based memories. It helps convert episodic memories and skills into stable, lasting forms, allowing the brain to "weed out" fleeting sensations or unnecessary details, so our mental garden remains fertile for future learning.

REM sleep, renowned for producing vivid dreams, plays a different yet equally essential role in memory. Emotional and skill-based memories are both robustly processed during REM. The brain integrates impressions, feelings, and even motor patterns to help us navigate emotional challenges and acquire new skills. The thalamus, typically quiet during non-REM sleep, springs to life—relaying sensory images to the cortex, where they're integrated into dreams and linked to earlier experiences. This cross-pollination fosters creativity, solves problems, and even helps regulate mood and stress.

Therefore, sleep is not just a time of rest, but an active period when the brain tends to the garden of memory, making sure that our sense of self remains strong and coherent. Sleep deprivation is akin to neglecting a garden. Without sleep, pruning halts; weeds spread. Experiments consistently show that students who sleep after studying recall information far better than those who stay awake cramming.

Furthermore, musicians are able to consolidate complex pieces more effectively after a night's sleep. Infants, whose brains are rapidly developing, also demonstrate increased learning after daytime naps. Sleep is no indulgence. It is cultivation. Without it, memories rot, identity frays.

~

As we drift into sleep, the boundaries between memory and imagination blur. Dreams assemble themselves from the raw materials of our minds: faces from childhood, places we have visited, fears and hopes that linger quietly in the background. The very brain regions that crystallize memory by day—the hippocampus, limbic system, and the visual cortex—become architects of the stories we experience at night. Sometimes, dreams help us process difficult emotions, rehearse for future challenges, or make sense of chaotic events. At other times, they serve as a playground for the imagination, blending fragments of memory into wild, unexpected combinations.

Keeping our garden metaphor alive, dreams work as pollinators. They carry fragments of memory from night to night, nourishing creativity and recombining familiar experiences in novel ways. This isn't just the stuff of famous stories like Mary Shelley's *Frankenstein* or Paul McCartney's *Yesterday*; it's something almost anyone can experience, even if only occasionally. For instance, plenty of people keep a notebook on their nightstand, ready to jot down a strange dream or an idea that pops up in the night, hoping to capture inspiration before it evaporates. Maybe it's a plot for a story, a solution to a work problem, or even a joke—like the classic Seinfeld episode where Jerry tries to decode his own midnight scribble, spending the day asking friends what his half-remembered joke could possibly mean.

Research shows there's good reason for this habit: sleep, and especially the transition into sleep, primes the brain for creative ideation. During these brief hypnagogic moments, the mind becomes less constrained, allowing connections between distant ideas that would never meet in waking life. When someone is prompted to think about a specific topic—such as trees—these images appeared in their dreams, and afterwards, their creativity scores increased on tests. Dreams don't just mix memory and imagination randomly; they actively help the brain incubate new ideas, expand associative networks, and generate fresh solutions. Neuroimaging studies confirm that during REM, associative brain areas light up, while the "editor" function of the prefrontal cortex relaxes its grip. This is why dreams can seem both vivid and bizarre, and also why some are particularly fertile for creative insight. Even if the details seem nonsensical the next morning, their emotional charge or unique juxtapositions might still stimulate a new direction for thought.

For the average person, maybe it's not a world-changing novel or a chart-topping song—perhaps it's a dream-inspired project, a new recipe, an impressive solution to a work problem, or just an entertaining story to share with friends. Even the wildest dreams, scientists believe, may strengthen emotional integration, helping the subconscious work through unresolved feelings or grief, whether or not they ever make sense at breakfast. That's why so many keep dream journals, sketchpads, or even voice recorders by their bed, hoping to harvest those pollinated seeds before they wilt in daylight.

~

Nightmares, on the other hand, differ from ordinary dreams in both their emotional impact and neurobiology. While regular dreams might be whimsical, odd, or even joyful, nightmares are dreams with a powerful negative emotional charge. These most often center on fear, terror, sadness, disgust, or confusion, and jolt the dreamer awake. They may linger in waking life.

Nightmares, like dreams, occur predominantly during REM sleep, but the brain regions involved exhibit heightened activity. The amygdala, which processes fear and threat, is especially active. The circuits responsible for memory, emotion, and internal imagery are also active. Interestingly, the visual cortex processes dream images generated from inside the brain, not through the eyes, which augments the vividness of nightmares.

Unlike typical dreams, which may simply process the day or knit random memories into strange imagery, nightmares are marked by vividness and emotional intensity. They are often linked to emotional memories—stressful life events, worries, or unresolved trauma may re-emerge in dream form, sometimes explicitly, sometimes symbolically. Researchers found, for example, that people closer to traumatic events like earthquakes tend to experience more nightmares in the weeks following the event.

Recent theories suggest nightmares of this kind might serve as an "overnight therapy". They provide the brain with a safe space to revisit distressing experiences and attempt to extinguish the fear associated with them. By replaying and reworking these memories, nightmares may assist in integrating and adapting emotional experiences into the broader narrative of self, though they can also unearth lingering pain. They can even evoke physical symptoms, such as rapid heartbeat and sweating, upon awakening. Many people report waking in the night, heart pounding, after a nightmare so intense they struggle to fall back asleep.

Most people have occasional nightmares, a small percentage experience them so frequently that their sleep and even daily life are disrupted, a condition known as nightmare disorder. Children often have recurring nightmares that fade with age, but even adults may experience them during periods of stress or change. Soldiers returning from deployments, survivors of trauma, or those in personal turmoil frequently see echoes of their waking worries in nightmares, reminding us how closely dreams are tied to lived experience.

Why does all this matter so deeply?

Because it is the narrative spine of the self, strip away episodic memory and the self unravels. Patients with hippocampal damage lose the ability to form new memories and have described feeling trapped as a result. One of the most famous examples is that of Henry Gustav Molaison, known to science for decades simply as "H.M."

He was an ordinary man whose life became a turning point in our understanding of memory. For years, Henry suffered from debilitating epileptic seizures that medications could not control, robbing him of independence and hope. In 1953, desperate for relief, he underwent an experimental surgery. Doctors removed large sections of his medial temporal lobes, including the hippocampus. The operation reduced his seizures—but it had an unintended, life-altering consequence.

H.M. could no longer form new long-term memories. His mind became stuck in an endless present. He was unable to remember conversations, new faces, or daily events just moments after they happened. If someone greeted him and then left the room, he would forget the encounter within minutes. Family, friends, and even the nurses who cared for him were strangers again each time they returned. He was left *"waking from a dream... every day alone in itself,"* as he once described it.

Older memories from childhood remained fairly stable, but the last decade before his operation was hazy—lost to retrograde amnesia. It was as if his narrative, the story that made him who he was, unraveled back to the recent past. His case illustrated to us that ultimately, memory, dreams, and nightmares are deeply intertwined with identity.

Our memories anchor us to the story of who we are, while our dreams allow us to revise, rehearse, and sometimes reinvent that story. The self is a living river. The stones of experience forever shape it, the currents of emotion, and the unseen hand of time. We are, each of us, both the author and the archive, the gardener and the garden, endlessly revising the story of who we are.

In the swirl of modern life—endless photographs, digital reminders, cloud storage—our memories often live outside our brains, housed in external "prosthetic" systems. Some worry that outsourcing memory dulls our natural recall; others suggest it frees mental bandwidth for richer, more abstract thinking. Despite all these technological advances, no algorithm yet replicates how the amygdala sears joy into recollection. No database encodes heartbreak. Our memory systems remain uniquely alive and uniquely human.

So, what practical steps can people take to strengthen their own "memory gardens"?

Science offers several evidence-based strategies that anyone can use. First and foremost, prioritize sleep. As we saw, sleep is the ultimate gardener of memory. Skimping on sleep not only leads to fuzzy recall but also disrupts the consolidation and pruning required for healthy, adaptive memory. You can also attach feelings and curiosity to what matters. Genuine interest or connecting facts to life events fertilizes deep roots. Of course, the other side of this emotional encoding could be safely processing your trauma. Difficult memories, when revisited with support, can be reconsolidated and reframed as integrated lessons. This process, used in therapies like cognitive reprocessing, was found to help people transform "thorns" into more manageable stories.

Additionally, you can challenge yourself to recall. Retrieval practice is one of the most robust ways to reinforce memory. Quizzing yourself, revisiting names and facts at spaced intervals, and using tests can tease information back into awareness. Flash cards, quick self-quizzes, and explaining concepts to others all help the memory "plants" grow stronger with each recollection.

Every choice, from a good night's sleep to a moment of genuine curiosity, is a way of tending your memory. So, try to remember: your memory is not a static archive. It is a landscape. A wild, resilient, living garden. Sleep is its caretaker. Emotion is its fertilizer. Time is its climate. But you—through choices, habits, attachments—are its gardener too. *Tend it well.*

PART SIX
A SOCIAL BRAIN

CHAPTER 16
FROM VILLAGE TO VIRAL: THE NEUROSCIENCE OF COMMUNITY

WE ARE NOT ISLANDS. We are archipelagos, bound by bridges of laughter, rivalry, and longing. From the flickering firelight of our ancestors' circles to the digital glow of today's screens, the architecture of community has shifted, multiplied, and become ever more intricate. Once, our tribes were small families and villages huddled together for warmth, safety, and the comfort of shared stories. Now, community is a mosaic: a crowded subway car, a comment thread, a viral dance challenge on TikTok.

We gather in coffee shops, in parks, in virtual chat rooms, each space stitched together by the same ancient longing: to belong, to be seen, to matter. Yet, for all our innovations, the ache remains unchanged. The need for connection is not a luxury. It is a necessity. It is as essential as bread or breath.

This longing for connection has been the subject of both scientific inquiry and philosophical reflection for centuries. Charles Darwin, in his *Descent of Man*, argued that our moral sense—our empathy, our urge to help, our capacity for love—evolved from the social instincts seen in animals. He saw in the bonds of sympathy and love the roots of morality, suggesting that the ability to cooperate and care for others was as vital to survival as strength or cunning. Darwin's observations of animal communities, such as the loyalty of dogs, the sacrifices of social insects, and the affection between apes and their young, revealed that the drama of belonging is not uniquely human. It is a thread through the fabric of life itself.

Philosophers, too, have long pondered the paradox of human existence: we are singular, yet we yearn for the plural. Aristotle declared that *"man is by nature a social animal,"* insisting that a complete human life requires the company of others, the shared pursuit of virtue, and the bonds of community. To live outside the city, he argued, was to be either a beast or a god, not a person.

In the modern era, thinkers like Martin Buber and Emmanuel Levinas have explored the idea that our encounters with others define our very humanity. This is the *"I-Thou"* relationship, where we meet another not as an object, but as a fellow subject, alive with hopes and fears. Even Jean-Paul Sartre, who saw conflict and alienation in human relations, left open the possibility of authentic connection. This freedom-enhancing encounter transcends mere rivalry.

Today, the modern landscape is a labyrinth of connections. Some deep and nourishing, others fleeting and hollow. We scroll through feeds. We are searching for echoes of ourselves in the lives of others, craving affirmation, fearing rejection. Social media has become the new village square. It is the place where stories are shared, alliances formed, and rivalries played out in public view.

Platforms like TikTok, Instagram, and Snapchat have made us more social than ever, at least in appearance. We can reach across continents in a heartbeat. We can also join communities built around the most niche interests. We can even find belonging in spaces our ancestors could not have even imagined.

However, this new web of connections comes with its complexities. Neuroscience reveals that our brains are exquisitely sensitive to social feedback. Studies show that habitual checking of social media, especially among adolescents, is linked to changes in the brain's reward circuits. The anticipation of likes, comments, or shares activates the same pathways as social acceptance in face-to-face encounters. This is making us hypersensitive to feedback from our peers. Each notification is a tiny pulse of dopamine. Always drawing us back for more, much like the rewards of food or touch.

The rapid-fire nature of platforms like TikTok, with their endless stream of short, stimulating videos, can have other, more profound effects on the brain. Recent research has found that compulsive use of these platforms is associated with increased activity in regions linked to emotional regulation and reward, as well as structural changes in areas responsible for attention and decision-making.

The constant barrage of novelty may make us better at rapid information processing. However, it also weakens the neural circuits required for deep focus, sustained attention, and meaningful reflection. The result is a paradox: we are more connected than ever, yet sometimes feel more alone, more distracted, more hungry for authentic connection.

~

The neurobiology of our social experiences is as intricate as all the other experiences, feelings, and emotions we've discussed so far. The hypothalamus monitors our social temperature. It's tracking the warmth of companionship as carefully as it tracks hunger or thirst. When we feel isolated, this tiny cluster of cells sounds an alarm. It releases chemical messengers that ripple outward. These activate the same pain circuits that flare when we stub a toe or burn a finger.

Loneliness, in the brain's language, is not just sadness. It is a kind of hurt, as real as any physical wound. The amygdala scans every encounter for hints of acceptance or exclusion. *Did that friend's smile linger a little too briefly? Was that text message a little too curt?*

The amygdala notices. When it senses rejection, it triggers a cascade of stress responses. These speed the heart, sharpen attention, and prime us to defend our place in the group. When the brain detects welcome, it quiets, letting us relax into the comfort of belonging.

Simultaneously, at the front of the brain, the prefrontal cortex helps us decide when to reach out, when to hold back, when to trust, and when to guard our hearts. This region is especially active during social interactions, juggling dozens of subtle cues—tone of voice, flicker of an eyebrow, the rhythm of conversation. It's the webspinner of our social lives, blending emotion and logic into the art of human connection.

When the web of connection frays—when we feel left out or ignored—the body responds as if under siege. The anterior cingulate cortex, nestled within the frontal lobes, lights up with the same intensity as if we had suffered a physical wound. The overlap is so striking that the sting of social rejection can even be eased by the same painkillers that dull a headache.

Stress hormones like cortisol surge, weakening our immune defenses and making the world seem colder, more hostile. Chronic loneliness can even leave fingerprints on our DNA, accelerating aging and increasing vulnerability to illness. This neural crossroads reminds us that the ache of loneliness is not imagined.

When we are welcomed, the brain's reward centers light up. When a friend's praise lands on our ears, or a loved one's hug wraps around us, the ventral striatum glows with pleasure. The ventral striatum transforms a smile, a compliment, or a gesture of affection into a rush of warmth and satisfaction. Oxytocin, the so-called "bonding hormone," floods the system.

This deepens trust and soothes anxiety. Dopamine also sparkles through neural pathways. It makes us feel alive, valued, and safe. These are more than fleeting feelings. There are measurable shifts in brain chemistry. They are our ancient signals that our place in the tribe is secure. They are the neural hearth where the joy of belonging is kindled, making us crave connection and cherish the bonds we build.

In every glance, every word, every act of kindness or rivalry, we enact the ancient drama of belonging. The modern world may have changed the stage, but the script is written in our bones and brains. To understand ourselves, we must look beyond the self to the networks that shape us, the emotions that bind us, and the stories we share. In the end, it is the connections we forge, the empathy we extend, and the love we dare to give that define us.

Step into a crowded café. You notice a stranger wince as hot coffee spills onto their hand. Instantly, a twinge shoots through your own body—a fleeting echo of their pain. This is empathy in action: the silent, invisible current that connects us, mind to mind, heart to heart. The question is: *what, exactly, is happening beneath your skull when you feel another's joy or sorrow?*

Empathy is a symphony, played by a network of brain regions working in harmony. The amygdala scans faces and voices for emotional signals—such as fear, anger, and delight—and assigns them meaning. It's the amygdala that makes your heart race when you see someone else's distress, or feel warmth when you witness a smile. The prefrontal cortex helps you imagine what others are thinking or feeling. It takes raw emotional signals and turns them into understanding. It allows you to *"put yourself in someone else's shoes."* Damage here can blunt empathy, making it hard to grasp the feelings of others.

The anterior cingulate cortex and insula light up when you see someone in pain, as if your own body is mirroring their experience. This mirroring is more than metaphor—it's a literal echo, with your brain simulating the other person's state. Scattered throughout are mirror neurons, special cells that fire both when you perform an action and when you see someone else perform it. They are the neural glue that lets you *"catch"* another's mood, mimic their expressions, and feel their feelings.

In this way, empathy has two main forms. Emotional empathy is the ability to feel what others feel. See a friend cry, and your own eyes may sting. This is a fast, automatic, and deeply rooted process, rooted in the older parts of the brain. Cognitive empathy is the ability to understand what others feel. This is the slower, thoughtful process of imagining another's perspective—what scientists call *"theory of mind."* It's what lets you comfort a friend even if you don't share their sadness.

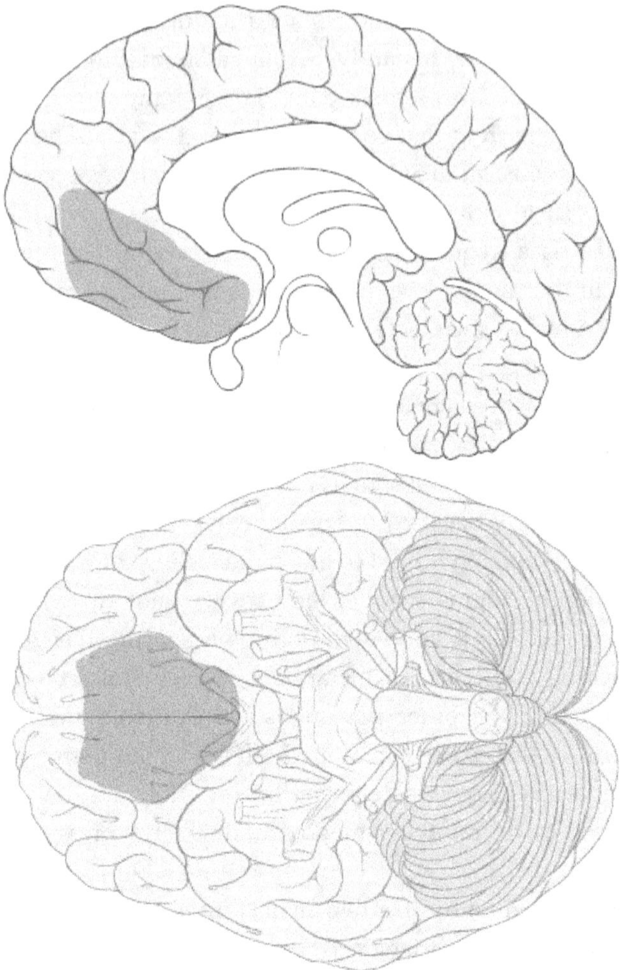

Figure 17. *The location of the ventromedial prefrontal cortex is shown on ventral and medial views of the brain.* Finereach on Wikimedia Commons

Not everyone experiences empathy in the same way. Some are flooded by others' feelings, while others sense only a trickle. Studies of people with brain injuries offer a window into why. Consider a man named John, once known for his kindness. After a car accident, he began to seem cold, missing social cues and failing to comfort friends in distress. Doctors discovered damage to his ventromedial prefrontal cortex—a region essential for blending emotion and logic. John could still recognize facts, but the feelings behind them slipped away. This case, echoed in scientific studies, shows how specific brain injuries can rob a person of empathy, altering their relationships and sense of self.

We've seen this pattern before. Recall Phineas Gage, the railroad foreman whose life and personality were forever changed when an iron rod pierced his skull. Once responsible and sociable, Gage became impulsive, indifferent, and emotionally disconnected after his accident. His story, as seen in the previous chapters, stands as an early and dramatic testament to how injuries to the brain's frontal regions can unravel the delicate balance of emotion, reason, and empathy. Both John and Gage remind us: the architecture of empathy is fragile, rooted in neural circuits.

Empathy is not just a soft skill—it's part of our biology. When you see someone stub their toe, your brain's pain centers flicker as if it's your own foot. When a friend laughs, your face muscles unconsciously mimic theirs, drawing you into shared joy. This uncanny resonance is the handiwork of mirror neurons. These specialized brain cells, discovered in the motor cortex, fire when we perform an action, and also when we observe someone else performing that same action.

It's as if the brain blurs the boundary between self and other. This allows us to simulate another's experience in our own neural circuitry. Mirror neurons are the silent mimics behind contagious yawns, empathetic tears, and the shared thrill of a victory. They let us "taste" another's joy, "flinch" at their pain, and "echo" their laughter, giving rise to the deep, embodied empathy that unites us. Empathy is the silent language of the brain that allows us to share, understand, and care. It is as ancient as the first human tribe, and as modern as a texted *"I'm here for you."* Though the pathways are complex, the outcome is simple: in feeling for others, we find what it means to be human.

Go back to our café from earlier. Every table holds a quiet drama. You watch as a woman's lips twitch into a half-smile, as a man's fingers drum a nervous rhythm on his cup. Words drift through the air, but meaning shimmers beneath the surface—hidden, layered, waiting to be uncovered. This is the art of reading others. It's not a matter of simple observation. It's a living puzzle of signals and secrets. We do not simply see a face or hear a voice; we sense the tremor in a laugh, the shadow behind a compliment, the weight of a pause. Here we can see that we are wired for even more than just empathetic feelings.

Our brains are ceaseless detectives. They are gathering fragments: a raised eyebrow, an averted gaze, the subtle tightening of a jaw. They shape them into stories. Each neuron seems to lean in, listening for the nuance that transforms a gesture into a confession. The room becomes a kaleidoscope of intentions: a friend's sudden quiet, a stranger's eager nod, a lover's lingering glance. Meaning emerges not in declarations, but in the spaces between.

Why did we develop this uncanny ability to read the unspoken?

The answer is written in the dust of ancient campsites and the echoes of our evolutionary past. Long before cities and screens, survival depended on our ability to sense danger, detect deception, and recognize trust. In the wild of early human life, those who could read the intentions of others—friend or foe, ally or rival—were more likely to survive and thrive. This skill, known as social inference, became our evolutionary superpower. Charles Darwin, through the lens of natural selection, saw that *"those communities which included the greatest number of the most sympathetic members would flourish best, and rear the greatest number of offspring."*

To read another's face was, in a very real sense, to glimpse the future. However, not everyone moves through the social world with the same ease. Some glide through crowds. They are attuned to every nuance. While others stumble, missing the cues that signal joy or sorrow, trust or suspicion. This variation is shaped by a blend of nature and nurture, encompassing genetic differences, early experiences, and the practice of socialization.

Children raised in rich social environments, with plenty of face-to-face interaction, tend to develop sharper social inference skills. Neuroscientific studies reveal that individuals who excel at reading emotions have stronger connections between regions, such as the amygdala and the prefrontal cortex. For some, though, the social world is a bewildering maze. Conditions like autism spectrum disorder can make it difficult to interpret facial expressions or infer intentions. In these individuals, brain scans often reveal differences in the "social brain" network. This is particularly evident in areas such as the fusiform face area, which is crucial for recognizing faces.

We have long been fascinated by our ability to read emotion from the human face. Seminal experiments by Paul Ekman and others presented participants with photographs of faces showing basic emotions—fear, anger, joy, disgust, surprise, and sadness. Even when shown only the eyes or the mouth, most people could identify the emotion with surprising accuracy. These studies revealed that the brain is exquisitely tuned to the micro-expressions that flicker across a face, sometimes lasting only a fraction of a second.

Further research using functional MRI has shown that when we look at faces, specialized brain regions allow for the decoding of subtle shifts in facial expressions. In individuals with social difficulties, these regions may be less active or may not communicate as effectively with other brain regions. This can explain why the silent riddle of social life and social inference can be so challenging to solve.

Social inference includes emotion recognition, theory of mind, social prediction, and deception detection. Each of these abilities draws on overlapping yet distinct neural circuits. Some people may excel in one area and struggle in another, depending on their unique brain wiring and life experiences.

The hippocampus remembers, the prefrontal cortex predicts, and the sensory regions decode the flood of information from faces, voices, and gestures. Together, they allow us to navigate the ever-shifting landscape of human relationships, to solve the living mystery of each encounter. We do not simply decode words or catalog expressions. We feel the pulse of the room, the currents of intention and emotion, the unspoken stories that bind us together. In this way, every social moment becomes an adventure. It's a testament to the collaborative power of the human mind.

We now understand why social connection is essential, what happens in our brain during connection, and how we empathize and recognize emotions. Next, let's explore what happens when we experience negative social interactions or emotions.

The story of human connection takes an intriguing turn here. Beneath the drama of rivalry and longing lies a quieter, more mysterious force —a desire to resonate with others. Our brains, shaped by thousands of years of communal living, are highly attuned to the rhythms of those around us. Our brainwaves, measured by neural oscillations, can sync with those of our companions.

Beneath the skin, the story of human connection is written in the language of cells and circuits. Our brains are built for both the warmth of the group and the solitude of the self. When we gather, something stirs—a resonance, a synchrony, as if our nervous systems are tuning forks, vibrating together in invisible harmony. This is not just poetry; it is biology.

In the hypothalamus, circuits monitor our social needs, much like a thermostat tracks temperature. Zoom in further, and you find bundles of nerve fibers, passing messages at lightning speed, allowing us to sense the mood of a room or the intentions of a friend in a heartbeat. When we feel lonely, these circuits send out signals. They urge us to reach out, to close the gap between ourselves and others.

Surprisingly, the story does not end with the brain. Our very DNA carries instructions for building the molecules that shape our social instincts. Genes influence our sensitivity to the emotions of others, our likelihood of cooperating or competing, and the depth of our feelings for friendship and love. Some genes affect the production of oxytocin, which surges when we hug, laugh, or share secrets. Others influence the wiring of brain circuits that underlie trust, empathy, and even rivalry. These genetic blueprints do not determine our destiny. They create the foundation on which the narrative of social life unfolds.

Modern science has also begun to map the networks of connection that stretch from the smallest scale—between individual brain cells—to the largest, linking whole societies. Inside the brain, neurons form webs of communication, with some acting as hubs, connecting many others, much like influential people in a community. These patterns of connectivity are echoed in our social networks, where friendships, alliances, and rivalries create intricate maps of influence and support. When scientists study how information or emotions ripple through a group, they find striking similarities to the way signals travel through neural circuits. The same principles that govern the spread of a rumor in a village can be seen in the way electrical impulses jump from neuron to neuron.

Across history and culture, the tension between the individual and the group has shaped our stories, our rituals, and our brains. Some societies celebrate the lone hero, the one who stands apart. Others prize the harmony of the collective, the safety of belonging. Yet, beneath these differences, the need for connection is universal. It is written into our biology and whispered in the language of our genes. Whether we gather around a fire, join a protest, or share a smile, we are enacting a script that is as old as humanity itself. This script binds us together, even as it allows us to stand apart.

~

We are all woven into a living web, each of us a single thread, yet none of us alone. The need for connection is not just a feeling—it is a force as ancient as our species. It is etched into our biology and echoed in the very architecture of our brains. When we look into another's eyes, share a laugh, or even clash in a moment of rivalry, our brains light up in patterns that have been shaped by millions of years of evolution. However, this web of connection is not just about biology; it is also about the stories we tell and the cultures we build.

From the earliest days, humans gathered in groups, sharing food, songs, and stories around the fire. These gatherings were not just for warmth or safety; they were for belonging. Our brains learned to recognize familiar faces, to remember who had helped us and who had hurt us, and to pass on the knowledge that held the group together. Over time, these patterns became traditions, rituals, and even the rules that guide our societies today. The networks we form—families, friendships, communities—are reflected in the very structure of our brains, with specific areas growing stronger and more connected the more we interact with others.

To truly understand who we are, we must look beyond the boundaries of our own minds. We must see ourselves as part of a larger network, shaped by the people around us and the emotions that pass between us. It is not the urge to compete or compare that makes us human, but the willingness to reach out, to listen, to care. Every act of kindness, every moment of empathy, every bond of love we form sends a signal through the web, strengthening the connections that hold us all together. In the end, our greatest strength is not in standing apart, but in daring to connect, to share, and to belong. Perhaps this is part of why loneliness can feel so insidious.

Loneliness is more than a passing mood or a shadow at the edge of a crowded room. It is a physical ache, a hunger that gnaws at the bones and echoes through the chambers of the mind. Imagine the quiet after a party, the hush when the last voice fades. That emptiness is more than a metaphor. The sensation of loneliness is as real as a scraped knee or a growling stomach. The brain's alarm bells ring out, urging us to seek connection, to close the gap between ourselves and the world. As we've touched on briefly earlier in this chapter, the body reacts physically to loneliness and isolation.

The amygdala, ever watchful, becomes more sensitive in times of isolation. It scans the environment for threats, amplifying feelings of anxiety and suspicion. The world seems colder, faces are less friendly, and every silence is a possible rejection. The prefrontal cortex, which helps us weigh risks and imagine the minds of others, struggles to quiet these alarms. It tries to reason, to remind us that solitude is sometimes safe, but the emotional tide is hard to stem.

Meanwhile, the reward centers of the brain—those that light up with laughter, touch, or the warmth of a friend's gaze—fall silent. Levels of dopamine and oxytocin, the chemicals that bring pleasure and bonding, dwindle. The world loses its color, food its flavor, music its joy. The hippocampus, keeper of memories, replays old hurts and missed connections, making the ache sharper, the sense of separation more profound.

Loneliness is not just a state of mind; it is a state of the body. Stress hormones like cortisol rise, weakening the immune system, clouding the mind, and making the heart beat a little faster, a little harder. Over time, chronic loneliness can carve grooves in the brain, changing the way nerve cells talk to each other, making it harder to reach out, to trust, to hope.

Yet, loneliness is not a sentence—it is a signal. It is the body's way of calling us back to the web of connection, to the warmth of another's presence. Just as hunger drives us to eat, loneliness drives us to seek out others, to rebuild the bonds that make us human. In every pang, there is a message: you are meant to belong, to be seen, to be held.

The cure for loneliness is not found in isolation, but in the courage to reach out, to touch, to speak, and to listen. In the end, the brain's longing for connection is a testament to the truth that we are, at our core, creatures of togetherness—wired not for solitude, but for the living, breathing company of others.

CHAPTER 17

NAVIGATING THE SOCIAL SCOREBOARD: COMPARISON AND COMPETITION IN THE BRAIN

PICTURE THE MIND as a vast stadium. At its center, the self moves through daily rituals—working, dressing, creating, loving—while unseen crowds fill the stands. Their silent cheers and jeers are felt as a constant undercurrent, a collective judgment that shapes our every move. This is the social scoreboard: an ever-present tally of how we measure up in the eyes of others.

Deep inside, the ventral striatum—a reward center—lights up when you win social approval, when praise lands, when you "score a goal" in others' eyes. The same circuits are ignited by money, chocolate, or music. Social triumph is wired into reward systems. However, when you lose status, when the scoreboard tilts against you, the brain registers failure and exclusion. Dopamine circuits dip, serotonin sync falters. Emotional lows arrive. This circuitry ensures that humans constantly calibrate themselves against others. *What am I worth? Am I above or below?* It is not vanity; it is wiring. Jealousy and envy are the subjective versions of these dips—the felt consequence of scoreboard tracking. They are the sharp tang in the air when you see a friend laughing with someone else, the hollow ache in your chest when love seems to drift beyond your reach.

Psychology draws a careful line between envy and jealousy, though in daily life the two often blur together. Envy is the discomfort that arises when we desire what another possesses—success, material goods, or even an air of confidence. It is a comparison of position: *where do I stand relative to others?* Jealousy, in contrast, is the fear of losing something already held—a cherished relationship, trust, or affection. Here, the comparison is about possession: *will what I value be taken from me?*

Both emotions are rooted in the social scoreboard, that persistent sense of who stands where. Neuroscience reveals that envy and jealousy activate similar brain circuits, but differ in emotional tone and the actions they inspire.

Jealousy often manifests as anger, suspicion, and a vigilant guarding of what one values—like a guard dog protecting its territory. Envy, on the other hand, can slip into resentment, feelings of inferiority, or, in some cases, even admiration. Both emotions can be toxic, sowing discord and pain, but both can also be motivating. Envy may spur self-improvement and growth, while jealousy, when recognized and managed, can strengthen bonds through honest repair. Their power is ambivalent: destructive or constructive, depending on whether we are aware of their signals and how we choose to respond to them.

Jealousy can feel deeply personal—a sharp, private ache—but in reality, it's a universal mammalian response, embroidered into our biology over millions of years. From primates fiercely guarding mates and defending territory, to dogs sulking when their human pays attention to another, even birds growing vigilant at the arrival of a rival, the threads of jealousy weave through the animal kingdom. Evolutionary biologists see these behaviors not as quirks but as "design features," evolved to safeguard precious social bonds, resources, and opportunities for reproduction. It's proof that if jealousy stings, it does so as an ancient warning: pay attention, protect what matters.

For early humans, hierarchy meant the difference between life and death. Imagine our ancestors huddled in small tribes. Anthropologists suggest that they were acutely aware of their social rank within tribes. To be excluded—to lose the affection of an ally or the attention of a partner—was not just sad. It was perilous. Being left alone meant a higher chance of starvation, predation, and failure to reproduce. This pain—the visceral ache of rejection—ensured no one casually risked expulsion. Furthermore, those who felt the sting of exclusion were more likely to fight for their place, to repair bonds, to stay close to the fire. Over generations, the brain's architecture evolved to treat threats to our social connections with the same urgency as threats to food or shelter.

To the brain, the loss of status or intimacy is not a metaphor, but a genuine threat. Neuroscience shows that social pain is processed as a bodily danger. The anterior cingulate cortex, which fires when you touch a hot stove, also activates during moments of social rejection. The insula, the brain's register of bodily sensation, responds whether you bite into a chili pepper or endure a romantic betrayal. Long before science mapped these circuits, our language captured their force: 'heartache,' 'gut-wrenching,' 'stabbed in the back.' These phrases are not mere figures of speech, but echoes of our neurobiology—evidence that social and physical pain are deeply intertwined.

~

The modern human inherits this wiring in a vastly different context. Our survival no longer hinges on our place in a dozen-person band, but our brains have not updated the code. The same neural machinery that once responded to whispered approval or frowns around a campfire now fires urgently for digital notifications: a "like" on a post, a message from a crush, an email about a raise, or the comparison with an online rival. Unlike our ancestors' dozen-person bands, our social world now spans hundreds or thousands of connections, floods of curated images, workplace hierarchies, and digital validation; the alarms ring louder, longer, and more relentlessly.

Social media platforms are engineered to tap directly into our reward pathways, especially the ventral striatum, delivering dopamine bursts with every heart, thumbs-up, or retweet. Each positive interaction brings a flicker of pleasure; each absence, a quiet pang of exclusion. These apps are meticulously designed to keep us engaged, exploiting unpredictable rewards and novelty in much the same way as slot machines or addictive substances. The endless scroll exposes us to a constant stream of others' highlight reels, amplifying envy, fueling anxiety, and often leaving us feeling as though we never quite measure up.

Research shows social media use is tied to rising rates of anxiety and depression, particularly among young people whose brains are super-sensitive to peer approval during adolescence. Adolescence is the peak time for ventral striatal reactivity. This means the teen brain is wired to care deeply about peer status. Now, instead of comparisons in just one classroom, young users face "scoreboards" of likes and comments from an entire planet. Neuroscientists warn that repeated, high-frequency dopamine surges can lead to dysregulation: brains become less sensitive to everyday joys and may experience a "dopamine deficit" outside the app, increasing risk for compulsive use, impulse control problems, and emotional instability.

Recognizing this risk, Instagram made a bold move to reduce the pressure of public scoring. Instead of showing the total number of likes on each post, the interface now displays *"Liked by [username] and others,"* with the actual count hidden from public view. Users can still view their own like counts privately, but others only see a list of users who have engaged, not the actual number. The goal is to shift focus away from popularity contests toward authentic self-expression and meaningful sharing. Early studies and user feedback suggest this reduces anxiety and self-comparison for some, helping people post what genuinely matters to them rather than chasing external validation.

Brands, influencers, and marketers have had to adjust to this change: instead of targeting posts for maximum likes, there is an increasing emphasis on comments, shares, and real conversation—metrics thought to reflect deeper engagement and connection. While not a perfect solution, Instagram's shift underscores the importance of supporting mental health and cultivating a healthier, less competitive digital environment. Ultimately, the real challenge is to use these platforms mindfully, prioritizing solidarity, creativity, and meaningful engagement over numbers on a scoreboard.

The challenge and opportunity of modern life is to make conscious choices in navigating social environments—both online and off. Modern platforms can foster affirmation, solidarity, and new friendships—many users share stories of finding support, communities, and inspiration online. The neural circuitry itself isn't good or bad; it's neutral hardware responding to the environment and social context. The outcomes depend on how platforms are navigated: mindful engagement, setting boundaries, and digital detoxes are increasingly recommended to prevent comparison and validation-seeking from becoming toxic. Recognizing these dynamics helps us reclaim agency and shape a more compassionate, resilient sense of self amid the constant buzz.

Despite how natural social comparison is, jealousy is often treated like a dirty secret—an embarrassing emotional weakness that "strong" people are supposed to hide, deny, or suppress. We are taught, sometimes from early childhood, that "strong" or "good" individuals suppress jealous feelings and never let them show. This cultural script can be so ingrained that admitting jealousy, even to oneself, feels like confessing a secret weakness.

Where does this stigma come from?

Several roots underlie this stigma. First, jealousy is linked to feelings we are taught to avoid: insecurity, fear of loss, and low self-esteem. Because jealousy exposes our most vulnerable places—the relationships and values we hold dear, and our anxiety that they might slip away—it threatens the image of control and confidence that many strive to maintain. Few want to be labeled 'ungrateful,' 'possessive,' or 'overly dramatic'—judgments that often attach to those who openly struggle with jealousy.

Second, the fear of judgment perpetuates silence. People worry that if they express jealousy, others will see them as petty or unstable, or worse, attach the emotion to their identity rather than viewing it as a passing state. Instead of acknowledging and letting feelings pass, many people swallow them, risking emotional isolation or resentment that lingers beneath the surface. Past experiences, trauma, and cultural taboos around emotional openness further deepen the sense that jealousy is something to hide, making honest dialogue harder.

Yet, everyone has felt jealousy's sting—over a friend's new job, a partner's lingering glance, or a sibling's moment in the spotlight. Jealousy is not merely a shadow in the background; it is a central player in art and culture, adding tension to relationships and depth to conflict.

Take, for example, the blockbuster musical *Wicked*. Elphaba and Glinda's friendship is colored at every turn by longing, rivalry, and the ache of wanting what someone else has. Elphaba watches Glinda bask in the adoration of their classmates, wishing for just a sliver of the spotlight. Glinda, for her part, envies Elphaba's powerful magic and unapologetic individuality. The "green-eyed monster" becomes literal —a force so potent it shapes nearly every word and gesture in their relationship, turning ordinary moments into emotional battlegrounds.

This unsparing honesty about jealousy is part of why stories like *Wicked* resonate so deeply. We see characters struggle not just with spells and politics, but with the urgent, persistent need to belong and be valued. This need is as timeless as humanity itself. When art and music shine a light on jealousy, they help us see our own feelings more clearly, reminding us that to envy is to be alive, hopeful, and searching for meaning in connection. Those moments of jealousy—while uncomfortable—are simply proof that we care, and that caring, for better or worse, is what ties us together.

~

It may surprise us, but a measure of jealousy is not only normal—it is necessary. Jealousy is the mind's signal that something matters, that a bond is worth defending. Though it can be painful, jealousy reveals what we value most. We do not envy what we do not care about; we do not feel jealousy where there is no love. In this way, jealousy acts as a compass, pointing us toward our deepest attachments and values.

In small doses, jealousy can also prompt honest conversations, rekindle affection, and reinforce the value of our relationships. It can also encourage healthy competition. Often understood as envy's cousin, competition is a foundational concept. In mammals, competition ensures the distribution of resources, mate selection, and dominance hierarchies. In humans, competition fuels innovation, striving, and growth. The dopamine system thrives on challenge, firing not only in response to rewards but also in pursuit of goals. Competing galvanizes concentration, effort, and risk-taking.

Throughout history, rivalry has sparked both brilliance and downfall. A powerful rivalry can shape the world as profoundly as any invention. Consider Steve Jobs and Bill Gates—the defining duel of the digital era. Born months apart, they built empires—Apple and Microsoft—that transformed how billions work, create, and connect. Their competition was more than a business contest; it was a clash of philosophies. Jobs championed design, intuition, and taste, while Gates built his legacy on scale, software, and relentless problem-solving.

This rivalry was far from just tech jargon or shareholder drama. Jobs and Gates traded public barbs. Jobs accused Microsoft of "no taste"; Gates dismissed the iPad as "okay". Yet they also learned from and occasionally leaned on one another, with Gates even investing $150 million to save Apple in its darkest hour. At home, the friction went so deep that Melinda Gates famously banned iPods and iPhones in the Gates household. Their story is familiar to anyone who's chosen —or been forced—to define themselves against a rival. Whether rooted in envy, admiration, or pride, their competition drove innovation, turned each defeat into fuel, and made each victory sweeter.

Beyond Silicon Valley, rivalry lights up headlines and group chats. Coke vs. Pepsi, Nike vs. Reebok, Serena vs. Venus, Beyoncé vs. Rihanna—even among celebrities, athletes, and brands, fans watch as competitive sparks ignite new music, world records, or billion-dollar ad wars. These duels become part of our cultural memory, each side sharpening the other, and all of us choosing favorites just as we've done since childhood.

Rivals can be both a thorn and a blessing. They push individuals, teams, and ideas to new heights, but also stir anxiety and doubt. For most, rivalry is not just a spectacle—it's a force encountered in workplaces, friendships, and families. Sometimes it inspires brilliance; other times, it unsettles peace of mind. In every era, the dance of rivals remains a stage for human complexity.

On a neurobiological level, rivalry activates the brain's dopaminergic pursuit circuits. When competition arises, the mesolimbic and mesocortical systems light up, enhancing drive, focus, and the determination to outperform a rival. The ventral tegmental area releases dopamine to the ventral striatum and prefrontal cortex, heightening motivation and reinforcing the urge to excel. Rivals, in this sense, act as powerful amplifiers, transforming ordinary effort into extraordinary ambition. Yet, the sharp edge of rivalry carries risk: intense competition also triggers the amygdala and anterior cingulate cortex, regions that signal threat, pain, and social distress.

Jealousy and envy are the emotional equivalent of a tornado siren—a warning, not a verdict. However, when the system misfires, when the amygdala's alarms sound too often or too loudly, they can become corrosive. Some people, due to genetics, early experiences, or differences in brain wiring, are more prone to these misfires. Their amygdala may be hypersensitive, their prefrontal cortex less able to quiet the storm. The result is a life lived on high alert, where every laugh, every glance, every text message is scrutinized for signs of betrayal. For others, the signals are muted. They move through relationships with a calm detachment. They feel less troubled by the shifting tides of attention and affection.

Most of us live somewhere in between, learning to navigate the surges and ebbs of jealousy as best we can. Neuroscientific studies reveal that the circuitry underlying jealousy overlaps with that of pain, reward, and fear. The same brain regions that light up when we experience physical pain are also activated when we feel social exclusion or romantic rivalry. This is why jealousy can feel so sharp, so physical, so hard to shake.

The pain of jealousy is an indication of the value we place on our relationships. It is not an emotion to be tamed or dismissed, but a signal to be understood. It's a message from the brain, urging us to pay attention to the ties that hold us together. Like Elphaba and Glinda, we are all haunted by the fear of being left behind, yet also driven by the hope of being loved. So, *can we turn down the volume of the endless scoreboard?*

Neuroscience suggests several practical ways to soften the sting of comparison and jealousy. One is reappraisal: the prefrontal cortex can reinterpret envy, shifting the mindset from *"I am less"* to *"I can learn."* This reframing reduces threat responses in the amygdala and helps cultivate a growth mindset. Gratitude and reflection are also powerful tools. By practicing gratitude, we activate circuits in the medial prefrontal cortex that counteract envy loops and help refocus our attention on abundance rather than scarcity.

Social connection is equally important. Genuine intimacy and close bonds can quiet our inner vigilance, buffering the signals in the anterior cingulate cortex that register social exclusion and pain. Mindfulness practices offer another path: by reducing habitual rumination and overactivation in the insula, mindfulness makes jealous pangs less overwhelming and more manageable. Finally, shifting our approach to competition—from striving to 'beat others' to aiming to 'contribute more'—can rewire the brain's reward system. Altruistic competition links feelings of reward to effort and meaning, rather than to surpassing others.

These strategies make it clear that the urge to compare cannot be erased; it is part of our wiring. Its sting can be softened, and its fire can be harnessed to fuel growth instead of corrosion. The choice, the conscious reframe, is whether you become a prisoner of scoreboards or a gardener of values. The brain may tally, but the self can guide interpretation.

In the end, competition, envy, and jealousy—these are neither flaws nor final verdicts. They are pressures that shape identity, hone desires, and demand reflection. They are invitations: to reaffirm connections, to direct ambition toward growth, to see the scoreboard not as a cage but as a mirror and then step beyond it into the wider field of shared humanity.

PART SEVEN
A CHANGING BRAIN

CHAPTER 18
FRAGILE MACHINERY: HOW DISEASE AND INJURY REVEAL THE MYSTERIES OF THE BRAIN

THE MIND'S workings are hidden in plain sight. Every movement, word, memory, and desire springs from a dense lattice of neurons, orchestrating our lives. We seldom notice this machinery until it falters. When disease, injury, or trauma disrupts this neural scaffolding, we see the mind's complexity, its vulnerability, and above all, its resilience through plasticity. This ability to adapt lies at the heart of understanding the brain.

On a bright January morning in 2011, U.S. Congresswoman Gabby Giffords stood to greet her constituents in Tucson, Arizona. The day unfolded as any other—shaking hands, exchanging smiles—when the unthinkable happened: a gunman opened fire, and a bullet tore through the left hemisphere of Giffords' brain. Instantly, her world changed. She was rushed to surgery, her brain swelling and battered.

Giffords awoke unable to speak, her movements halting, her most basic abilities, like walking, talking, remembering, locked away by trauma. Each relearned word and regained step marked a victory over loss. Her recovery required not only medical expertise and determination, but also the slow, painstaking rewiring of her neural circuits—a vivid demonstration of the brain's plasticity. In reclaiming speech and movement, Giffords showed that identity can persist, even after profound injury. Her journey is a testament to human resilience and the brain's capacity to adapt.

Gabby Giffords' story, like the stories of countless others whose minds have been altered by injury or illness, reveals the machinery behind the curtain. When brokenness cracks the façade, the true marvels and mysteries of consciousness and self come to light. This is why we turn our attention to what fails, what fractures, what fades.

By studying malfunction, we uncover the principles that govern adaptation. Through celebrated cases and everyday stories, neuroscience reveals both possibility and vulnerability, with plasticity underpinning this balance. The machinery of the mind is robust yet poised on a knife-edge. It balances cognition and confusion, emotion and emptiness, movement and rigidity. Ultimately, being human is not defined by flawless machinery but by our capacity to adapt and reshape ourselves. Disease and injury do not simply reduce identity. They can reveal unexpected strengths and new rhythms of life. Let us look behind the curtain and explore how brain plasticity teaches us about resilience and the pursuit of meaning.

~

From these high-profile cases to quiet domestic scenes, the consequences of neural breakdown play out in countless ways. Imagine a sunlit kitchen. A grandmother pauses, searching for a word, her stories circling back on themselves. Her eyes linger on family photographs, tracing faces she once knew by name. Alzheimer's disease advances quietly, a slow and silent storm. Early signs, such as misplaced keys and forgotten appointments, are often dismissed as a simple part of aging. Only when these lapses impact daily life do we recognize the true weight of what is unfolding.

For Mark and his mother Sylvia, that storm came one night when Sylvia forgot the details of a family dinner, something she'd always cherished. As months passed, once-ordinary routines became uncertain terrain. Sylvia repeated questions. She lost track of schedules and sometimes mistook her own son for her late husband. Mark watched as the person he'd always known—quick-witted, affectionate, fiercely independent—slowly retreated behind a veil of memory loss.

Alzheimer's begins its assault in the hippocampus, the seahorse-shaped hub of memory. Here, plaques and tangled proteins gradually choke the neural pathways that once carried the stories of a lifetime. The landscape of memory becomes fractured, its contours jagged and incomplete. Subtle losses accumulate, giving way to deeper erosion: learning falters, cherished stories dissolve, and even the faces of loved ones may become unfamiliar.

Alzheimer's does more than cloud thought; it unravels the very narrative of identity. As the hippocampus withers and its capacity ebbs, the machinery that sequences, recalls, and projects our lives begins to fail. Memory, we learn, is not a decorative flourish. It is the central beam that supports every relationship and the story we tell ourselves about who we are.

Yet even in decline, islands of self remain. For many, childhood songs linger when conversation fades; such melodies reside in brain areas beyond the hippocampus. Emotional bonds remain strong; caregivers find that a gentle touch or a smile can prompt recognition, a spark in the haze.

"Though she had no concept I was her daughter, she knew me to be familiar and safe," writes Laury about her mother's early-onset Alzheimer's. This is the paradox: memory's machinery is persistently emotional, not just cognitive. So Alzheimer's is more than forgetting—it is the slow fading of self, witnessed by families daily. In these shadows, the need for human warmth becomes clear.

While Alzheimer's erodes the self from within, Parkinson's disease offers a different lesson: here, the body falters before the mind. Picture a grandfather at breakfast, his hand trembling as he lifts a spoon, his steps slow and deliberate, pausing at each threshold as if bracing for unseen obstacles. Parkinson's targets the substantia nigra, a narrow band in the midbrain that produces dopamine. As these neurons die, muscles stiffen, and tremors emerge. Once-simple tasks—tying shoelaces, pouring coffee—become daily trials of patience and resolve.

Yet within, many people with Parkinson's retain sharp minds and quick wit. The irony is stark. Thought and memory endure even as the body's freedom of movement slips away. Parkinson's shows us that motion is a symphony of coordination, chemistry, and resilience. Patients describe the "on-off" phenomenon. These are moments when medication restores movement, followed by sudden returns to rigidity. The machinery runs, then stalls, but the human spirit adapts, discovering new rhythms for living.

~

As we move from degenerative diseases to injuries, the pace and nature of neural disruption change. We shift from gradual decline to abrupt disruption—a sudden jolt that can fracture the self in an instant. Not all damage is dramatic. Some wounds seep quietly into daily life, subtly altering routines and relationships. These are the quiet catastrophes: injuries that hide beneath the surface, revealed only in moments of forgetfulness or fatigue, when a person no longer seems quite themselves.

Traumatic brain injury, for example, comes in countless forms: car accidents, falls, sports collisions, military blasts. The effects are unpredictable and uniquely personal. Memory blurs, confusion reigns, and familiar personality traits fade or warp, replaced by irritability, impulsivity, fatigue, or frustration that feels alien. It's not chosen but imposed by the altered landscape of the brain. One survivor described waking after a car accident, knowing his name but suddenly struggling to remember the simplest tasks or conversations. Others report feeling lost at work or unable to manage emotions.

Stroke offers another perspective. A clot or ruptured vessel can upend daily life in an instant. Words disappear mid-sentence, limbs refuse to move, perceptions fragment. Yet recovery can be remarkable. With determination and focused rehabilitation, the brain often remaps its functions, recruiting new networks when old ones fail. Survivors speak of the relentless, humbling work required to regain language or movement—a process that exemplifies neuroplasticity, the brain's remarkable capacity for renewal and reorganization.

Some injuries leave no visible scars, yet they rewire the mind's machinery just as profoundly. Psychiatric conditions—depression, schizophrenia, PTSD—do not always stem from a single lesion, but from subtle disruptions in the brain's interconnected networks. The result can be emotional or cognitive dissociation as real and disabling as any physical wound. For some, trauma strikes deepest in the realm of meaning and morality: soldiers, first responders, caregivers who witness events that fracture their sense of justice or self. Moral injury can slice through the narrative of identity, leaving guilt, shame, and alienation that fragment not only mood but the very story that holds a person together.

All these forms of injury reveal a universal truth. The machinery of self is distributed, interconnected, and vulnerable, but also plastic. Language, impulse control, emotion, movement, and memory are woven together, each thread essential to the whole. When disease or injury disrupts one domain, ripples spread, reminding us that the self is not a single entity but a network. The brain's plasticity means that it is capable of both adaptation and extraordinary renewal.

Understanding injury and disease lays the groundwork for exploring how the brain can recover and adapt. For much of modern history, scientists viewed the adult brain as fixed—hardwired in youth, then set for life. Under this belief, damage was destiny. Stroke, trauma, or degenerative disease were thought to leave permanent marks with little hope for repair. Yet, over the past fifty years, this view has undergone a steady change. Researchers have revealed that the nervous system is also remarkably adaptable. The brain and its networks can be pruned, reshaped, and rewired. In crisis or repetition, they bend rather than break. This quiet capacity, called neuroplasticity, has rewritten our understanding of resilience.

Consider the experience of an amputee. Those who lose an arm or leg frequently report phantom pains—ghostly sensations that feel as though they emanate from a missing body part. Such symptoms arise from the brain's "body maps," dynamic blueprints that track the spatial arrangement of our limbs. When an amputation occurs, neighboring cortical areas may encroach on the territory once dedicated to the absent limb, blurring distinctions. Mirror therapy, which uses reflections of intact limbs to trick the brain into "seeing" the missing one, can recalibrate these maps over time, reducing pain and confusion. What was once pathology becomes an opportunity for creative rewiring.

This principle reaches beyond sudden trauma to chronic illness. In Alzheimer's disease, activities such as listening to music, creating art, or repeating familiar routines can activate these surviving neural circuits. While such engagement cannot stop decline, it can preserve autonomy. Here, plasticity serves as a buffer, enriching the quality of life even as time grows short.

Meditation and mindfulness shift the focus from clinical recovery to everyday flourishing. Neuroimaging studies reveal that sustained contemplative practice strengthens brain regions associated with emotion regulation, attention, and self-awareness. For those facing depression, trauma, or anxiety, such training can reshape not only experience but also the architecture of neural networks. In some cases, practitioners reverse patterns of stress-induced atrophy. Here, plasticity is not just a tool for compensation, but a means for growth—the brain becomes what it practices.

Community also shapes the brain deeply. Relationships and social engagement play a crucial role in maintaining brain health throughout life. Loneliness accelerates decline, while friendships and vibrant communities foster new connections and support. Even late in life, making new bonds or engaging socially can slow deterioration and enliven circuits of empathy and belonging. Plasticity grows not just in solitude, but in connection.

~

Taken together, these examples reveal that plasticity is more than a biological curiosity—it is the hidden engine of hope and adaptation. It does not undo every injury or guarantee full recovery, but it reframes our minds as built not just to endure damage but to continually remake themselves. Brokenness initiates adaptation, and plasticity is at the center of that story.

The question for scientists is no longer whether the brain can change, but how we might guide that change with intention. New tools and therapies aim to direct plasticity, not simply wait for it to occur. Brain-computer interfaces already allow paralyzed individuals to control robotic arms with their thoughts, translating faint neural signals into movement. These devices restore agency and point toward futures where lost functions may be bypassed or replaced. Neuroprosthetics are redefining what it means to repair the brain.

At the same time, stem cell therapies and genetic engineering offer another path to renewal—not just rerouting signals, but regrowing tissue itself. Transplanted stem cells in damaged brain regions show promise for replacing lost neurons, while genetic tools target the mutations behind some neurodegenerative diseases. Though still experimental, these approaches suggest that even the cellular foundations of thought may one day be rebuilt.

Digital technologies add a new dimension. Cognitive training programs and virtual reality therapies are being evaluated to help rebuild memory, sharpen attention, and restore language function after injury or decline. Unlike passive rehabilitation, these methods utilize repetition and active engagement to intentionally sculpt neural circuits. They mark a shift from general recovery to targeted retraining of the brain's architecture.

Precision medicine takes this approach even further. By tailoring treatments to each person's unique genetic and neural profile, physicians can develop highly specific therapies for conditions once thought to be uniform. Therapy becomes sculpting: each intervention reinforces, prunes, or bypasses the brain's wiring with purpose.

However, perhaps soft, human therapies most clearly reveal the paradox of plasticity: resilience lies in narrative and relationship as much as in technology. Art, music, storytelling, mindfulness, and community engagement enrich the inner lives of those at risk of disorder. They stimulate neural circuits and bring meaning. In shaping the brain, they shape the self.

The future of the brain is neither the bleak determinism of the past nor a utopian vision of total regeneration. The machinery will fail in time—entropy, age, and chance guarantee it. Yet between permanence and collapse lies a broad landscape of possibility, where adaptation and renewal surpass what was once thought possible.

Hope endures: selfhood is not fixed, but ever-changing. Through brain plasticity, we can rebuild, reroute, and redefine ourselves. The so-called broken brain becomes a window into how the machinery truly works and what is possible when adaptation takes center stage. Illness and injury will leave their marks, but new selves can emerge—tender and remarkable—reshaping what it means to be resiliently human.

CHAPTER 19
LIFELONG LEARNING: RECOVERY, GROWTH AND THE BRAIN THAT HEALS

CAN *you really teach an old dog new tricks?*

For much of the twentieth century, science insisted the adult brain was fixed. Once organized in childhood, its structure was believed to be permanent. Neurons died, connections faded, and losses were seen as irretrievable. Stroke, Alzheimer's, or injury seemed irreversible. The brain, in this view, was an organ of unyielding permanence.

Yet in recent decades, a different picture has emerged. Contrary to older beliefs, the brain is not a machine of frozen wires but a living, dynamic system—constantly reshaping itself in response to experience and learning. This remarkable adaptability is known as neuroplasticity. Far from being confined to childhood, plasticity is a lifelong companion, quietly overturning the old adage that you can't teach an old dog new tricks. In truth, you can.

Neuroplasticity is the brain's capacity to alter its structure and function in response to experience. Each time you practice a skill, summon a memory, repeat a phrase, or adjust a habit, the connections between your neurons are subtly rewired. They are strengthened, weakened, or rerouted. Imagine your brain as clay, molded by the repeated touch of daily life. This is not just poetic imagery; it is a biological fact. Learning leaves tangible footprints in the architecture of your neural networks.

For children, this process is especially intense, laying the groundwork for future growth. At birth, a newborn arrives with roughly 100 billion neurons, but what matters more than sheer numbers are the connections between them. During the first years of life, synapses proliferate at a furious pace. A toddler's brain is making hundreds of thousands of new connections per second, sculpted by voices, faces, textures, and light. By the age of three, each neuron may host thousands of synapses. As childhood progresses, these neural patterns begin to shift from explosive creation to more selective refinement.

Then comes refinement. Circuits that are engaged repeatedly are reinforced; those neglected wither and vanish. This process of "pruning" establishes solid networks for language, motor skills, and the foundations of self. Some capabilities—such as the cadence of a native language or the perception of musical pitch—are especially sensitive in these early years, when neural pathways are malleable. Yet the existence of critical periods does not mean that growth later in life is forbidden. The groundwork laid in early childhood is expanded and extended over the course of decades. The next distinct remodeling phase arrives with adolescence, when the brain's priorities and capacities undergo dramatic shifts.

Adolescence marks a significant period of further transformation, highlighting the brain's ongoing adaptability. The brain's frontal regions, especially the prefrontal cortex, undergo dramatic change. Responsible for judgment, impulse control, long-term planning, and abstract reasoning, this area thickens with new growth before gradually thinning and refining into its adult state. Teenagers often appear reckless, spontaneous, and voraciously curious, and in many ways, they are. However, research shows that this volatility is not simply a social phenomenon; it reflects a genuine neurological architecture. The adolescent brain thrives on exploration. Mistakes, risks, and experimentation drive the construction of higher-order skills. Error itself becomes an educator. By early adulthood, the brain continues changing, but with a subtler rhythm and different opportunities.

In adulthood, neuroplasticity persists, though its tempo changes—shifting the focus from rapid growth to refinement and adaptation. Learning a new language leaves a lasting impact on the regions governing grammar and vocabulary. Musicians, even those who start later in life, show growth in areas tied to motor skills and auditory processing. London taxi drivers, who master the city's labyrinthine streets, develop enlarged hippocampi, the brain's center for navigation. These examples reveal an adult brain that remains capable of architectural refinement through sustained effort and practice.

Even emotional and regulatory processes adapt. Mindfulness and meditation, once seen as cultural practices, increase cortical thickness in the prefrontal cortex. They strengthen attention networks and rebalance those linked to anxiety and stress. Adults who practice reflection and attention reshape the very organ they use to think and feel.

Aging brings wear. Synapses falter, white matter develops microtears, and neurotransmitter production drops. Aging means slower recall, less concentration, and weaker coordination. Diseases like Alzheimer's and Parkinson's increase these losses. Still, new discoveries about neurogenesis in the aging brain offer hope.

One of the most transformative discoveries in neuroscience is that the hippocampus. It continues to generate new neurons well into old age. This idea was once controversial, but the evidence is now compelling. Physical activity, social connection, and mental challenge all stimulate the birth of new neurons and help maintain resilient neural networks. Aerobic exercise, whether walking, jogging, or cycling, has been shown to increase the size of the hippocampus in older adults, thereby improving memory. Engaging in novel learning—puzzles, games, crafts—can guard against cognitive decline. Older adults who embrace new skills, from bridge to digital technology, demonstrate measurable gains in neural efficiency. In short, the aging brain retains its capacity for growth.

What, at the cellular level, underlies these changes?

Neurons communicate through synapses, sending electrical and chemical signals. When a pathway is used repeatedly—such as reciting a fact or practicing a movement—it becomes more efficient. More neurotransmitters are released. Receptors multiply, and signals travel more swiftly. This process, known as long-term potentiation, is the cellular basis of learning and memory. Over time, dendrites branch out, axons sprout new terminals, and myelin sheaths thicken. Glial cells proliferate, supporting and maintaining the neural environment. In essence, repeated use strengthens networks. The adage 'neurons that fire together wire together' is not just a saying; it is visible under the microscope.

Meaning is the catalyst for change. Moving from cellular mechanics to lived experience, studies show that learning driven by purpose and emotion forges deeper neural connections than rote repetition. Older adults who pursue passions—singing in choirs, learning new languages, creating art—achieve greater neural gains than those who approach learning as a medical chore. Social relationships are equally powerful. Long-term studies of centenarians and so-called Blue Zone elders reveal that social connection is the strongest predictor of healthy cognitive aging, surpassing even diet and exercise. Loneliness erodes resilience, while friendship, family, and community nourish it.

Biology and behavior intersect in daily habits that sustain neuroplasticity. Physical activity triggers the release of growth factors, such as brain-derived neurotrophic factor, which nourish synapses and strengthen connections. Intellectual challenges—like coding, chess, or career changes—expand neural circuits and keep the brain adaptable.

Creativity—through music, art, or writing—sparks new combinations in the mind and activates networks left untouched by routine. Social engagement is vital; interacting with others exercises memory and attention, demanding empathy and flexible thinking. Mindfulness and meditation rewire connectivity patterns, especially for self-reflection and emotional balance. By integrating these into daily life, we help the brain stay adaptable and grow at any age.

Even brief immersion in unfamiliar environments, such as traveling to new places, engaging with different cultures, and exploring museums, leaves lasting neural traces. A variety of experiences is a powerful engine of resilience. The rules are clear but deceptively simple. Start small, repeat often, explore broadly, and prioritize meaning and connection. Mistakes are not failures, but mechanisms for growth, revealing where circuits need strengthening. And while not every deficit can be fully repaired, adaptation is often possible in ways earlier scientists considered impossible. Key takeaway: Lifelong learning and adaptability are supported by the brain's design.

Looking ahead, medicine continues to expand possibilities through technology. Beyond biological and lifestyle interventions, technology adds a new dimension. Brain-computer interfaces enable individuals with paralysis to control robotic limbs, translating neural signals into movement. Stem cell therapies aim to regenerate lost neurons. Digital tools, such as cognitive training and virtual reality rehabilitation, target brain circuits to support recovery and improve outcomes. Precision medicine uses genetics to tailor interventions for neurodegenerative diseases. These innovations do not replace the core principles of neuroplasticity; instead, they enhance the brain's natural capacity for change.

Yet the most profound implication is human, not technological. After surveying science and new frontiers, we return to the central insight: understanding the brain's changeability means your habits, memories, and thinking do not have to harden with age. The potential for renewal is greater than once believed. Recovery after injury, later-life breakthroughs, and adapting to new roles are not wishful thinking but realities supported by evidence.

You are not a static entity. With intention, your brain shapes itself in response to what you do, what you feel, and with whom you connect. Each day offers choices—movements, words, practices, encounters—that leave lasting impressions in the tissue of thought. Whether you are eighteen or eighty, your neural landscape awaits the imprint of tomorrow's experiences. The myth of a rigid brain has faded. The essential lesson: *at every stage of life, neuroplasticity enables change and renewal.*

CHAPTER 20
THE ARCHITECT OF BECOMING: PRACTICES FOR TRANSFORMATION AND GROWTH

THE BRAIN IS a living metropolis at dusk. Imagine it: the sky is streaked with lavender and indigo, the last light of day glinting off glass towers. Down below, neon pulses in the labyrinth of alleyways and along the sweep of grand boulevards. Windows blaze to life, one after another. Behind the glass, dramas unfold: a memory replayed in sepia tones, a sudden surge of longing, a decision teetering on the edge of action. Some rooms are crowded with noise and light, others shadowed and secretive, their stories whispered behind drawn curtains. The aroma of rain on warm pavement mingles with the metallic tang of city air, and somewhere, the scent of something sweet—nostalgia, perhaps, or hope—drifts by.

You walk these streets daily. Sometimes you are a tourist, marveling at the unfamiliar corners of your own mind. Sometimes you are a fugitive, ducking down side streets to escape old regrets or urgent cravings. Always, you are a resident. Your feet on the cobblestones, heart attuned to the city's restless rhythms. Every alley you explore, every boulevard you cross, is a journey through the living, breathing architecture of thought and feeling. Here, in this metropolis of dusk, the brain is not merely a map—it is the city itself, alive with possibility, waiting for you to wander and to wonder.

For centuries, philosophers and poets have wandered these streets, asking: *Are we mere prisoners of our own circuitry, shackled to the rails of habit and instinct? Or can we redraw the map—can we, through will or wisdom, reroute the traffic of our minds?*

Modern neuroscience answers: *Yes, change is possible.*

Our exploration has illustrated how the brain's reward system, once honed for seeking food and shelter, now responds to modern pleasures—chocolate, smartphones—with dopamine reinforcing paths to pleasure, regardless of moral implication. Yet, excess desire can lead to overconsumption and cravings that overshadow fullness. This makes moderation a formidable challenge.

The struggle between the self-regulating prefrontal cortex and the impulsive limbic system complicates the breaking of habits. Unmet desires trigger emotional turmoil, as the amygdala and hippocampus react to stress and setbacks. Motivation, too, is fickle. Dopamine can sharpen focus or scatter it. Above all, our social nature emerges: connection, comparison, and empathy are vital in building communities.

Through these discoveries, it becomes clear that our desires are deeply human, normal, even, but that does not mean we must surrender to them. The brain is not a stone monument, cold and unyielding. It is reshaped by experience. This is neuroplasticity: the brain's ability to rewire itself in response to learning, practice, and intention. Each time you reach for a new skill or resist an old temptation, you are a mason at work, laying fresh cobblestones.

Beneath the metaphor, neuroplasticity is a team of chemical messengers and molecular switches. When you practice a new skill or resist a familiar urge, neurons converse in bursts of neurotransmitters, dopamine, glutamate, and GABA, each one an agent of change. Dopamine, that restless herald of reward, marks moments of surprise and pleasure. This reinforces the neural pathways that led you there.

It is not a passive process. It is an active, dynamic dance, where repetition tips the balance and some synapses grow robust while others wither from neglect. Long-term potentiation—strengthening connections through repeated use—and its counterpart, long-term depression—weakening unused connections—are the twin sculptors of our neural landscape. In certain corners, such as the hippocampus, new neurons even spring to life, adding fresh potential for adaptation.

Yet, this remodeling is not uniform across the brain's geography. The cerebral cortex, seat of thought and voluntary action, is especially malleable. Here, practice thickens the gray matter, as seen in musicians whose brains bear the fingerprints of years of training. Neurons sprout new dendritic spines—tiny branches reaching for connection—when challenged by learning or enriched environments.

The brain's highways of white matter, too, become more insulated with use. While specific times in childhood are especially fertile for change, the adult brain retains a surprising capacity for remodeling. This is especially true when driven by focused attention and motivation.

From a neuroscience perspective, neuroplasticity is both a gift and a paradox. The same mechanisms that allow us to master a new language or recover from injury can also entrench habits, biases, or addictions. The brain does not judge; it simply strengthens the paths most traveled.

"Neurons that fire together, wire together"—the adage of Hebb's Rule —explains how habits form and why they can be so persistent. Every experience, every challenge, every triumph and setback sculpts the brain's architecture, not just genetics. Even deeply ingrained patterns can be altered with sustained effort. Stroke survivors, for example, can regain some lost functions by recruiting new neural circuits through intensive rehabilitation.

Throughout this journey, we have seen that desire is not destiny. The brain's plasticity is a source of hope—a reminder that change is not only possible, but inevitable. Whether learning a new skill, overcoming compulsion, or reshaping the stories we tell ourselves, each act of intention is a brick in the ever-evolving architecture of the self. You are not a prisoner of your wiring. You are the architect, the mason, the city planner—laying new roads, rerouting old ones, and expanding the map of your own becoming.

All that said, you may now be thinking... *okay, but how? How do you change?*

~

There are days when the struggle feels like a storm. Days when cravings or compulsions feel as if they belong to someone else entirely. In these moments, remember: just as a seasoned navigator consults the stars when the seas grow wild, so too can you consult therapists and physicians. They offer evidence-based interventions and, for some, new pharmacological tools that gently recalibrate the brain's circuits of appetite and desire. These are not shortcuts; they are simply offering new vantage points and strategies for change.

To embark on the journey of self-modification, begin with intention. In the hush of early morning, or the velvet quiet before sleep, sit with yourself. Reflect honestly. Take pen to paper and write down what you wish to change. Do not write as a judge, but as a witness.

Begin with precision. Identify the specific craving, habit, or behavior you wish to change. Name it aloud or write it down. The act of naming transforms the abstract into the tangible, making it something you can work with, not just something you endure.

Remember, change is rarely one and done. It is the slow accumulation of small victories—a skipped snack, a mindful pause, a single walk taken instead of a cigarette. The brain, ever the diligent archivist, records these moments. Each small win is a signal flare, lighting a new path through the neural thicket.

To this end, harness the power of digital tools: a habit-tracking app that turns progress into a visible pattern, a calendar where each day of success becomes a badge, a simple checklist that transforms intention into action. Let your phone become a companion, not a distraction—a gentle nudge toward your goal. Remember: no victory is too minor.

Did you pause before reaching for the snack? Did you take a single mindful breath before replying in anger?

These are the bricks and mortar of transformation. Over time, the accumulation of these moments becomes a fortress—strong, resilient, uniquely yours.

Furthermore, know that your surroundings are not neutral. They whisper to your habits, coaxing old routines to life. Rearrange your environment to support your intentions. Remove triggers where possible—clear the pantry of tempting snacks, silence notifications that lure you into distraction, or set out your running shoes the night before. Small changes in your environment can tip the scales in your favor.

Desire is energy, and energy can be redirected. When you feel a craving rise, pause. Notice its texture—the tightness in your chest, the quickening of thought. Rather than suppressing it, substitute a healthier action: a glass of water, a brief walk, a call to a friend. Over time, these substitutions become new habits, new default responses. This is often known as mindfulness.

Mindful awareness is the art of watching the mind without trying to steer it. Picture yourself as a lighthouse keeper, observing the restless tides of craving and compulsion as they rise and fall against the rocks. The urge arrives, insistent, electric, but you do not leap into the surf. You watch, you wait, you breathe.

Set aside a few minutes each day for this practice. Sit quietly. When an urge appears—a desire for sugar, a flash of irritation, the itch of distraction—notice it.

Where does it live in your body? How does it move? Does it build, crest, and then dissolve?

Resist the reflex to act. Instead, become a witness. Modern neuroscience reveals that this act of observation is not passive. The brain's default mode network, the circuitry responsible for self-reflection and wandering thought, is plastic. With each repetition, you widen the space between impulse and action. The urge becomes weather—real, but passing. You become the sky, vast and untroubled, able to choose your response.

In daily life, this practice offers freedom. The next time you feel the pull of habit, pause. Take a single breath. Remind yourself: *"This is an urge. It will pass."* Over weeks and months, you may notice the cravings lose their sharpness, the compulsions their urgency. You are not at the mercy of your desires. With mindful awareness, you become both observer and architect, shaping your inner landscape with patience and skill.

Also know and accept that setbacks will occur. The old patterns are persistent, and lapses are not failures but feedback. When you stumble, respond with curiosity, not criticism.

Ask: *What triggered this? How can I prepare differently next time?*

Self-compassion is not indulgence; it is the soil in which resilience grows. Make reflection a ritual. Each week, revisit your intentions and your progress. Adjust your strategies as needed. The process of change is dynamic—a dance, not a march. With each cycle of reflection and adjustment, you become more adept at steering your own course.

Of course, change is hard in solitude. In the architecture of transformation, no scaffold is more intricate or more powerful than the web of human connection. As we saw previously, the brain, for all its solitary brilliance, is fundamentally social. Its circuits were forged in the fires of tribe and kin, shaped by the need to belong, to imitate, to be seen and understood. When you seek to change, you do not simply rewrite your own neural pathways; you tap into a collective current, a shared field of influence that can amplify or undermine your efforts.

Within your cortex, mirror neurons fire not only when you act, but when you watch another perform the same action. This is the neural basis of imitation, empathy, and social learning. When you witness a friend resisting temptation or forging a new habit, your brain rehearses the same pathways, priming you for change.

Behavior is contagious. In groups, new norms emerge—what is praised, what is expected, what is possible. If your peers value healthy habits, generosity, or resilience, your brain adapts, recalibrating its expectations and desires. This is social neuroplasticity in action: the rewiring of your brain in response to the behaviors and attitudes of those around you.

Furthermore, social networks act as external regulators of behavior. Declaring your intentions to a friend or group transforms a private wish into a public commitment. The brain's reward system, especially the release of dopamine, responds to personal achievement and to social recognition and approval. A word of encouragement, a nod of acknowledgment, or even a shared struggle can make the difference between persistence and relapse.

It is also important to realize that the same mechanisms that make positive behaviors contagious can spread habits that undermine your goals. If your social circle normalizes procrastination, cynicism, or unhealthy routines, your brain's plasticity works against you, reinforcing unhelpful patterns. Social pressure can subtly or overtly sabotage your intentions. Also, constant comparison, especially in the age of curated social media, can breed envy, shame, or a sense of inadequacy. These emotions activate stress circuits in the brain, narrowing your capacity for flexible thinking and making change feel more daunting.

All that being said, when it comes to our social brains, here are the main takeaways on how we can effectively use them to adopt healthy habits:

Surround yourself with people who embody the changes you seek. Let their habits, language, and mindset become the template your brain mirrors. Make your intentions visible. Mark progress—yours and others'—with rituals of acknowledgment. This strengthens both neural pathways and social bonds. Limit exposure to negative influences, whether in person or online. Curate your networks as you would your environment. Offer support, not just seek it. Helping others change reinforces your own pathways of empathy, resilience, and self-control.

And so, as dusk deepens and the city of the mind prepares for rest, we move from the bright marketplace of social exchange into the hush of night. Here, in the silent theater where dreams are made, sleep stands as our next aspect of transformation.

~

Too often, in our culture of relentless striving, rest is treated as an afterthought—a luxury to be trimmed away in pursuit of more hours, more hustle. Yet science and history share another truth: sleep is not a thief of time, but its guardian.

Imagine sleep as a walled garden, its gates swinging shut against the clamor of unfinished tasks and the blue glow of midnight notifications. Inside, the air is cool and fragrant with possibility. Here, the brain is not dormant. It is a silent artisan, replaying the day's encounters, sculpting memory and understanding. Each night, as you surrender to darkness, your mind is busy at work—chiseling away what is unneeded, reinforcing what is vital, and pruning the tangles of habit and desire.

Cultures across centuries have honored the rituals of sleep. The particulars shift, but the need for deep, restorative slumber is universal. When sleep is neglected, the mind's resolve grows brittle. Fatigue seeps in, eroding intention, and the old patterns find their way back, emboldened by your exhaustion.

If we need sleep for change, what happens when the gates to this sanctuary refuse to close?

Insomnia is more than a restless night. When sleep is fragmented or elusive, the brain's nightly work is left unfinished. Memories remain jumbled, emotional wounds unhealed, and the neural scaffolding that supports new habits is left fragile and incomplete. Insomnia blunts the tools of neuroplasticity. The brain's ability to forge new pathways, to adapt and rewire in response to intention and effort, is intimately tied to the quality of sleep.

Without sufficient rest, the chemical messengers that enable learning and memory falter. The hippocampus struggles to file away new lessons. The prefrontal cortex grows sluggish, its signals dulled by fatigue. In this state, cravings grow louder, impulses harder to resist, and the will to change is sapped at its root. Chronic insomnia is not merely an inconvenience; it is a barrier to transformation. The mind becomes reactive, prone to anxiety and rumination. The emotional storms that accompany setbacks become harder to weather, and setbacks themselves become more frequent. Even the body conspires against change, as stress hormones rise and inflammation smolders, making every effort feel heavier.

To live with intention is to defend your sleep as fiercely as any precious resource. Treat bedtime as a sacred threshold. Dim the lights an hour before you wish to drift off, signaling to your body that night is near. Let the bedroom become a haven—calm, uncluttered, free from the digital glare and the demands of the day. Establish a gentle rhythm: a book, a warm drink, a moment of quiet reflection. These are not indulgences, but investments, each one a brick in the foundation of lasting change. Sometimes, the path to transformation begins not with another act of will, but with the simple, radical act of rest.

If insomnia shadows your nights, approach it with curiosity and compassion. Notice patterns: *Is it worry, caffeine, or the blue light of screens that keeps you awake?* Experiment with small adjustments, and if sleep remains elusive, seek support.

Speaking of seeking support, in the labyrinth of habit and desire, there are moments when the walls seem to close in—when cravings roar louder than reason, and old routines feel immovable. In these moments, seeking professional guidance is not a retreat, but an act of courage. Therapists and physicians are navigators in this terrain, equipped with scientific tools that can illuminate the path out of compulsion. Every year, new treatments—both behavioral and pharmacological—emerge, offering fresh hope and practical strategies for those feeling overwhelmed.

Recall our image from before: your mind as a sprawling city—a place of glittering skylines and shadowed alleys, bustling intersections and forgotten dead ends. Habits are the well-worn roads winding through this metropolis, some smooth and efficient, others cracked and overgrown, leading you in circles or toward places you'd rather not revisit. Sometimes, the city's infrastructure is tangled with detours and blockages, old patterns that slow your progress or steer you off course.

When you work with a trained therapist, cognitive behavioral therapy becomes both the city planner's blueprint and the demolition crew's jackhammer. Under professional guidance, you identify the crumbling overpasses of negative thought patterns—those mental routes that always seem to lead to the same dead ends. Through structured sessions and expert-led exercises, your therapist helps you close off these unhelpful roads, reroute traffic, and lay down new thoroughfares. Each time you challenge an automatic thought or recognize a trigger, you're supported in redirecting the flow of mental traffic. Over time, these guided renovations reinforce healthier pathways. These changes make it easier to travel the routes of self-control and intention.

Wearables and biofeedback devices, when used in partnership with healthcare professionals, become the city's sensors and monitors. In a clinical setting, these tools bring hidden rhythms—heart rate, sleep, stress—into the light for both you and your provider to observe. Just as city officials interpret traffic cameras and weather alerts, the data from these devices is reviewed by clinicians who can help you spot trouble before it snarls the flow. Noticing a spike in stress during a therapy session, for example, allows your provider to guide you through a mindful pause, rerouting energy before a pile-up of cravings or frustration occurs. Over time, this professional oversight helps you regain control over your responses, giving you agency over your city's pulse.

Pharmacological interventions, prescribed and monitored by physicians, are the engineers working deep beneath the streets, adjusting the city's foundational wiring. Medications such as GLP-1 agonists are not self-serve solutions; they require the expertise of a medical professional to assess, prescribe, and monitor. These treatments recalibrate the appetite circuits, dampening signals that fuel compulsive behaviors—not just for food, but for other urges as well. With the support of your healthcare provider, these medications can enhance feelings of fullness, slow the rush of impulses, and reduce the brain's response to tempting cues, offering a biochemical ally in the struggle for change.

Meanwhile, scientists and clinicians are developing new molecular tools—experimental therapies designed to help the city "unlearn" entrenched routes and reinforce healthier ones. Some, like psychedelic-assisted therapy or drugs targeting specific neurotransmitters, are available only in clinical trials or specialized medical settings. Their use is strictly supervised by professionals, ensuring safety and maximizing potential benefit. Early results suggest that, under expert care, these therapies may one day make the mind's infrastructure even more adaptable and resilient.

If you find yourself lost in your city's labyrinth—stuck in gridlock, circling the same blocks—*remember: you do not have to navigate alone.*

Professionals are there to help you choose the right tools, whether it's a new route, a digital guide, or a structural upgrade. The science of self-modification is evolving, but its core message remains: change is possible, and you are worthy of the support needed to achieve it. Every detour, every new street you pave with the help of experts, is a signal to your mind that a better map is being drawn... one choice, one intersection, one day at a time.

Yet even with the best maps and the guidance of seasoned city planners, progress through the maze of change is never just a matter of direction or technique. What propels us forward—what turns hesitation into momentum and possibility into reality—is the quiet engine of motivation.

~

Motivation is the force that animates every choice, the inner current that pushes us to seek out new streets and persist through detours. It is the difference between wandering aimlessly and moving with purpose. Picture yourself at the crossroads of habit, with one path worn smooth by repetition and the other overgrown, leading toward the unknown. The question is not only which path to take, but why you wish to walk at all.

What compels you to leave the comfort of the known? What vision shimmers on the horizon, drawing you forward?

Begin by asking yourself—not just how you might change, but why. Set aside a quiet moment, free from the clamor of obligation. Sit with a notebook, or simply close your eyes. *What values pulse beneath your desire for change? Is it the longing for health, for freedom, for deeper connection?*

Perhaps it is the wish to be present for your children, to reclaim a sense of agency, to live in harmony with the earth or your own body. Let these values rise, unhurried, like lanterns in the dusk. Write them down. Name them. This act of articulation is not mere sentimentality; it is the forging of a compass. When your efforts are aligned with your core values, the work of change transforms. It becomes less a daily skirmish and more a pilgrimage—an ongoing journey toward a life that feels authentic and whole.

Imagine the difference: to diet for the sake of a number on the scale, versus eating well to improve the health of a body that carries you through the world to quit smoking, not out of shame, but out of love for the breath that fills your lungs and the laughter you share with friends. Motivation rooted in values is resilient. It endures setbacks, weathers boredom, and finds renewal in meaning.

Revisit your motivations often. Let them evolve as you do. When the inevitable resistance arises, when the old habits beckon with their siren song, return to your "*why.*" Remind yourself: this is not just about discipline, but about devotion. You are not merely changing habits; you are shaping a life that reflects your deepest convictions. In this way, reflection becomes both anchor and sail. It grounds you in purpose and propels you forward, turning the daily work of change from a burden into a sacred journey—one step, one choice, one day at a time.

What does it mean to change ourselves?

The optimism of science casts long shadows. For every new tool that lets us rewrite the script of our biology, there is an ancient echo: caution, wonder, and the uneasy wisdom that not all that can be done should be done. Imagine, for a moment, standing before a mirror that shows not just your reflection, but your potential selves—each shaped by choices, by interventions, by the quiet or dramatic reworking of your appetites and fears. The power to change is thrilling, but it is also weighty. To tame a hunger, to soften a compulsion, is to reach into the most private chambers of the self.

Is this an act of nobility, a triumph of reason over impulse? Or does it risk hubris, the arrogance of rewriting what nature, culture, and history have inscribed in our bones?

History offers both inspiration and warning. The quest for purity, for mastery over the body and mind, has often led to excess—eugenics, forced sterilizations, and the demonization of "unnatural" interventions. Yet, the same arc of history bends toward healing: vaccines, antibiotics, and therapies once branded as heresy now save lives. The boundary between wisdom and folly is rarely bright; it is a shifting line, drawn anew by each generation.

Let us pause and consider three questions that haunt the ethics of self-modification.

Who decides what a "healthy" or "unhealthy" desire is?

In the privacy of your own mind, the urge to change may feel like liberation. When society, family, or commerce begin to dictate which desires are acceptable, autonomy frays. The danger is not only in the tools themselves, but in who wields them, and for what purpose. True freedom lies not just in the ability to change, but in the right to choose whether, how, and why to do so.

Will the fruits of scientific progress be shared, or hoarded?

As new technologies emerge—pills that quiet cravings, apps that nudge behavior, therapies that rewire the brain—there is a risk that only the privileged will access them. The gap between those who can afford to sculpt their desires and those who cannot may widen, turning self-modification into yet another axis of inequality. Justice demands that we ask: Who is left behind?

If we change our cravings, do we change who we are?

Desire is not merely a glitch in the system; it is a thread woven through our stories, our cultures, our sense of self. To edit our hungers is to edit the narrative of our lives. Some changes may bring relief and freedom; others may leave us feeling estranged from our own history. The line between healing and erasure is delicate, and each person must walk it with care.

There are no easy answers, only deeper invitations to reflect. This is not a puzzle to be solved, but a landscape to be explored—one that asks us to weigh possibility against wisdom, freedom against responsibility, and transformation against authenticity. Perhaps the truest guide is humility: a willingness to question not just what is possible, but what is right, what is just, and what is true to the story we wish to live.

In the end, the power to change ourselves is both a gift and a burden. It asks us not only to dream of who we might become, but to honor the complexity of who we are and to tread carefully, with both courage and care, as we shape the next chapter of our becoming. Change, then, is not a single act but a continual unfolding—a dialogue between intention and biology, between the old self and the new. Your brain is not a prison, but a landscape awaiting cultivation. With patience, knowledge, and compassion, you can redraw its map. The city of your mind is alive with possibility, its lights flickering in the dusk, waiting for you to choose which ones to kindle.

CHAPTER 21

IMPERFECT AND EVOLVING: SELF-COMPASSION AND THE PATH FORWARD

WHEN YOU FIRST OPENED THESE pages, we asked: *What is this power that can so easily unseat reason?*

We began our journey in a crowded room, where a single glance could ignite a storm within; a moment when the pulse of desire drowned out the measured voice of reason. We have wandered through the tangled forest of the brain, tracing the ancient, electric pathways that shape our cravings, our choices, our very sense of self. Now, as the final curtain falls, we pause to ask: *What have we learned? And what, in the end, does it mean to be a creature of desire?*

To stand at the crossroads of appetite and aspiration is to be human. It is to feel the wild horses of impulse straining at the reins, even as the charioteer of reason clings for balance—a drama as old as consciousness itself. Plato's chariot, Zen's restless monkey, Darwin's dog with eyes shining in wordless affection: these metaphors are not relics, but living companions, guiding us as we peer into the mirror of our own minds.

Desire is not a flaw to be cured, but the unmistakable watermark of our species. It is a signature pressed deep into the marrow of our bones and the winding grooves of our brains. It is as ancient as the first heartbeat, as persistent as the tides. Before the first spark of reason flickered in the human mind, before we spoke in words or carved our stories into stone, we felt. Emotion was our original language: a primal pulse that guided our ancestors through the wild, whispering warnings and promises, shaping every choice and every chance encounter.

Emotion is not the adversary of thought, but its ancestor and lifelong companion. It is the fertile soil from which all intention grows. Imagine the mind as a vast, tangled forest: roots of feeling stretch deep beneath the surface, anchoring every towering trunk of logic and every delicate branch of reflection. As neuroscientist Antonio Damasio observed, *"We are not thinking beings that feel, but feeling beings that think."*

The brain is not a battlefield where reason and passion clash, but a living manuscript. Each page is inscribed with the looping script of instinct and the careful edits of intellect, entwined and inseparable. Within the labyrinthine folds of the cortex, the limbic system pulses quietly. It is a conductor guiding the symphony of hunger, fear, joy, and longing.

Picture the amygdala firing bursts of raw, electric code: the jolt of anxiety when shadows gather, the rush of elation at a lover's touch, the ache of yearning that refuses to be silenced. These are not random sparks but ancient instincts, handed down through a thousand generations, each one a survival strategy etched into our neural circuitry. The cortex does not write the story from scratch. Instead, it interprets the wild weather of the inner world, storms of anger, surges of love, the tidal pull of longing. It also translates them into the language of memory and meaning. It is the storyteller, the archivist, the one who makes sense of chaos and weaves it into a narrative.

To truly understand this is to stand humbled before our biology. The brain does not pit reason against instinct; it marries them in a restless, creative union. Our noblest aspirations—art, invention, compassion—rise not despite desire's heat, but because of it. The same neural pathways that once propelled our ancestors to flee predators or cradle their young now drive us to create symphonies, to seek connection, to reach for meaning in a universe that offers no guarantees.

We are not fallen creatures, forever at war with our impulses. We are living archives, walking testaments to the brutal, beautiful alchemy of endurance. Every longing, every hope, every ache is a chapter in the story of our survival; a reminder that to feel deeply is not a weakness, but the very engine of our becoming.

~

The self is not a statue carved in marble, unmoved by the winds of time. It is a living, breathing story—restless, ever-changing, as fluid as a river winding through the landscape of memory, imagination, and choice. Picture your life not as a single snapshot, but as a film reel, each frame stitched together by unseen hands, flickering with moments of joy, regret, hope, and wonder.

Recall that deep within the parietal lobe, the precuneus works quietly, almost like a film editor in a darkened studio. It pieces together the scenes of our lives, blending the lessons of yesterday with the dreams of tomorrow. The hippocampus, meanwhile, acts as the library's archivist, carefully cataloging our joys and sorrows, preserving the raw material of our experiences. And then there is the prefrontal cortex forever weighing our options, nudging us toward growth or retreat, daring us to imagine a better self, or warning us of the risks ahead.

To know oneself is to wander through a forest of shifting trails. Some paths lead to sunlit clearings of fulfillment, where pride swells, and contentment settles in the chest. Others wind into tangled thickets of frustration, where shame and doubt cast long shadows. Yet the footprints of desire mark each trail, those restless urges that propel us forward or pull us back. The stories we tell about who we are—the pride that buoys us, the shame that shrinks us, the longing that keeps us moving—are all written in the neural script of the brain, inscribed in the language of synapse and signal.

Memory is not a locked vault where the past gathers dust. It is a garden, alive and ever-changing, pruned and reshaped by time, sleep, and emotion. Each night, as we surrender to dreams, the brain tends to the roots of our identity. It strengthens the branches that serve us, letting go of those that no longer fit our evolving story. Like a gardener, we are constantly cultivating, weeding, and replanting the landscape of who we are.

We are, each of us, both the gardener and the garden—endlessly revising, nurturing, and sometimes uprooting the story of who we are becoming. To be human is to live within this dynamic, ever-unfolding narrative. We are not the sum of our past mistakes or our proudest achievements, but the ongoing process of becoming, shaped by the interplay of memory, imagination, and the choices we make each day. The self is not a monument to be admired from afar, but a living forest to be explored, tended, and cherished. Every day, with every thought and every action, we write the next chapter.

We are not solitary islands, adrift and self-contained. We are archipelagos, clusters of experience and memory, bound together by invisible bridges of laughter, rivalry, longing, and love. Across these bridges flow the vital currents of connection, as necessary to our survival as bread or breath. To be human is to be woven into a tapestry of relationships, each thread shimmering with the promise of acceptance or the sting of rejection.

Our brains are sculpted by evolution for communion. The need for connection is not a modern indulgence; it is a fundamental human need. It is an ancient imperative, encoded in the very circuits that govern our survival. Within the amygdala, each encounter is scanned for the faintest signals: a glance that lingers, a smile that falters, a tone that betrays suspicion or trust. The prefrontal cortex, that master juggler, weighs these subtle cues, calculating the risks and rewards of vulnerability. Every moment, we are reading and being read, deciphering the silent language of belonging.

Loneliness is not a mere shadow passing across the mind; it is a physical ache, a visceral alarm that reverberates through the body. When the web of connection frays, the brain cries out in protest. Chronic isolation does not simply dampen the spirit—it carves grooves in the neural landscape, making it harder to reach out, to trust, to hope. The ache of loneliness is as real as hunger, as urgent as thirst. It is the body's plea for reconnection, a biological summons to reconnect.

Yet, when we are welcomed, when a hand clasps ours, when laughter rings out in shared delight, the brain's reward centers ignite. Oxytocin, the so-called "bonding hormone," floods our system, dissolving barriers and reminding us, in a rush of warmth, that to be human is to belong. In these moments, the world feels safer, brighter, and more meaningful.

Empathy is the silent current that runs beneath the surface of every interaction, stitching us together in ways both subtle and profound. Within the folds of the brain, mirror neurons fire not only when we act, but when we witness another's joy or pain. Through these neural echoes, we "catch" each other's moods, our bodies unconsciously mimicking the postures, expressions, and rhythms of those around us. This is the ancient dance of attunement, the choreography of shared feeling.

To empathize is to step into another's shoes, to feel their sorrow as a heaviness in our chest, their laughter as a lightness in our breath. Empathy is not just a moral virtue; it is a biological imperative, a thread that binds us to the fate of others. In the act of feeling with, rather than simply for, we discover what it means to be fully human.

Our lives are tapestries, each strand colored by the people we love, the rivals who challenge us, the strangers who become friends. The need for connection is not a weakness, but our greatest strength—a force that has shaped our brains, our cultures, our very sense of self. We are, each of us, both the weaver and the woven, endlessly creating and recreating the fabric of belonging.

To reach out is to affirm our place in this intricate web of relationships. To listen, to laugh, to grieve together is to honor the ancient truth that we are not meant to walk alone. Ultimately, the measure of our humanity is not found in isolation. It is found in the bridges we build—bridges of empathy, trust, and shared hope—that carry us across the ever-shifting waters of life.

Change is not a thunderclap that splits the sky, transforming us in a single, blinding instant. It is quieter, more patient—a slow, persistent accumulation of small victories. Imagine the mind not as a fortress of stone, but as a living forest: roots stretching deep, branches reaching for light, leaves trembling in the wind of every new experience. Growth here is not sudden, but seasonal. Each act of intention, a skipped dessert, a gentle breath before anger, a solitary walk in place of an old craving, plants a seed, carves a new trail, or clears a tangled path through the neural undergrowth.

This is the miracle of neuroplasticity—the brain's astonishing ability to reshape itself in response to what we do, think, and feel. The forest is never fixed. Each moment of reflection, every deliberate practice, lays down fresh pathways in the thicket of neurons. The act of choosing, again and again, is the sunlight that coaxes new growth from the soil of the self.

Habits are the well-worn tracks of this living forest. Some are sunlit avenues, lined with the flowers of joy and accomplishment. Others are shadowed ruts, carved by repetition and avoidance, so familiar they feel inevitable. Even avoidance itself is a habit. A path we tread so often that it becomes the only way we know. But the forest is not static. With conscious effort and the gentle persistence of daily practice, we can forge new trails, step by step, breath by breath.

Every experience, every challenge, every triumph, and setback is a gardener's hand, sculpting the architecture of the brain. Genetics may set the landscape, but our choices—however small—shape the terrain.

In this ever-shifting forest, self-awareness is the compass that keeps us from getting lost. To pause, to notice, to name what stirs within us—these are not acts of weakness, but of quiet courage. Mindful awareness is the ancient art of observing the mind without trying to control it. It is the willingness to stand still among the trees, to listen for the rustle of old fears and the whisper of new hopes.

Each time we pause before reacting, we widen the space between impulse and action. In that space, we become the architects of our becoming. We choose the next step, the next word, the next breath. We decide whether to follow the old path or strike out in a new direction.

Change, then, is not a destination but a journey—an ongoing exploration of the forest within. It is the slow, patient work of tending to our becoming, of honoring each small victory and forgiving every misstep. The forest grows not by force, but by the steady rhythm of sun and rain, intention and reflection.

To change is to trust in the possibility of new growth, to believe that the smallest acts of care can transform the landscape of the mind. In this way, we are all gardeners of the self, shaping the living forest of who we are, one mindful step at a time.

To change ourselves is to stand at the threshold of a vast and trembling mystery. The promise of science gleams like a lantern in the dusk, illuminating new paths through the tangled forest of our biology. Each breakthrough—a pill, a gene edit, a neural interface—offers the tantalizing prospect of rewriting our own script. Yet, for every bright possibility, there is a shadow: a hushed reminder from the depths of human history that not all that can be done should be done.

Picture the scene: a laboratory humming with the quiet confidence of progress, glass vials catching the morning light. In the next room, a philosopher paces, haunted by the echoes of old stories—Prometheus stealing fire, Icarus soaring too close to the sun. The optimism of science is real, but so is the weight of caution. We are reminded that every tool, every discovery, reverberates with questions as old as myth.

Who, in this new world, decides what is "healthy" or "unhealthy" desire? Is it the physician with a prescription pad, the ethicist with a code, the legislator with a gavel, or the individual with their own aching heart?

The boundaries blur. What was once vice becomes virtue; what was once forbidden becomes fashionable. The fruits of scientific progress—be they therapies for addiction, enhancements for memory, or dampeners for longing—raise the specter of inequality.

Will these gifts be shared, or hoarded behind high walls? Will they liberate, or divide? If we change our cravings, do we change who we are?

The question is not a riddle to be solved, but a landscape to be wandered. Imagine standing in a field at dawn, the mist curling around your ankles. Each step forward is a negotiation between possibility and wisdom, freedom and responsibility, transformation and authenticity. The terrain is uneven, the path uncertain.

The tension between possibility and wisdom often shapes our journeys. The lure of what could be tempts us onward, inviting us to explore new horizons and opportunities. Yet, wisdom quietly reminds us of the unintended consequences that may arise, warning us that stories do not always end as we expect them to. Similarly, the balance between freedom and responsibility is a delicate one.

While the right to shape our minds is a precious gift, we must also recognize our duty to consider the ripples our choices send through our families, communities, and future generations. Lastly, the desire for transformation is exhilarating, offering the chance to become someone new. However, we must ask ourselves what we owe to the person we have been and to the history that is written in our bones, honoring the journey that brought us to this moment.

The power to change is both a shimmering gift and a heavy burden. It asks us to dream boldly of who we might become, to reach for the next branch in the forest of possibility. Yet it also demands that we honor the intricate complexity of who we already are—the scars, the stories, the contradictions that make us human.

To step forward is to walk a tightrope strung between hope and humility. It is to move with both courage and care, knowing that each decision shapes not just our own lives, but the unfolding story of our species. We are the authors and the experiment, the gardeners and the garden.

So we return, as all great journeys do, to a question rather than an answer. As we peer into the shimmering pool of our potential, we must ask: *How do we strike a balance between the urge to transcend our limitations and the wisdom to cherish our imperfections? Where does the path of progress lead—and who do we become, if we follow it to its end?*

The edge of becoming is not a place of certainty, but of wonder. It is here, in the half-light between what is and what might be, that we are called to shape the next chapter of our story—together, and with care.

The journey through desire is not a relentless march toward an unreachable summit of perfection. It is a dance—sometimes graceful, sometimes stumbling—with the beautiful, inescapable imperfections that make us human. In this dance, our struggles are not failures to be hidden or shamed, but invitations to be acknowledged. Each misstep, each pang of longing or regret, is a beckoning hand, urging us to look more closely at the intricate choreography of our minds.

There exists a gap between who we wish to be and who we are—a space often mistaken for a chasm, a place of judgment and self-reproach. *What if, instead, we saw this space as a bridge?*

A living, breathing structure where growth, compassion, and transformation are not only possible but inevitable. On this bridge, we learn to honor our contradictions, to find meaning in the tension between aspiration and reality. It is here, in the crossing, that our deepest learning takes root.

Throughout these pages, we have advocated for a radical shift: from judgment to understanding. The old story—that our behaviors, our cravings, our moments of weakness define us as "bad"—no longer serves us. Instead, we are invited to ask more profound questions.

What stories, told and retold in the quiet chambers of our minds, shape our inclinations?

Which desires, ancient and urgent, propel us toward confident choices?

How can we live not in denial of our wildness, but in partnership with it —intentional, awake, and alive?

This is not a call to abandon responsibility, but to replace shame with curiosity. To see each urge, each stumble, as a clue in the unfolding mystery of who we are. To embrace the science of the self is to accept both our inheritance and our possibility. Our brains are not blank slates, nor are they prisons. They are living archives, shaped by millions of years of evolution—by the struggles and triumphs of ancestors who learned, again and again, to adapt, to connect, to hope.

Every day, we are handed the pen. With each breath, each choice, we write the following line in the story of our lives. Self-awareness is the ink; reflection, the paper. We are not bound to repeat old scripts, nor is our biology a hindrance. Instead, we are offered the chance to edit, revise, and imagine new endings.

To live intentionally is to step onto the dance floor of imperfection, to move with both humility and hope. It is to recognize that our wildness is not an enemy, but a wellspring—a source of creativity, resilience, and connection. In embracing this, we become more than our cravings, more than our mistakes. We become the authors of a story still unfolding, alive to the possibility of change.

So let us move forward—not as judges, but as curious explorers. Let us honor the bridge between who we are and who we wish to be, and walk it with courage. In doing so, we discover that the journey itself—messy, unpredictable, and wondrous—is where growth, compassion, and transformation truly flourish.

As you close this book, picture yourself standing before a mirror within the heart of an ancient forest. The sunlight filters through the canopy in dappled patches, and the air is rich with the earthy scent of moss and rain-soaked leaves. In this quiet, sacred space, you see yourself—not as a battleground where sin and virtue wage endless war, but as a wondrous, evolving being. You are shaped by the intricate dance of biology, memory, and feeling, a living story unfolding with every breath.

Here, desire is not an enemy to be subdued or banished. It is the vital pulse that courses through the core of what it means to be alive. It is the current that moves through your veins, the fire that kindles your creativity, your connection, your very will to live. Desire is the heartbeat of existence itself, a force neither to be feared nor denied, but to be recognized and embraced.

Yet, this moment of reflection is not an ending. The forest around you stretches endlessly, its winding trails disappearing into shadows and sunlight alike. The path ahead is uncharted, full of mystery and possibility. The next step is yours alone to choose. May your journey through the tangled forest of existence be one of discovery, compassion, and wonder. *The story continues—and so do you.*

BIBLIOGRAPHY

This book's referencing is organized in order of appearance.

1. Sescousse G, Caldú X, Segura B, Dreher JC. Processing of primary and secondary rewards: A quantitative meta-analysis and review of human functional neuroimaging studies. *Neuroscience & Biobehavioral Reviews*. 2013;37(4):681-696. doi:https://doi.org/10.1016/j.neubiorev.2013.02.002
2. Zeki S. The neurobiology of love. *FEBS Letters*. 2007;581(14):2575-2579. doi:https://doi.org/10.1016/j.febslet.2007.03.094
3. Roney JR, Simmons ZL. Hormonal predictors of sexual motivation in natural menstrual cycles. *Hormones and Behavior*. 2013;63(4):636-645. doi:https://doi.org/10.1016/j.yhbeh.2013.02.013
4. Willis J, Todorov A. First impressions: Making up your mind after a 100-ms exposure to a face. *Psychological Science*. 2006;17(7):592-598. doi:https://doi.org/10.1111/j.1467-9280.2006.01750.x
5. Georgiadis JR, Kringelbach ML. The human sexual response cycle: Brain imaging evidence linking sex to other pleasures. *Progress in Neurobiology*. 2012;98(1):49-81. doi:https://doi.org/10.1016/j.pneurobio.2012.05.004
6. Acevedo BP, Aron A, Fisher HE, Brown LL. Neural correlates of long-term intense romantic love. *Social Cognitive and Affective Neuroscience*. 2011;7(2):145-159. doi:https://doi.org/10.1093/scan/nsq092
7. Berke JD. What does dopamine mean? *Nature Neuroscience*. 2018;21(6):787-793. doi:https://doi.org/10.1038/s41593-018-0152-y
8. Aron A, Fisher H, Mashek DJ, Strong G, Li H, Brown LL. Reward, Motivation, and Emotion Systems Associated with Early-Stage Intense Romantic Love. *Journal of Neurophysiology*. 2005;94(1):327-337. doi:https://doi.org/10.1152/jn.00838.2004
9. Heatherton TF, Wagner DD. Cognitive neuroscience of self-regulation failure. *Trends in Cognitive Sciences*. 2011;15(3):132-139. doi:https://doi.org/10.1016/j.tics.2010.12.005
10. Wang Y, Song X, Chen X, et al. Integrating reproductive states and social cues in the control of sociosexual behaviors. *Cell*. 2025;188(13):3530-3549.e24. doi:https://doi.org/10.1016/j.cell.2025.04.035
11. Pfaus JG. REVIEWS: Pathways of Sexual Desire. *The Journal of Sexual Medicine*. 2009;6(6):1506-1533. doi:https://doi.org/10.1111/j.1743-6109.2009.01309.x
12. Wiktor Bogacki-Rychlik, Katarzyna Gawęda, Bialy M. Neurophysiology of male sexual arousal—Behavioral perspective. *Frontiers in behavioral neuroscience*. 2024;17. doi:https://doi.org/10.3389/fnbeh.2023.1330460
13. Sander D, Grafman J, Zalla T. The Human Amygdala: An Evolved System

for Relevance Detection. *Reviews in the Neurosciences*. 2003;14(4). doi:https://doi.org/10.1515/revneuro.2003.14.4.303

14. Phelps EA. Human emotion and memory: interactions of the amygdala and hippocampal complex. *Current Opinion in Neurobiology*. 2004;14(2):198-202. doi:https://doi.org/10.1016/j.conb.2004.03.015
15. Dennerstein L, Goldstein I. GUEST EDITORIAL: Postmenopausal Female Sexual Dysfunction: At a Crossroads. *The Journal of Sexual Medicine*. 2005;2:116-117. doi:https://doi.org/10.1111/j.1743-6109.2005.00127.x
16. Meston CM, Frohlich PF. The neurobiology of sexual function. *Archives of general psychiatry*. 2000;57(11):1012-1030. doi:https://doi.org/10.1001/archpsyc.57.11.1012
17. Šimić G, Tkalčić M, Vukić V, et al. Understanding Emotions: Origins and Roles of the Amygdala. *Biomolecules*. 2021;11(6):823. doi:https://doi.org/10.3390/biom11060823
18. Goel M, Mittal A, Vijaya Raje Jain, et al. Integrative Functions of the Hypothalamus: Linking Cognition, Emotion and Physiology for Well-being and Adaptability. *Annals of neurosciences*. 2024;32(2). doi:https://doi.org/10.1177/09727531241255492
19. Hiller-Sturmhöfel S, Bartke A. The Endocrine System: An Overview. *Alcohol Health and Research World*. 1998;22(3):153. https://pmc.ncbi.nlm.nih.gov/articles/PMC6761896/
20. MOTOFEI IG, ROWLAND DL. The physiological basis of human sexual arousal: neuroendocrine sexual asymmetry. *International Journal of Andrology*. 2005;28(2):78-87. doi:https://doi.org/10.1111/j.1365-2605.2004.00514.x
21. Cleveland Clinic. Parasympathetic nervous system (PSNS): What it is & function. Cleveland Clinic. Published June 6, 2022. https://my.clevelandclinic.org/health/body/23266-parasympathetic-nervous-system-psns
22. Lorenz TA, Harte CB, Hamilton LD, Meston CM. Evidence for a curvilinear relationship between sympathetic nervous system activation and women's physiological sexual arousal. *Psychophysiology*. 2011;49(1):111-117. doi:https://doi.org/10.1111/j.1469-8986.2011.01285.x
23. Goldstein I. The Central Mechanisms of Sexual Function» Sexual Medicine» BUMC. www.bumc.bu.edu. https://www.bumc.bu.edu/sexualmedicine/publications/the-central-mechanisms-of-sexual-function/
24. Purves D, Augustine GJ, Fitzpatrick D, et al. Autonomic Regulation of Sexual Function. *Neuroscience 2nd edition*. Published online 2001. https://www.ncbi.nlm.nih.gov/books/NBK11157/
25. Calabrò RS, Cacciola A, Bruschetta D, et al. Neuroanatomy and function of human sexual behavior: A neglected or unknown issue? *Brain and Behavior*. 2019;9(12). doi:https://doi.org/10.1002/brb3.1389
26. Lewis RG, Florio E, Punzo D, Borrelli E. The Brain's Reward System in Health and Disease. *Advances in Experimental Medicine and Biology*. 2021;1344(1344):57-69. doi:https://doi.org/10.1007/978-3-030-81147-1_4

27. Oei NYL, Rombouts SA, Soeter RP, van Gerven JM, Both S. Dopamine Modulates Reward System Activity During Subconscious Processing of Sexual Stimuli. *Neuropsychopharmacology*. 2012;37(7):1729-1737. doi:https://doi.org/10.1038/npp.2012.19
28. Komisaruk BR, Rodriguez del Cerro MC. How Does Our Brain Generate Sexual Pleasure? *International Journal of Sexual Health*. 2021;33(4):1-10. doi:https://doi.org/10.1080/19317611.2021.1989534
29. Schreyach M. *History and Desire: A Short Introduction to the Art of Cy Twombly* .; 2017. https://digitalcommons.trinity.edu/cgi/viewcontent.cgi?article=1065&context=mono
30. Laios K;Tsoucalas G;Kontaxaki MI;Karamanou M;Sgantzos M;Androutsos G. Mental health and sexual activity according to ancient Greek physicians. *Psychiatrike = Psychiatriki*. 2015;26(3). https://pubmed.ncbi.nlm.nih.gov/26480224/
31. Stephen D, Chang T. *THE BOOK of INFINITE WISDOM*. Accessed July 21, 2025. https://www.obafemio.com/uploads/5/1/4/2/5142021/tao_of_sexology.pdf
32. Cohut M. Sex: How does it impact brain activity? www.medicalnewstoday.com. Published April 6, 2018. https://www.medicalnewstoday.com/articles/321428
33. Pawluski JL, Kokras N, Charlier TD, Dalla C. Sex matters in neuroscience and neuropsychopharmacology. *European Journal of Neuroscience*. 2020;52(1):2423-2428. doi:https://doi.org/10.1111/ejn.14880
34. Fuchshuber J, Jauk E, Hiebler-Ragger M, Unterrainer HF. The Affective Neuroscience of Sexuality: Development of a LUST Scale. *Frontiers in Human Neuroscience*. 2022;16. doi:https://doi.org/10.3389/fnhum.2022.853706
35. Inoue S. Hormonal and circuit mechanisms controlling female sexual behavior. *Frontiers in neural circuits*. 2024;18. doi:https://doi.org/10.3389/fncir.2024.1409349
36. Sisk CL, Zehr JL. Pubertal hormones organize the adolescent brain and behavior. *Frontiers in Neuroendocrinology*. 2005;26(3-4):163-174. doi:https://doi.org/10.1016/j.yfrne.2005.10.003
37. Arnold AP. The organizational–activational hypothesis as the foundation for a unified theory of sexual differentiation of all mammalian tissues. *Hormones and Behavior*. 2009;55(5):570-578. doi:https://doi.org/10.1016/j.yhbeh.2009.03.011
38. Puts DA. Cyclic variation in women's preferences for masculine traits. *Human Nature*. 2006;17(1):114-127. doi:https://doi.org/10.1007/s12110-006-1023-x
39. Roney JR, Simmons ZL. Women's estradiol predicts preference for facial cues of men's testosterone. *Hormones and Behavior*. 2008;53(1):14-19. doi:https://doi.org/10.1016/j.yhbeh.2007.09.008
40. Dreher JC, Schmidt PJ, Kohn P, Furman D, Rubinow D, Berman KF. Menstrual cycle phase modulates reward-related neural function in women. *Proceedings of the National Academy of Sciences of the United States of America*. 2007;104(7):2465-2470. doi:https://doi.org/10.1073/pnas.0605569104

41. Grebe NM, Sarafin RE, Strenth CR, Zilioli S. Pair-bonding, fatherhood, and the role of testosterone: A meta-analytic review. *Neuroscience & Biobehavioral Reviews*. 2019;98:221-233. doi:https://doi.org/10.1016/j.neubiorev.2019.01.010
42. Babak R, Rasmus B, Saad E. Marital Status and Serum Level of Testosterone: In Relation to Serum Level of Cortisol. *Archive of Urological Research*. 2024;8(2):018-022. doi:https://doi.org/10.17352/aur.000052
43. Gettler LT, McDade TW, Feranil AB, Kuzawa CW. Longitudinal evidence that fatherhood decreases testosterone in human males. *Proceedings of the National Academy of Sciences*. 2011;108(39):16194-16199. doi:https://doi.org/10.1073/pnas.1105403108
44. Muller MN, Marlowe FW, Bugumba R, Ellison PT. Testosterone and paternal care in East African foragers and pastoralists. *Proceedings of the Royal Society B: Biological Sciences*. 2008;276(1655):347-354. doi:https://doi.org/10.1098/rspb.2008.1028
45. Komisaruk BR, Whipple B, Crawford A, et al. Brain activation during vaginocervical self-stimulation and orgasm in women with complete spinal cord injury: fMRI evidence of mediation by the Vagus nerves. *Brain Research*. 2004;1024(1-2):77-88. doi:https://doi.org/10.1016/j.brainres.2004.07.029
46. Georgiadis JR, Reinders AATS, Paans AMJ, Renken R, Kortekaas R. Men versus women on sexual brain function: Prominent differences during tactile genital stimulation, but not during orgasm. *Human Brain Mapping*. 2009;30(10):3089-3101. doi:https://doi.org/10.1002/hbm.20733
47. Wise NJ, Frangos E, Komisaruk BR. Brain Activity Unique to Orgasm in Women: An fMRI Analysis. *The Journal of Sexual Medicine*. 2017;14(11):1380-1391. doi:https://doi.org/10.1016/j.jsxm.2017.08.014
48. Pfaus JG. Orgasms, sexual pleasure, and opioid reward mechanisms. *Sexual Medicine Reviews*. Published online May 8, 2025. doi:https://doi.org/10.1093/sxmrev/qeaf023
49. Coria-Avila GA, Herrera-Covarrubias D, Ismail N, Pfaus JG. The role of orgasm in the development and shaping of partner preferences. *Socioaffective Neuroscience & Psychology*. 2016;6(1):31815. doi:https://doi.org/10.3402/snp.v6.31815
50. Komisaruk BR, Beyer C, Whipple B. Orgasm. BPS. Published 2008. https://www.bps.org.uk/psychologist/orgasm
51. Alonso-Alonso M, Woods SC, Pelchat M, et al. Food reward system: current perspectives and future research needs. *Nutrition Reviews*. 2015;73(5):296-307. doi:https://doi.org/10.1093/nutrit/nuv002
52. Rupp HA, James TW, Ketterson ED, Sengelaub DR, Janssen E, Heiman JR. The role of the anterior cingulate cortex in women's sexual decision making. *Neuroscience Letters*. 2009;449(1):42-47. doi:https://doi.org/10.1016/j.neulet.2008.10.083
53. Brody S, Krüger THC. The post-orgasmic prolactin increase following intercourse is greater than following masturbation and suggests greater satiety. *Biological Psychology*. 2006;71(3):312-315. doi:https://doi.org/10.1016/j.biopsycho.2005.06.008

54. Margolis E. Women with persistent genital arousal disorder: "People hear orgasm and they think it's a good thing." the Guardian. Published April 14, 2014. Accessed July 21, 2025. https://www.theguardian.com/lifeandstyle/2014/apr/14/women-persistent-genital-arousal-disorder-orgasm-pgad-pain
55. Jewell T. Persistent Genital Arousal Disorder (PGAD) Explained. Healthline. Published June 26, 2023. Accessed July 21, 2025. https://www.healthline.com/health/persistent-genital-arousal-disorder
56. McCoy D. Scientists uncover neurobiological basis for romantic love, trust, and self. EurekAlert! Published November 10, 2003. Accessed July 21, 2025. https://www.eurekalert.org/news-releases/612778
57. Fisher HE, Aron A, Brown LL. Romantic love: a mammalian brain system for mate choice. *Philosophical Transactions of the Royal Society B: Biological Sciences*. 2006;361(1476):2173-2186. doi:https://doi.org/10.1098/rstb.2006.1938
58. Seshadri KG. The neuroendocrinology of love. *Indian Journal of Endocrinology and Metabolism*. 2016;20(4):558-563. doi:https://doi.org/10.4103/2230-8210.183479
59. LeWine H. Oxytocin: The love hormone. Harvard Health. Published June 13, 2023. https://www.health.harvard.edu/mind-and-mood/oxytocin-the-love-hormone
60. Johnson MC, Zweig JA, Zhang Y, et al. Effects of oxytocin receptor agonism on acquisition and expression of pair bonding in male prairie voles. *Translational Psychiatry*. 2024;14(1). doi:https://doi.org/10.1038/s41398-024-02993-x
61. Insel TR, Winslow JT, Wang Z, Young LJ. Oxytocin, Vasopressin, and the Neuroendocrine Basis of Pair Bond Formation. *Advances in Experimental Medicine and Biology*. Published online 1998:215-224. doi:https://doi.org/10.1007/978-1-4615-4871-3_28
62. Winslow JT, Hastings N, Carter CS, Harbaugh CR, Insel TR. A role for central vasopressin in pair bonding in monogamous prairie voles. *Nature*. 1993;365(6446):545-548. doi:https://doi.org/10.1038/365545a0
63. MARAZZITI D, AKISKAL HS, ROSSI A, CASSANO GB. Alteration of the platelet serotonin transporter in romantic love. *Psychological Medicine*. 1999;29(3):741-745. doi:https://doi.org/10.1017/s0033291798007946
64. Meghna R. International Journal of Scientific Research and Technology. *International Journal of Scientific Research and Technology*. 2025;03(01):1-1. doi:https://doi.org/10.5281/zenodo.14680744
65. Song H, Zou Z, Kou J, et al. Love-related changes in the brain: a resting-state functional magnetic resonance imaging study. *Frontiers in Human Neuroscience*. 2015;9(9). doi:https://doi.org/10.3389/fnhum.2015.00071
66. Wang C, Song S, d'Oleire Uquillas F, et al. Altered brain network organization in romantic love as measured with resting-state fMRI and graph theory. *Brain Imaging and Behavior*. 2020;14(6):2771-2784. doi:https://doi.org/10.1007/s11682-019-00226-0

67. Stony Brook University. Love Can Last: SBU Imaging Study Shows Brain Activity Of Those In Love Long Term Similar To Those Newly In Love - SBU News. SBU News - News & Features at Stony Brook University. Published January 7, 2011. https://news.stonybrook.edu/newsroom/press-release/general/010711lovecanlast/
68. Li L, Huang X, Xiao J, et al. Neural synchronization predicts marital satisfaction. *Proceedings of the National Academy of Sciences of the United States of America*. 2022;119(34):e2202515119. doi:https://doi.org/10.1073/pnas.2202515119
69. Pauly T, Michalowski VI, Drewelies J, et al. LINKS BETWEEN PARTNER INTERACTIONS, EMPATHY, AND EVERYDAY PHYSIOLOGICAL SYNCHRONY IN OLDER COUPLES. *Innovation in Aging*. 2019;3(Supplement_1):S435-S436. doi:https://doi.org/10.1093/geroni/igz038.1629
70. Schneiderman I, Zagoory-Sharon O, Leckman JF, Feldman R. Oxytocin during the initial stages of romantic attachment: Relations to couples' interactive reciprocity. *Psychoneuroendocrinology*. 2012;37(8):1277-1285. doi:https://doi.org/10.1016/j.psyneuen.2011.12.021
71. Ortigue S, Bianchi-Demicheli F. Why is your spouse so predictable? Connecting mirror neuron system and self-expansion model of love. *Medical Hypotheses*. 2008;71(6):941-944. doi:https://doi.org/10.1016/j.mehy.2008.07.016
72. Eckstein M, Stößel G, Gerchen MF, Bilek E, Kirsch P, Ditzen B. Neural responses to instructed positive couple interaction: an fMRI study on compliment sharing. *Social Cognitive and Affective Neuroscience*. 2023;18(1). doi:https://doi.org/10.1093/scan/nsad005
73. Pfaus JG, Safron A, Zakreski E. From distal to proximal to interactive: behavioral and brain synchrony during attraction, courtship, and sexual interaction—implications for clinical assessments of relationship style and quality. *Sexual Medicine Reviews*. 2023;11(4):312-322. doi:https://doi.org/10.1093/sxmrev/qead034
74. Coutinho J, Pereira A, Oliveira-Silva P, Meier D, Lourenço V, Tschacher W. When our hearts beat together: Cardiac synchrony as an entry point to understand dyadic co-regulation in couples. *Psychophysiology*. 2020;58(3). doi:https://doi.org/10.1111/psyp.13739
75. Sened H, Zilcha-Mano S, Shamay-Tsoory S. Inter-brain plasticity as a biological mechanism of change in psychotherapy: A review and integrative model. *Frontiers in Human Neuroscience*. 2022;16. doi:https://doi.org/10.3389/fnhum.2022.955238
76. Trovão JN, Serefoglu EC. Neurobiology of male sexual dysfunctions in psychiatric disorders: the cases of depression, anxiety, mania and schizophrenia. *International Journal of Impotence Research*. 2018;30(6):279-286. doi:https://doi.org/10.1038/s41443-018-0077-8
77. Simonsen U, Comerma-Steffensen S, Andersson KE. Modulation of Dopaminergic Pathways to Treat Erectile Dysfunction. *Basic & Clinical Pharmacology & Toxicology*. 2016;119:63-74. doi:https://doi.org/10.1111/bcpt.12653

78. Yang JC. Functional Neuroanatomy in Depressed Patients with Sexual Dysfunction: Blood Oxygenation Level Dependent Functional MR Imaging. *Korean Journal of Radiology*. 2004;5(2):87. doi:https://doi.org/10.3348/kjr.2004.5.2.87
79. Ferranti EP, Dunbar SB, Dunlop AL, Corwin EJ. 20 Things you Didn't Know About the Human gut Microbiome. *The Journal of Cardiovascular Nursing*. 2014;29(6):479-481. doi:https://doi.org/10.1097/jcn.0000000000000166
80. Campos A, Port JD, Acosta A. Integrative Hedonic and Homeostatic Food Intake Regulation by the Central Nervous System: Insights from Neuroimaging. *Brain Sciences*. 2022;12(4):431. doi:https://doi.org/10.3390/brainsci12040431
81. Lutter M, Nestler EJ. Homeostatic and Hedonic Signals Interact in the Regulation of Food Intake. *The Journal of Nutrition*. 2009;139(3):629-632. doi:https://doi.org/10.3945/jn.108.097618
82. Rossi MA, Stuber GD. Overlapping Brain Circuits for Homeostatic and Hedonic Feeding. *Cell Metabolism*. 2018;27(1):42-56. doi:https://doi.org/10.1016/j.cmet.2017.09.021
83. Gunnars K. Leptin and Leptin Resistance: Everything You Need to Know. Healthline. Published December 4, 2018. https://www.healthline.com/nutrition/leptin-101
84. Näslund E, Bogefors J, Skogar S, et al. GLP-1 slows solid gastric emptying and inhibits insulin, glucagon, and PYY release in humans. *American Journal of Physiology-Regulatory, Integrative and Comparative Physiology*. 1999;277(3):R910-R916. doi:https://doi.org/10.1152/ajpregu.1999.277.3.r910
85. Peikin SR. Role of cholecystokinin in the control of food intake. *Gastroenterology clinics of North America*. 2021;18(4). https://pubmed.ncbi.nlm.nih.gov/2693351/
86. Picó C, Palou M, Pomar CA, Rodríguez AM, Palou A. Leptin as a key regulator of the adipose organ. *Reviews in Endocrine and Metabolic Disorders*. 2021;23(1). doi:https://doi.org/10.1007/s11154-021-09687-5
87. Moran TH, Kinzig KP. Gastrointestinal satiety signals II. Cholecystokinin. *American Journal of Physiology-Gastrointestinal and Liver Physiology*. 2004;286(2):G183-G188. doi:https://doi.org/10.1152/ajpgi.00434.2003
88. Nauck MA, Niedereichholz U, Ettler R, et al. Glucagon-like peptide 1 inhibition of gastric emptying outweighs its insulinotropic effects in healthy humans. *The American Journal of Physiology*. 1997;273(5):E981-988. doi:https://doi.org/10.1152/ajpendo.1997.273.5.E981
89. Cork SC. The role of the vagus nerve in appetite control: Implications for the pathogenesis of obesity. *Journal of Neuroendocrinology*. 2018;30(11):e12643. doi:https://doi.org/10.1111/jne.12643
90. Ueno H, Nakazato M. Mechanistic relationship between the vagal afferent pathway, central nervous system and peripheral organs in appetite regulation. *Journal of Diabetes Investigation*. 2016;7(6):812-818. doi:https://doi.org/10.1111/jdi.12492
91. Madison A, Kiecolt-Glaser JK. Stress, depression, diet, and the gut microbiota: human–bacteria interactions at the core of

psychoneuroimmunology and nutrition. *Current Opinion in Behavioral Sciences*. 2019;28(3):105-110. doi:https://doi.org/10.1016/j.cobeha.2019.01.011

92. Epel E, Lapidus R, McEwen B, Brownell K. Stress may add bite to appetite in women: a laboratory study of stress-induced cortisol and eating behavior. *Psychoneuroendocrinology*. 2001;26(1):37-49. doi:https://doi.org/10.1016/s0306-4530(00)00035-4
93. Sominsky L, Spencer SJ. Eating behavior and stress: a pathway to obesity. *Frontiers in Psychology*. 2014;5(434). doi:https://doi.org/10.3389/fpsyg.2014.00434
94. Min S, Than N, Shin YC, et al. Live probiotic bacteria administered in a pathomimetic Leaky Gut Chip ameliorate impaired epithelial barrier and mucosal inflammation. *Scientific Reports*. 2022;12(1). doi:https://doi.org/10.1038/s41598-022-27300-w
95. Federica Di Vincenzo, Angelo Del Gaudio, Petito V, Loris Riccardo Lopetuso, Franco Scaldaferri. Gut microbiota, intestinal permeability, and systemic inflammation: A narrative review. *Internal and Emergency Medicine*. 2023;19(2):275-293. doi:https://doi.org/10.1007/s11739-023-03374-w
96. McKlveen JM, Morano RL, Fitzgerald M, et al. Chronic Stress Increases Prefrontal Inhibition: A Mechanism for Stress-Induced Prefrontal Dysfunction. *Biological Psychiatry*. 2016;80(10):754-764. doi:https://doi.org/10.1016/j.biopsych.2016.03.2101
97. Tryon MS, Carter CS, DeCant R, Laugero KD. Chronic stress exposure may affect the brain's response to high calorie food cues and predispose to obesogenic eating habits. *Physiology & Behavior*. 2013;120:233-242. doi:https://doi.org/10.1016/j.physbeh.2013.08.010
98. Elzinga SE, Henn R, Murdock BJ, et al. cGAS/STING and innate brain inflammation following acute high-fat feeding. *Frontiers in immunology*. 2022;13:1012594. doi:https://doi.org/10.3389/fimmu.2022.1012594
99. Pursey KM, Contreras-Rodriguez O, Collins CE, Stanwell P, Burrows TL. Food Addiction Symptoms and Amygdala Response in Fasted and Fed States. *Nutrients*. 2019;11(6):1285. doi:https://doi.org/10.3390/nu11061285
100. Nakamura Y, Koike S. Daily fat intake is associated with basolateral amygdala response to high-calorie food cues and appetite for high-calorie food. *Nutritional neuroscience*. Published online September 20, 2023:1-9. doi:https://doi.org/10.1080/1028415x.2023.2260585
101. de Pablos RM. Stress Increases Vulnerability to Inflammation in the Rat Prefrontal Cortex. *Journal of Neuroscience*. 2006;26(21):5709-5719. doi:https://doi.org/10.1523/jneurosci.0802-06.2006
102. Laugero K. USDA ARS Online Magazine Vol. 62, No. 10. Usda.gov. Published 2025. Accessed July 21, 2025. https://agresearchmag.ars.usda.gov/2014/nov/foods
103. Iikuni N, Kwan Lam Q, Lu L, Matarese G, Cava A. Leptin and Inflammation. *Current Immunology Reviews*. 2008;4(2):70-79. doi:https://doi.org/10.2174/157339508784325046

104. Pérez-Pérez A, Sánchez-Jiménez F, Vilariño-García T, Sánchez-Margalet V. Role of Leptin in Inflammation and Vice Versa. *International Journal of Molecular Sciences*. 2020;21(16). doi:https://doi.org/10.3390/ijms21165887

105. Gómez WA, Humeres G, Orozco-Castaño CA, et al. Leptin Signaling and Its Relationship with Obesity-induced Insulin Resistance: A Bioinformatics-assisted Review. *Gene Expression*. 2024;000(000). doi:https://doi.org/10.14218/ge.2024.00039

106. Chao AM, Jastreboff AM, White MA, Grilo CM, Sinha R. Stress, cortisol, and other appetite-related hormones: Prospective prediction of 6-month changes in food cravings and weight. *Obesity*. 2017;25(4):713-720. https://dx.doi.org/10.1002%2Foby.21790

107. Hall KD. Ultra-Processed Diets Cause Excess Calorie Intake and Weight Gain: An Inpatient Randomized Controlled Trial of Ad Libitum Food Intake. *Cell Metabolism*. 2019;30(1). doi:https://doi.org/10.1016/j.cmet.2019.05.008

108. Bettadapura S, Dowling K, Jablon K, Al-Humadi AW, le Roux CW. Changes in food preferences and ingestive behaviors after glucagon-like peptide-1 analog treatment: techniques and opportunities. *International Journal of Obesity*. Published online March 7, 2024:1-9. doi:https://doi.org/10.1038/s41366-024-01500-y

109. B. C. Brain scans reveal junk food damages hunger control centers, fueling overeating – NaturalNews.com. NaturalNews.com. Published July 2025. Accessed July 21, 2025. https://www.naturalnews.com/2025-07-01-brain-scans-junk-food-hunger-overeating.html

110. Filip Morys, Arsene Kanyamibwa, Fängström D, et al. Ultra-processed food consumption affects structural integrity of feeding-related brain regions independent of and via adiposity. *npj Metabolic Health and Disease*. 2025;3(1). doi:https://doi.org/10.1038/s44324-025-00056-3

111. Bairqdar A, Shakhtshneider E, Dinara Ivanoshchuk, et al. Rare Variants of Obesity-Associated Genes in Young Adults with Abdominal Obesity. *Journal of Personalized Medicine*. 2023;13(10):1500-1500. doi:https://doi.org/10.3390/jpm13101500

112. Melhorn SJ, Askren MK, Chung WK, et al. FTO genotype impacts food intake and corticolimbic activation. *The American Journal of Clinical Nutrition*. 2018;107(2):145-154. doi:https://doi.org/10.1093/ajcn/nqx029

113. Szalanczy AM, Key CCC, Solberg Woods LC. Genetic variation in satiety signaling and hypothalamic inflammation: merging fields for the study of obesity. *The Journal of Nutritional Biochemistry*. 2022;101:108928. doi:https://doi.org/10.1016/j.jnutbio.2021.108928

114. Czogała W, Strojny W, Schab M, et al. FTO and PLAG1 Genes Expression and FTO Methylation Predict Changes in Circulating Levels of Adipokines and Gastrointestinal Peptides in Children. *Nutrients*. 2021;13(10):3585. doi:https://doi.org/10.3390/nu13103585

115. Jesús Gustavo Ponce-González, Á. Martínez-Ávila, Velázquez-Díaz D, et al. Impact of the FTO Gene Variation on Appetite and Fat Oxidation in Young

Adults. *Nutrients*. 2023;15(9):2037-2037. doi:https://doi.org/10.3390/nu15092037

116. Loos RJF, Yeo GSH. The genetics of obesity: from discovery to biology. *Nature Reviews Genetics*. 2021;23(23):1-14. doi:https://doi.org/10.1038/s41576-021-00414-z
117. Wardle J, Carnell S, Haworth CMA, Farooqi IS, O'Rahilly S, Plomin R. Obesity Associated Genetic Variation inFTOIs Associated with Diminished Satiety. *The Journal of Clinical Endocrinology & Metabolism*. 2008;93(9):3640-3643. doi:https://doi.org/10.1210/jc.2008-0472
118. Luengo N, Goldfield GS, Obregón AM. Association between dopamine genes, adiposity, food addiction, and eating behavior in Chilean adult. *Frontiers in Nutrition*. 2024;11. doi:https://doi.org/10.3389/fnut.2024.1466384
119. Romer AL, Su Kang M, Nikolova YS, Gearhardt AN, Hariri AR. Dopamine genetic risk is related to food addiction and body mass through reduced reward-related ventral striatum activity. *Appetite*. 2019;133:24-31. doi:https://doi.org/10.1016/j.appet.2018.09.010
120. Obregón AM, Valladares Vega MA, Goldfield G, Llewellyn C. Genetic variation of the dopamine D2 receptor gene: association with the reinforcing value of food and eating in the absence of hunger in Chilean children. *Nutrición Hospitalaria*. Published online 2020. doi:https://doi.org/10.20960/nh.02897
121. Godoy M. NPR Choice page. Npr.org. Published 2019. https://www.npr.org/sections/thesalt/2019/05/16/723693839/its-not-just-salt-sugar-fat-study-finds-ultra-processed-foods-drive-weight-gain
122. Thompson D. Temptation Alley: Checkout Counters Are Prime Spots for Unhealthy Food Piedmont Orthopedics | OrthoAtlanta. Edreamz Echo Demo. Published 2023. Accessed July 21, 2025. https://www.orthoatlanta.com/health-news/temptation-alley-checkout-counters-are-prime-spots-for-unhealthy-food
123. Nikos KM. Temptation at the Checkout: 70% of Food, Drinks Within Arm's Reach Are Unhealthy. UC Davis. Published June 7, 2023. https://www.ucdavis.edu/curiosity/news/temptation-checkout-70-food-drinks-within-arms-reach-are-unhealthy
124. DeJarnette P. Temptation over time: Delays help. *Journal of Economic Behavior & Organization*. 2020;177:752-761. doi:https://doi.org/10.1016/j.jebo.2020.06.027
125. Hall KD. Ultra-Processed Diets Cause Excess Calorie Intake and Weight Gain: An Inpatient Randomized Controlled Trial of Ad Libitum Food Intake. *Cell Metabolism*. 2019;30(1). doi:https://doi.org/10.1016/j.cmet.2019.05.008
126. Führer D, Zysset S, Stumvoll M. Brain Activity in Hunger and Satiety: An Exploratory Visually Stimulated fMRI Study. *Obesity*. 2008;16(5):945-950. doi:https://doi.org/10.1038/oby.2008.33
127. Alexandre Pastor-Bernier, Stasiak A, Schultz W. Reward-specific satiety affects subjective value signals in orbitofrontal cortex during

multicomponent economic choice. *Proceedings of the National Academy of Sciences*. 2021;118(30). doi:https://doi.org/10.1073/pnas.2022650118

128. Simon JJ, Müller T, Schöner F, Bendszus M, Friederich HC. Savoring Satiety: The Neural Correlates of Sensory Specific Satiety. Published online 2024. doi:https://doi.org/10.2139/ssrn.5046338
129. Embling R, Pink AE, Gatzemeier J, Price M, D Lee M, Wilkinson LL. Effect of food variety on intake of a meal: a systematic review and meta-analysis. *The American Journal of Clinical Nutrition*. 2021;113(3):716-741. doi:https://doi.org/10.1093/ajcn/nqaa352
130. Steenhuis IH, Vermeer WM. Portion size: review and framework for interventions. *International Journal of Behavioral Nutrition and Physical Activity*. 2009;6(1):58. doi:https://doi.org/10.1186/1479-5868-6-58
131. Robinson E, Aveyard P, Daley A, et al. Eating attentively: a systematic review and meta-analysis of the effect of food intake memory and awareness on eating. *The American Journal of Clinical Nutrition*. 2013;97(4):728-742. doi:https://doi.org/10.3945/ajcn.112.045245
132. Garg D, Smith E, Attuquayefio T. Watching Television While Eating Increases Food Intake: A Systematic Review and Meta-Analysis of Experimental Studies. *Nutrients*. 2025;17(1):166. doi:https://doi.org/10.3390/nu17010166
133. Hendriks AEM, Nederkoorn C, van Lier IMJ, van Belkom B, Bast A, Havermans RC. Sensory-specific satiety, the variety effect and physical context: Does change of context during a meal enhance food intake? *Appetite*. 2021;163:105179. doi:https://doi.org/10.1016/j.appet.2021.105179
134. Minère M, Wilhelms H, Bojana Kuzmanovic, et al. Thalamic opioids from POMC satiety neurons switch on sugar appetite. *Science*. 2025;387(6735):750-758. doi:https://doi.org/10.1126/science.adp1510
135. Max Planck Institute for Metabolism Research. Dessert stomach emerges in the brain. Www.mpg.de. Published 2025. https://www.mpg.de/24159607/0211-neur-dessert-stomach-emerges-in-the-brain-153735-x
136. Arcego DM, Krolow R, Lampert C, et al. Chronic high-fat diet affects food-motivated behavior and hedonic systems in the nucleus accumbens of male rats. *Appetite*. 2020;153:104739. doi:https://doi.org/10.1016/j.appet.2020.104739
137. Slomp M. *UvA-DARE (Digital Academic Repository) Decoding the Control of Food Intake.*; 2024. Accessed July 21, 2025. https://pure.uva.nl/ws/files/149956260/8.pdf
138. Stamatakis AM, Van Swieten M, Basiri ML, Blair GA, Kantak P, Stuber GD. Lateral Hypothalamic Area Glutamatergic Neurons and Their Projections to the Lateral Habenula Regulate Feeding and Reward. *Journal of Neuroscience*. 2016;36(2):302-311. doi:https://doi.org/10.1523/jneurosci.1202-15.2016
139. Gazit Shimoni, Neta, Tose AJ, Seng C, et al. Changes in neurotensin signalling drive hedonic devaluation in obesity. *Nature*. Published online March 26, 2025:1-10. doi:https://doi.org/10.1038/s41586-025-08748-y
140. Wu Y, Chen C, Chen M, et al. The anterior insular cortex unilaterally controls feeding in response to aversive visceral stimuli in mice. *Nature*

Communications. 2020;11(1):640. doi:https://doi.org/10.1038/s41467-020-14281-5

141. Kayyal H, Yiannakas A, Kolatt Chandran S, Khamaisy M, Sharma V, Rosenblum K. Activity of Insula to Basolateral Amygdala Projecting Neurons is Necessary and Sufficient for Taste Valence Representation. *The Journal of Neuroscience*. 2019;39(47):9369-9382. doi:https://doi.org/10.1523/jneurosci.0752-19.2019
142. Haley MS, Bruno S, Fontanini A, Maffei A. LTD at amygdalocortical synapses as a novel mechanism for hedonic learning. *eLife*. 2020;9. doi:https://doi.org/10.7554/elife.55175
143. Cubero I, Thiele TE, Bernstein IL. Insular cortex lesions and taste aversion learning: effects of conditioning method and timing of lesion. *Brain Research*. 1999;839(2):323-330. doi:https://doi.org/10.1016/s0006-8993(99)01745-x
144. Schafe GE, Thiele TE, Bernstein IL. Conditioning Method Dramatically Alters the Role of Amygdala in Taste Aversion Learning. *Learning & Memory*. 1998;5(6):481. Accessed July 21, 2025. https://pmc.ncbi.nlm.nih.gov/articles/PMC311265/
145. Max Planck Institute . Thirst and hunger neurons. Www.mpg.de. Published 2025. Accessed July 21, 2025. https://www.mpg.de/24427625/0331-psy-what-drives-our-cravings-for-food-and-drink-155111-x
146. Morris JS, Dolan RJ. Involvement of Human Amygdala and Orbitofrontal Cortex in Hunger-Enhanced Memory for Food Stimuli. *The Journal of Neuroscience*. 2001;21(14):5304-5310. doi:https://doi.org/10.1523/jneurosci.21-14-05304.2001
147. Montagrin A, Martins-Klein B, Sander D, Mather M. Effects of hunger on emotional arousal responses and attention/memory biases. *Emotion*. 2021;21(1):148-158. doi:https://doi.org/10.1037/emo0000680
148. Spector N. The science behind being “hangry.” NBC News. Published 2018. https://www.nbcnews.com/better/pop-culture/science-behind-being-hangry-ncna887806
149. Gometz E. Neuroscience Can Explain Why We Get Hangry. Science Friday. Published March 15, 2024. Accessed July 21, 2025. https://www.sciencefriday.com/articles/balanced-brain-book-excerpt-hangry/
150. News N. How Hunger Influences Decision-Making - Neuroscience News. Neuroscience News. Published November 16, 2023. https://neurosciencenews.com/ghrelin-decision-making-25228/
151. Dance A. The neurons that make us feel “hangry”: A new path to treating anorexia and overeating. EL PAÍS English. Published July 6, 2023. Accessed July 21, 2025. https://english.elpais.com/science-tech/2023-07-06/the-neurons-that-make-us-feel-hangry-a-new-path-to-treating-anorexia-and-overeating.html
152. Holsen L. Probing the Neurobiology of Emotional Eating. Harvard Brain Science Initiative. https://brain.harvard.edu/hbi_news/probing-the-neurobiology-of-emotional-eating/
153. Adam TC, Epel ES. Stress, eating and the reward system. *Physiology &*

Behavior. 2007;91(4):449-458. doi:https://doi.org/10.1016/j.physbeh.2007.04.011

154. Giddens E, Noy B, Steward T, Verdejo-García A. The influence of stress on the neural underpinnings of disinhibited eating: a systematic review and future directions for research. Published online June 13, 2023. doi:https://doi.org/10.1007/s11154-023-09814-4
155. Circadian Fasting: Heart & Metabolic Health Effects | The Institute for Functional Medicine. Ifm.org. Published 2024. Accessed July 21, 2025. https://www.ifm.org/articles/circadian-fasting-precursors-to-heart-health
156. Charlot A, Hutt F, Sabatier E, Zoll J. Beneficial Effects of Early Time-Restricted Feeding on Metabolic Diseases: Importance of Aligning Food Habits with the Circadian Clock. *Nutrients*. 2021;13(5):1405. doi:https://doi.org/10.3390/nu13051405
157. Queiroz J do N, Macedo RCO, Tinsley GM, Reischak-Oliveira A. Time-restricted eating and circadian rhythms: the biological clock is ticking. *Critical Reviews in Food Science and Nutrition*. 2020;61(17):1-13. doi:https://doi.org/10.1080/10408398.2020.1789550
158. Christensen S, Robinson K, Thomas S, Williams DR. Dietary intake by patients taking GLP-1 and dual GIP/GLP-1 receptor agonists: A narrative review and discussion of research needs. *Obesity Pillars*. 2024;11:100121-100121. doi:https://doi.org/10.1016/j.obpill.2024.100121
159. Wei S, Jin W, Zhu W, et al. Greed Personality Trait Links to Negative Psychopathology and Underlying Neural Substrates. *Social Cognitive and Affective Neuroscience*. 2022;18(1). doi:https://doi.org/10.1093/scan/nsac046
160. Li W, Wang H, Xie X, Li J. Neural mediation of greed personality trait on economic risk-taking. *eLife*. 2019;8. doi:https://doi.org/10.7554/elife.45093
161. Deng K, Jin W, Jiang K, et al. Reactivity of the ventromedial prefrontal cortex, but not the amygdala, to negative emotion faces predicts greed personality trait. *Behavioral and Brain Functions*. 2023;19(1). doi:https://doi.org/10.1186/s12993-023-00223-w
162. Dolan EW. The neuroscience of greed: A glimpse into our brain's reaction to fear and desire. PsyPost - Psychology News. Published February 27, 2024. https://www.psypost.org/the-neuroscience-of-greed-a-glimpse-into-our-brains-reaction-to-fear-and-desire/
163. Day JJ, Carelli RM. The Nucleus Accumbens and Pavlovian Reward Learning. *The Neuroscientist*. 2007;13(2):148-159. doi:https://doi.org/10.1177/1073858406295854
164. Xu Y, Lin Y, Yu M, Zhou K. The nucleus accumbens in reward and aversion processing: insights and implications. *Frontiers in Behavioral Neuroscience*. 2024;18. doi:https://doi.org/10.3389/fnbeh.2024.1420028
165. Life Kit - NPR. Too much pleasure can lead to addiction. How to break the cycle and find balance : Life Kit. NPR. Published April 4, 2022. https://www.npr.org/transcripts/1090009509
166. Koob GF. Hedonic homeostatic dysregulation as a driver of drug-seeking behavior. *Drug Discovery Today: Disease Models*. 2008;5(4):207-215. doi:https://doi.org/10.1016/j.ddmod.2009.04.002

167. Katzman M, Sternat T. Neurobiology of hedonic tone: the relationship between treatment-resistant depression, attention-deficit hyperactivity disorder, and substance abuse. *Neuropsychiatric Disease and Treatment*. 2016;Volume 12:2149-2164. doi:https://doi.org/10.2147/ndt.s111818

168. addiction-ssa. Dopamine and the pleasure–pain balance. SSA. Published February 8, 2023. https://www.addiction-ssa.org/features/book-excerpt/dopamine-and-the-pleasure-pain-balance/

169. Day JJ, Carelli RM. The Nucleus Accumbens and Pavlovian Reward Learning. *The Neuroscientist*. 2007;13(2):148-159. doi:https://doi.org/10.1177/1073858406295854

170. Mussel P, Hewig J. A neural perspective on when and why trait greed comes at the expense of others. *Scientific Reports*. 2019;9(1). doi:https://doi.org/10.1038/s41598-019-47372-5

171. Frenette H. How Social Media Affects Your Brain | Neuline. NeuLine Health. Published 2021. https://neulinehealth.com/how-social-media-affects-your-brain/

172. The Jed Foundation. Understanding Social Comparison on Social Media. The Jed Foundation. Published 2023. https://jedfoundation.org/resource/understanding-social-comparison-on-social-media/

173. Apps Matthew AJ, Rushworth Matthew FS, Chang Steve WC. The Anterior Cingulate Gyrus and Social Cognition: Tracking the Motivation of Others. *Neuron*. 2016;90(4):692-707. doi:https://doi.org/10.1016/j.neuron.2016.04.018

174. Kedia G, Mussweiler T, Linden DEJ. Brain mechanisms of social comparison and their influence on the reward system. *Neuroreport*. 2014;25(16):1255-1265. doi:https://doi.org/10.1097/WNR.0000000000000255

175. Lee D. Decision Making: From Neuroscience to Psychiatry. *Neuron*. 2013;78(2):233-248. doi:https://doi.org/10.1016/j.neuron.2013.04.008

176. Rosenbloom MH, Schmahmann JD, Price BH. The Functional Neuroanatomy of Decision-Making. *The Journal of Neuropsychiatry and Clinical Neurosciences*. 2012;24(3):266-277. doi:https://doi.org/10.1176/appi.neuropsych.11060139

177. Jones DT, Graff-Radford J. Executive Dysfunction and the Prefrontal Cortex. *CONTINUUM: Lifelong Learning in Neurology*. 2021;27(6):1586-1601. doi:https://doi.org/10.1212/con.0000000000001009

178. Guy-Evans O. The Role of Dopamine as a Neurotransmitter in the Human Brain - Simply Psychology. Simply Psychology. Published February 22, 2022. https://www.simplypsychology.org/the-role-of-dopamine-as-a-neurotransmitter-in-the-human-brain.html

179. Sebastian A, Jung P, Krause-Utz A, Lieb K, Schmahl C, TÃ¼scher O. Frontal Dysfunctions of Impulse Control â€" A Systematic Review in Borderline Personality Disorder and Attention-Deficit/Hyperactivity Disorder. *Frontiers in Human Neuroscience*. 2014;8. doi:https://doi.org/10.3389/fnhum.2014.00698

180. Henley C. Motivation and Reward. *openbookslibmsuedu*. Published online

January 1, 2021. https://openbooks.lib.msu.edu/neuroscience/chapter/motivation-and-reward/

181. Lewis RG, Florio E, Punzo D, Borrelli E. The Brain's Reward System in Health and Disease. *Advances in Experimental Medicine and Biology.* 2021;1344(1344):57-69. doi:https://doi.org/10.1007/978-3-030-81147-1_4

182. Dennison JB, Sazhin D, Smith DV. Decision neuroscience and neuroeconomics: Recent progress and ongoing challenges. *WIREs Cognitive Science.* 2022;13(3). doi:https://doi.org/10.1002/wcs.1589

183. Bromberg-Martin ES, Matsumoto M, Hikosaka O. Dopamine in motivational control: Rewarding, aversive, and alerting. *Neuron.* 2010;68(5):815-834. doi:https://doi.org/10.1016/j.neuron.2010.11.022

184. McCarthy G. Lecture 23 Dopamine Reward | The Human Brain. Yale.edu. Published 2024. Accessed July 22, 2025. https://campuspress.yale.edu/humanbrain/appendix-notes/Lecture_23_Dopamine_Reward/

185. Yin HH, Ostlund SB, Balleine BW. Reward-guided learning beyond dopamine in the nucleus accumbens: the integrative functions of cortico-basal ganglia networks. *European Journal of Neuroscience.* 2008;28(8):1437-1448. doi:https://doi.org/10.1111/j.1460-9568.2008.06422.x

186. Rogers RD. The Roles of Dopamine and Serotonin in Decision Making: Evidence from Pharmacological Experiments in Humans. *Neuropsychopharmacology.* 2010;36(1):114-132. doi:https://doi.org/10.1038/npp.2010.165

187. Duerler P, Vollenweider FX, Preller KH. A neurobiological perspective on social influence: Serotonin and social adaptation. *Journal of Neurochemistry.* 2022;162(1). doi:https://doi.org/10.1111/jnc.15607

188. Salvan P, Fonseca M, Winkler AM, Beauchamp A, Lerch JP, Johansen-Berg H. Serotonin regulation of behavior via large-scale neuromodulation of serotonin receptor networks. *Nature Neuroscience.* 2022;26(1):53-63. doi:https://doi.org/10.1038/s41593-022-01213-3

189. Bakkour A, Palombo DJ, Zylberberg A, et al. The hippocampus supports deliberation during value-based decisions. *eLife.* 2019;8. doi:https://doi.org/10.7554/elife.46080

190. Yu JY, Frank LM. Hippocampal–cortical interaction in decision making. *Neurobiology of Learning and Memory.* 2015;117:34-41. doi:https://doi.org/10.1016/j.nlm.2014.02.002

191. Wassum KM. Amygdala-cortical collaboration in reward learning and decision making. *eLife.* 2022;11. doi:https://doi.org/10.7554/elife.80926

192. Gupta R, Koscik TR, Bechara A, Tranel D. The amygdala and decision-making. *Neuropsychologia.* 2011;49(4):760-766. doi:https://doi.org/10.1016/j.neuropsychologia.2010.09.029

193. Shields GS, Sazma MA, Yonelinas AP. The effects of acute stress on core executive functions: A meta-analysis and comparison with cortisol. *Neuroscience & Biobehavioral Reviews.* 2016;68(68):651-668. doi:https://doi.org/10.1016/j.neubiorev.2016.06.038

194. Tucker AM, Whitney P, Belenky G, Hinson JM, Van Dongen HPA. Effects of

Sleep Deprivation on Dissociated Components of Executive Functioning. *Sleep*. 2010;33(1):47-57. doi:https://doi.org/10.1093/sleep/33.1.47

195. Endocrine Society. "Hunger hormone" ghrelin affects monetary decision making. Endocrine.org. Published March 20, 2021. Accessed July 22, 2025. https://www.endocrine.org/news-and-advocacy/news-room/featured-science-from-endo-2021/hunger-hormone-ghrelin-affects-monetary-decision-making
196. The Endocrine Society. "Hunger hormone" ghrelin affects monetary decision making. ScienceDaily. Published 2021. https://www.sciencedaily.com/releases/2021/03/210321215443.htm
197. Dickson SL. Ghrelin at the interface of hunger, reward and obesity. *European Psychiatry*. 2023;66(S1):S5-S5. doi:https://doi.org/10.1192/j.eurpsy.2023.34
198. News N. How Hunger Influences Decision-Making - Neuroscience News. Neuroscience News. Published November 16, 2023. https://neurosciencenews.com/ghrelin-decision-making-25228/
199. NiLSSON S, ARIESÖDERSTRÖM M, KARLSSON S, et al. *Less Effective Executive Functioning after One Night's Sleep Deprivation*. Accessed July 22, 2025. https://schoolstarttime.org/wp-content/uploads/2011/04/nilsson-et-al-less-effective-executive-functioning-after-one-nights-sleep-deprivation.pdf
200. Lima NC, Kirov R, de Almondes KM. Impairment of executive functions due to sleep alterations: An integrative review on the use of P300. *Frontiers in Neuroscience*. 2022;16. doi:https://doi.org/10.3389/fnins.2022.906492
201. Ordali E, Marcos-Prieto P, Avvenuti G, et al. Prolonged exertion of self-control causes increased sleep-like frontal brain activity and changes in aggressivity and punishment. *Proceedings of the National Academy of Sciences*. 2024;121(47). doi:https://doi.org/10.1073/pnas.2404213121
202. Wu JC, Gillin JC, Buchsbaum MS, et al. Frontal Lobe Metabolic Decreases with Sleep Deprivation not Totally Reversed by Recovery Sleep. *Neuropsychopharmacology*. 2006;31(12):2783-2792. doi:https://doi.org/10.1038/sj.npp.1301166
203. Muzur A, Pace-Schott EF, Hobson JAllan. The prefrontal cortex in sleep. *Trends in Cognitive Sciences*. 2002;6(11):475-481. doi:https://doi.org/10.1016/s1364-6613(02)01992-7
204. Pignatiello GA, Martin RJ, Hickman RL. Decision fatigue: A conceptual analysis. *Journal of Health Psychology*. 2018;25(1):135910531876351. doi:https://doi.org/10.1177/1359105318763510
205. LeWine HE. Understanding the stress response. Harvard Health. Published 2024. https://www.health.harvard.edu/staying-healthy/understanding-the-stress-response
206. Blum K. The Impact of Chronic Stress on Brain Function and Structure. *Neuroscience and Psychiatry: Open Access*. 2024;7(5):262-264. doi:https://doi.org/10.47532/npoa.2024.7(5).262-264
207. Shields GS, Hunter CL, Trudell EV, et al. Acute stress influences the emotional foundations of executive control: Distinct effects on control-

related affective and cognitive processes. *Psychoneuroendocrinology*. 2024;162:106942. doi:https://doi.org/10.1016/j.psyneuen.2023.106942

208. Wei, W, Rubin JE, Wang XJ. Role of the Indirect Pathway of the Basal Ganglia in Perceptual Decision Making. Jneurosci.org. Published 2014. https://www.jneurosci.org/content/35/9/4052

209. Kim HF, Hikosaka O. Parallel basal ganglia circuits for voluntary and automatic behaviour to reach rewards. *Brain*. 2015;138(7):1776-1800. doi:https://doi.org/10.1093/brain/awv134

210. Boas G. "It's All in the Eyes": The role of the amygdala in the experience and perception of fear | Martinos Center. Martinos Center | Revolutionizing imaging for the advancement of science and medicine. Published August 21, 2018. Accessed July 22, 2025. https://www.martinos.org/its-all-in-the-eyes-the-role-of-the-amygdala-in-the-experience-and-perception-of-fear/

211. Kamigaki T. Prefrontal circuit organization for executive control. *Neuroscience Research*. 2019;140:23-36. doi:https://doi.org/10.1016/j.neures.2018.08.017

212. Bevilacqua L, Goldman D. Genetics of impulsive behaviour. *Philosophical Transactions of the Royal Society B: Biological Sciences*. 2013;368(1615):20120380-20120380. doi:https://doi.org/10.1098/rstb.2012.0380

213. Hall A, Weaver SR, Compton LJ, Byblow WD, Jenkinson N, MacDonald HJ. Dopamine genetic risk score predicts impulse control behaviors in Parkinson's disease. *Clinical Parkinsonism & Related Disorders*. 2021;5:100113. doi:https://doi.org/10.1016/j.prdoa.2021.100113

214. Ekelund J, Lichtermann D, Järvelin MR, Peltonen L. Association between novelty seeking and the type 4 dopamine receptor gene in a large Finnish cohort sample. *The American Journal of Psychiatry*. 1999;156(9):1453-1455. doi:https://doi.org/10.1176/ajp.156.9.1453

215. Lesch KP. Linking emotion to the social brain. The role of the serotonin transporter in human social behaviour. *EMBO reports*. 2007;8:S24-S29. doi:https://doi.org/10.1038/sj.embor.7401008

216. Diamond A. Consequences of Variations in Genes that affect Dopamine in Prefrontal Cortex. *Cerebral Cortex*. 2007;17(suppl 1):i161-i170. doi:https://doi.org/10.1093/cercor/bhm082

217. Arnsten AFT. The emerging neurobiology of attention deficit hyperactivity disorder: The key role of the prefrontal association cortex. *The Journal of Pediatrics*. 2009;154(5):I-S43. doi:https://doi.org/10.1016/j.jpeds.2009.01.018

218. Andersen SL. Neuroinflammation, Early-Life Adversity, and Brain Development. *Harvard Review of Psychiatry*. 2022;30(1):24-39. doi:https://doi.org/10.1097/hrp.0000000000000325

219. Bick J, Nelson CA. Early adverse experiences and the developing brain. *Neuropsychopharmacology*. 2015;41(1):177-196. doi:https://doi.org/10.1038/npp.2015.252

220. Michaels TI, Stone E, Singal S, Novakovic V, Barkin RL, Barkin S. Brain reward circuitry: The overlapping neurobiology of trauma and substance

use disorders. *World Journal of Psychiatry*. 2021;11(6):222-231. doi:https://doi.org/10.5498/wjp.v11.i6.222

221. News N. Sweets Change Our Brain: Why Sweet Foods Are Irresistible - Neuroscience News. Neuroscience News. Published March 22, 2023. Accessed April 12, 2025. https://neurosciencenews.com/sweet-food-brain-changes-22847/
222. Mattson MP. An Evolutionary Perspective on Why Food Overconsumption Impairs Cognition. *Trends in Cognitive Sciences*. 2019;23(3):200-212. doi:https://doi.org/10.1016/j.tics.2019.01.003
223. Creativity: Following Your Creative Impulses. GCFGlobal.org. https://edu.gcfglobal.org/en/creativity/following-your-creative-impulses/1/
224. Fadelli I. Risk preference is governed by different hypothalamus–habenula circuits, study finds. Medicalxpress.com. Published January 23, 2025. Accessed July 22, 2025. https://medicalxpress.com/news/2025-01-hypothalamushabenula-circuits.html
225. UCL. The bit of your brain that signals how bad things could be. UCL News. Published July 29, 2014. Accessed July 22, 2025. https://www.ucl.ac.uk/news/2014/jul/bit-your-brain-signals-how-bad-things-could-be
226. Dolan EW. Neuroscientists discover distinct brain circuit that drives risk preference. PsyPost - Psychology News. Published February 25, 2025. Accessed July 22, 2025. https://www.psypost.org/neuroscientists-discover-distinct-brain-circuit-that-drives-risk-preference/
227. Groos D, Reuss AM, Rupprecht P, et al. A distinct hypothalamus–habenula circuit governs risk preference. *Nature Neuroscience*. Published online January 8, 2025. doi:https://doi.org/10.1038/s41593-024-01856-4
228. Groos D. Lateral Habenula Circuitry Governs Value-Guided and Risky Decision-Making. *Zorauzhch*. Published online 2022. doi:https://www.zora.uzh.ch/id/eprint/226449/1/Groos_Thesis_master_file_revisited.pdf
229. OpenStax. 2.2 How the Brain Processes Information to Make Decisions: Reflective and Reactive Systems - Principles of Management | OpenStax. openstax.org. Published March 20, 2019. https://openstax.org/books/principles-management/pages/2-2-how-the-brain-processes-information-to-make-decisions-reflective-and-reactive-systems
230. Fessenden M. Important Brain Regions for Decision-Making. www.brainfacts.org. Published May 8, 2023. https://www.brainfacts.org/thinking-sensing-and-behaving/thinking-and-awareness/2023/decision-making
231. Wikipedia Contributors. The Expression of the Emotions in Man and Animals. Wikipedia. Published March 21, 2019. https://en.wikipedia.org/wiki/The_Expression_of_the_Emotions_in_Man_and_Animals
232. Darwin C. *Charles Darwin: The Expression of the Emotions in Man and Animals: Chapter 14.*; 1872. https://brocku.ca/MeadProject/Darwin/Darwin_1872_14.html
233. Darwin C. *Charles Darwin: The Expression of the Emotions in Man and Animals: Chapter 1.*; 1872. https://brocku.ca/MeadProject/Darwin/Darwin_1872_01.html

234. Zschucke E, Renneberg B, Dimeo F, Wüstenberg T, Ströhle A. The stress-buffering effect of acute exercise: Evidence for HPA axis negative feedback. *Psychoneuroendocrinology*. 2015;51:414-425. doi:https://doi.org/10.1016/j.psyneuen.2014.10.019
235. Dimitroff SJ, Kardan O, Necka EA, Decety J, Berman MG, Norman GJ. Physiological dynamics of stress contagion. *Scientific Reports*. 2017;7(1). doi:https://doi.org/10.1038/s41598-017-05811-1
236. Oberle E, Schonert-Reichl KA. Stress contagion in the classroom? The link between classroom teacher burnout and morning cortisol in elementary school students. *Social Science & Medicine*. 2016;159(159):30-37. doi:https://doi.org/10.1016/j.socscimed.2016.04.031
237. Sterley TL, Baimoukhametova D, Füzesi T, et al. Social transmission and buffering of synaptic changes after stress. *Nature Neuroscience*. 2018;21(3):393-403. doi:https://doi.org/10.1038/s41593-017-0044-6
238. Brandl HB, Pruessner JC, Farine DR. The social transmission of stress in animal collectives. *Proceedings of the Royal Society B: Biological Sciences*. 2022;289(1974). doi:https://doi.org/10.1098/rspb.2021.2158
239. Arnsten AFT. Stress signalling pathways that impair prefrontal cortex structure and function. *Nature Reviews Neuroscience*. 2009;10(6):410-422. doi:https://doi.org/10.1038/nrn2648
240. Lupien SJ, McEwen BS, Gunnar MR, Heim C. Effects of stress throughout the lifespan on the brain, behaviour and cognition. *Nature Reviews Neuroscience*. 2009;10(6):434-445. doi:https://doi.org/10.1038/nrn2639
241. Chen C, Nakagawa S, An Y, Ito K, Kitaichi Y, Kusumi I. The exercise-glucocorticoid paradox: How exercise is beneficial to cognition, mood, and the brain while increasing glucocorticoid levels. *Frontiers in neuroendocrinology*. 2017;44:83-102. doi:https://doi.org/10.1016/j.yfrne.2016.12.001
242. Arvidson E, Dahlman AS, Börjesson M, Gullstrand L, Jonsdottir IH. The effects of exercise training on hypothalamic-pituitary-adrenal axis reactivity and autonomic response to acute stress—a randomized controlled study. *Trials*. 2020;21(1). doi:https://doi.org/10.1186/s13063-020-04803-3
243. Davidson K. 11 Natural Ways to Lower Your Cortisol Levels. Healthline. Published 2017. https://www.healthline.com/nutrition/ways-to-lower-cortisol
244. Schüler J, Haufler A, Ditzen B. Social Support as a Stress Buffer or Stress Amplifier and the Moderating Role of Implicit Motives: Protocol for a Randomized Study (Preprint). *JMIR Research Protocols*. Published online May 12, 2022. doi:https://doi.org/10.2196/39509
245. Stress-buffering effect of social support on immunity and infectious risk during chemotherapy for breast cancer. *Brain, Behavior, & Immunity - Health*. 2021;10:100186. doi:https://doi.org/10.1016/j.bbih.2020.100186
246. Troy AS, Wilhelm FH, Shallcross AJ, Mauss IB. Seeing the silver lining: Cognitive reappraisal ability moderates the relationship between stress and depressive symptoms. *Emotion*. 2010;10(6):783-795. doi:https://doi.org/10.1037/a0020262

247. Troy AS, Shallcross AJ, Brunner A, Friedman R, Jones MC. Cognitive Reappraisal and acceptance: Effects on emotion, physiology, and Perceived Cognitive costs. *Emotion*. 2018;18(1):58-74. doi:https://doi.org/10.1037/emo0000371
248. Kim SH. Mindfulness-Based Stretching and Deep Breathing Exercises Normalize Serum Cortisol Levels and Reverse Symptoms of PTSD: A Prospective Randomized-Controlled Trial. UNM Digital Repository. Published 2016. Accessed July 22, 2025. https://digitalrepository.unm.edu/educ_hess_etds/21/
249. Örün D, Karaca S, Arıkan Ş. The Effect of Breathing Exercise on Stress Hormones. *Cyprus Journal of Medical Sciences*. 2021;6(1):22-27. doi:https://doi.org/10.4274/cjms.2021.2020.2390
250. Wang Y, Yin B. A new understanding of the cognitive reappraisal technique: An extension based on the schema theory. *Frontiers in Behavioral Neuroscience*. 2023;17(1). doi:https://doi.org/10.3389/fnbeh.2023.1174585
251. Rogerson O, Wilding S, Prudenzi A, O'Connor DB. Effectiveness of stress management interventions to change cortisol levels: a systematic review and meta-analysis. *Psychoneuroendocrinology*. 2023;159(159):106415-106415. doi:https://doi.org/10.1016/j.psyneuen.2023.106415
252. Sell A, Tooby J, Cosmides L. Formidability and the logic of human anger. *Proceedings of the National Academy of Sciences*. 2009;106(35):15073-15078. doi:https://doi.org/10.1073/pnas.0904312106
253. Williams R. Anger as a Basic Emotion and Its Role in Personality Building and Pathological Growth: The Neuroscientific, Developmental and Clinical Perspectives. *Frontiers in psychology*. 2017;8:1950. doi:https://doi.org/10.3389/fpsyg.2017.01950
254. Govindan R, Anjanappa S, Munivenkatappa M, Bhaskarapillai B. Effectiveness of anger management program on anger level, problem solving skills, communication skills, and adjustment among school-going adolescents. *Journal of Education and Health Promotion*. 2023;12(1):90. doi:https://doi.org/10.4103/jehp.jehp_1216_22
255. Kim MJ, Elliott ML, d'Arbeloff TC, et al. Microstructural integrity of white matter moderates an association between childhood adversity and adult trait anger. *Aggressive Behavior*. 2019;45(3):310-318. doi:https://doi.org/10.1002/ab.21820
256. Teicher MH, Samson JA, Anderson CM, Ohashi K. The effects of childhood maltreatment on brain structure, function and connectivity. *Nature Reviews Neuroscience*. 2016;17(10):652-666. doi:https://doi.org/10.1038/nrn.2016.111
257. Thijssen S, Ringoot AP, Wildeboer A, et al. Brain morphology of childhood aggressive behavior: A multi-informant study in school-age children. *Cognitive, Affective & Behavioral Neuroscience*. 2015;15(3):564-577. doi:https://doi.org/10.3758/s13415-015-0344-9
258. Cross D, Fani N, Powers A, Bradley B. Neurobiological Development in the Context of Childhood Trauma. *Clinical Psychology: Science and Practice*. 2019;24(2):111-124. doi:https://doi.org/10.1111/cpsp.12198

259. Blair RJR. Considering anger from a cognitive neuroscience perspective. *Wiley Interdisciplinary Reviews: Cognitive Science*. 2011;3(1):65-74. doi:https://doi.org/10.1002/wcs.154
260. Siep N, Tonnaer F, van de Ven V, Arntz A, Raine A, Cima M. Anger provocation increases limbic and decreases medial prefrontal cortex connectivity with the left amygdala in reactive aggressive violent offenders. *Brain Imaging and Behavior*. 2018;13(5):1311-1323. doi:https://doi.org/10.1007/s11682-018-9945-6
261. Månsson KNT, Salami A, Frick A, et al. Neuroplasticity in response to cognitive behavior therapy for social anxiety disorder. *Translational Psychiatry*. 2016;6(2):e727-e727. doi:https://doi.org/10.1038/tp.2015.218
262. Okun M, Lampl I. Instantaneous correlation of excitation and inhibition during ongoing and sensory-evoked activities. *Nature Neuroscience*. 2008;11(5):535-537. doi:https://doi.org/10.1038/nn.2105
263. Omura M, Maguire J, Levett-Jones T, Stone TE. Effectiveness of assertive communication training programs for health professionals and students. *JBI Database of Systematic Reviews and Implementation Reports*. 2016;14(10):64-71. doi:https://doi.org/10.11124/jbisrir-2016-003158
264. Startup M, Startup S, Sedgman A. Immediate source-monitoring, self-focused attention and the positive symptoms of schizophrenia. *Behaviour Research and Therapy*. 2008;46(10):1176-1180. doi:https://doi.org/10.1016/j.brat.2008.07.003
265. Jiang Q, Hou L, Wang H, Li C. The Effect of Cognitive Reappraisal on Reactive Aggression: An fMRI Study. *Frontiers in Psychology*. 2018;9. doi:https://doi.org/10.3389/fpsyg.2018.01903
266. Hart T, Brockway JA, Maiuro RD, et al. Anger Self-Management Training for Chronic Moderate to Severe Traumatic Brain Injury. *Journal of Head Trauma Rehabilitation*. 2017;32(5):319-331. doi:https://doi.org/10.1097/htr.0000000000000316
267. Kübra Kayaoğlu, Mustafa Köse. Effect of Cognitive-Behavioral Therapy–Based Anger Management Training on Anger and Aggression Levels of Individuals Convicted of Violent Crimes. *Journal of psychosocial nursing and mental health services*. 2024;62(10):1-8. doi:https://doi.org/10.3928/02793695-20240509-02
268. Wells SY, Patel TA, Halverson TF, et al. The impact of trauma-focused psychotherapies on anger: A systematic review and meta-analysis. *Psychological trauma*. Published online March 28, 2024. doi:https://doi.org/10.1037/tra0001697
269. Henwood KS, Chou S, Brownev K. A Systematic Review and Meta-Analysis on the Effectiveness of CBT Informed Anger Management. Office of Justice Programs. https://www.ojp.gov/library/publications/systematic-review-and-meta-analysis-effectiveness-cbt-informed-anger
270. Luca Piretti, Edoardo Pappaianni, Garbin C, Rumiati RI, Job R, Alessandro Grecucci. The Neural Signatures of Shame, Embarrassment, and Guilt: A Voxel-Based Meta-Analysis on Functional Neuroimaging Studies. *Brain Sciences*. 2023;13(4):559-559. doi:https://doi.org/10.3390/brainsci13040559

271. Vaish A, Carpenter M, Tomasello M. The Early Emergence of Guilt-Motivated Prosocial Behavior. *Child Development*. 2016;87(6):1772-1782. doi:https://doi.org/10.1111/cdev.12628

272. Scaffidi Abbate C, Misuraca R, Roccella M, Parisi L, Vetri L, Miceli S. The Role of Guilt and Empathy on Prosocial Behavior. *Behavioral Sciences*. 2022;12(3):64. doi:https://doi.org/10.3390/bs12030064

273. Michl P, Meindl T, Meister F, et al. Neurobiological underpinnings of shame and guilt: a pilot fMRI study. *Social Cognitive and Affective Neuroscience*. 2014;9(2):150-157. doi:https://doi.org/10.1093/scan/nss114

274. Basile B, Mancini F, Macaluso E, Caltagirone C, Frackowiak RSJ, Bozzali M. Deontological and altruistic guilt: Evidence for distinct neurobiological substrates. *Human Brain Mapping*. 2010;32(2):229-239. doi:https://doi.org/10.1002/hbm.21009

275. Shin LM, Dougherty DD, Orr SP, et al. Activation of anterior paralimbic structures during guilt-related script-driven imagery. *Biological Psychiatry*. 2000;48(1):43-50. doi:https://doi.org/10.1016/s0006-3223(00)00251-1

276. Piretti L, Pappaianni E, Lunardelli A, et al. The Role of Amygdala in Self-Conscious Emotions in a Patient With Acquired Bilateral Damage. *Frontiers in Neuroscience*. 2020;14. doi:https://doi.org/10.3389/fnins.2020.00677

277. Uddin LQ, Nomi JS, Hébert-Seropian B, Ghaziri J, Boucher O. Structure and Function of the Human Insula. *Journal of Clinical Neurophysiology*. 2017;34(4):300-306. doi:https://doi.org/10.1097/wnp.0000000000000377

278. Deem MJ, Ramsey G. Guilt by association? *Philosophical Psychology*. 2016;29(4):570-585. doi:https://doi.org/10.1080/09515089.2015.1126706

279. Vaish A. The prosocial functions of early social emotions: the case of guilt. *Current Opinion in Psychology*. 2018;20:25-29. doi:https://doi.org/10.1016/j.copsyc.2017.08.008

280. Rotge JY, Lemogne C, Hinfray S, et al. A meta-analysis of the anterior cingulate contribution to social pain. *Social Cognitive and Affective Neuroscience*. 2014;10(1):19-27. doi:https://doi.org/10.1093/scan/nsu110

281. Lieberman MD, Eisenberger NI. The dorsal anterior cingulate cortex is selective for pain: Results from large-scale reverse inference. *Proceedings of the National Academy of Sciences*. 2015;112(49):15250-15255. doi:https://doi.org/10.1073/pnas.1515083112

282. Meyer ML, Williams KD, Eisenberger NI. Why Social Pain Can Live on: Different Neural Mechanisms Are Associated with Reliving Social and Physical Pain. Urgesi C, ed. *PLOS ONE*. 2015;10(6):e0128294. doi:https://doi.org/10.1371/journal.pone.0128294

283. Price RB, Duman R. Neuroplasticity in cognitive and psychological mechanisms of depression: An integrative model. *Molecular Psychiatry*. 2019;25(3). doi:https://doi.org/10.1038/s41380-019-0615-x

284. Zhang X, Wang J, Wang Y, Wang J, Luo F. The Effects of Mindfulness on Shame: Exploring Mediation by Cognitive Flexibility and Self-Compassion in a Chinese Adult Population. *PsyCh Journal*. Published online December 10, 2024. doi:https://doi.org/10.1002/pchj.817

285. Woods H, Proeve M. Relationships of Mindfulness, Self-Compassion, and Meditation Experience With Shame-Proneness. *Journal of Cognitive Psychotherapy*. 2014;28(1):20-33. doi:https://doi.org/10.1891/0889-8391.28.1.20

286. LeDoux JE. As soon as there was life, there was danger: the deep history of survival behaviours and the shallower history of consciousness. *Philosophical Transactions of the Royal Society B: Biological Sciences*. 2021;377(1844). doi:https://doi.org/10.1098/rstb.2021.0292

287. Bennett MS. Five Breakthroughs: A First Approximation of Brain Evolution From Early Bilaterians to Humans. *Frontiers in Neuroanatomy*. 2021;15. doi:https://doi.org/10.3389/fnana.2021.693346

288. Sun Y, Gooch H, Sah P. Fear conditioning and the basolateral amygdala. *F1000Research*. 2020;9(1). doi:https://doi.org/10.12688/f1000research.21201.1

289. Knight DC, Nguyen HT, Bandettini PA. The role of the human amygdala in the production of conditioned fear responses. *NeuroImage*. 2005;26(4):1193-1200. doi:https://doi.org/10.1016/j.neuroimage.2005.03.020

290. Ressler K. Understanding the Neural Basis of Fear to Transform our Anxieties. adaa.org. Published 2017. https://adaa.org/learn-from-us/from-the-experts/blog-posts/professional/understanding-neural-basis-fear-transform

291. Goldin PR, Manber T, Hakimi S, Canli T, Gross JJ. Neural Bases of Social Anxiety Disorder. *Archives of General Psychiatry*. 2009;66(2):170. doi:https://doi.org/10.1001/archgenpsychiatry.2008.525

292. Yu X, Ruan Y, Zhang Y, et al. Cognitive Neural Mechanism of Social Anxiety Disorder: A Meta-Analysis Based on fMRI Studies. *International Journal of Environmental Research and Public Health*. 2021;18(11):5556. doi:https://doi.org/10.3390/ijerph18115556

293. Kim JJ, Jung MW. Neural circuits and mechanisms involved in Pavlovian fear conditioning: A critical review. *Neuroscience & Biobehavioral Reviews*. 2006;30(2):188-202. doi:https://doi.org/10.1016/j.neubiorev.2005.06.005

294. Black R. Glossophobia (Fear of public speaking): Are you Glossophobic? www.healthcentral.com. Published September 12, 2019. https://www.healthcentral.com/condition/anxiety/glossophobia-fear-of-public-speaking

295. Heeren A, Ceschi G, Dethier V, Philippot P, Valentiner D. Assessing public speaking fear with the short form of the Personal Report of Confidence as a Speaker scale: confirmatory factor analyses among a French-speaking community sample. *Neuropsychiatric Disease and Treatment*. Published online May 2013:609. doi:https://doi.org/10.2147/ndt.s43097

296. Luchkina NV, Bolshakov VY. Mechanisms of fear learning and extinction: synaptic plasticity–fear memory connection. *Psychopharmacology*. 2018;236(1):163-182. doi:https://doi.org/10.1007/s00213-018-5104-4

297. Bouras NN, Mack NR, Gao W. Prefrontal modulation of anxiety through a lens of noradrenergic signaling. *Frontiers in Systems Neuroscience*. 2023;17. doi:https://doi.org/10.3389/fnsys.2023.1173326

298. Hamati R. Insights into the Neurobiology of Anxiety and a Potential Target for Pharmacotherapy. *The Journal of Neuroscience*. 2018;38(42):8919-8921. doi:https://doi.org/10.1523/jneurosci.1461-18.2018

299. Bremner JD, Krystal JH, Southwick SM, Charney DS. Noradrenergic mechanisms in stress and anxiety: I. preclinical studies. *Synapse*. 1996;23(1):28-38. doi:https://doi.org/10.1002/(sici)1098-2396(199605)23:1%3C28::aid-syn4%3E3.0.co;2-j

300. Morilak DA, Barrera G, Echevarria DJ, et al. Role of brain norepinephrine in the behavioral response to stress. *Progress in Neuro-Psychopharmacology and Biological Psychiatry*. 2005;29(8):1214-1224. doi:https://doi.org/10.1016/j.pnpbp.2005.08.007

301. Hauner KK, Mineka S, Voss JL, Paller KA. Exposure therapy triggers lasting reorganization of neural fear processing. *Proceedings of the National Academy of Sciences*. 2012;109(23):9203-9208. doi:https://doi.org/10.1073/pnas.1205242109

302. Zhu X, Suarez-Jimenez B, Lazarov A, et al. Exposure-based therapy changes amygdala and hippocampus resting-state functional connectivity in patients with posttraumatic stress disorder. *Depression and Anxiety*. 2018;35(10):974-984. doi:https://doi.org/10.1002/da.22816

303. Stojek MM, McSweeney LB, Rauch SAM. Neuroscience Informed Prolonged Exposure Practice: Increasing Efficiency and Efficacy Through Mechanisms. *Frontiers in Behavioral Neuroscience*. 2018;12. doi:https://doi.org/10.3389/fnbeh.2018.00281

304. Wardenaar KJ, Lim CCW, Al-Hamzawi AO, et al. The cross-national epidemiology of specific phobia in the World Mental Health Surveys. *Psychological Medicine*. 2017;47(10):1744-1760. doi:https://doi.org/10.1017/s0033291717000174

305. Schaefer HS, Larson CL, Davidson RJ, Coan JA. Brain, body, and cognition: Neural, physiological and self-report correlates of phobic and normative fear. *Biological Psychology*. 2014;98:59-69. doi:https://doi.org/10.1016/j.biopsycho.2013.12.011

306. Zauderer S. 31 Fear Of Public Speaking Statistics (Prevalence). www.crossrivertherapy.com. Published January 11, 2023. https://www.crossrivertherapy.com/public-speaking-statistics

307. Heshmati M, Russo SJ. Anhedonia and the Brain Reward Circuitry in Depression. *Current Behavioral Neuroscience Reports*. 2015;2(3):146-153. doi:https://doi.org/10.1007/s40473-015-0044-3

308. School MM. The Serotonin Basis of Depression: Unraveling the Neurochemical Web. Louis A. Faillace, MD, Department of Psychiatry and Behavioral Sciences. Published December 11, 2023. https://med.uth.edu/psychiatry/2023/12/11/the-serotonin-basis-of-depression-unraveling-the-neurochemical-web/

309. Cooney RE, Joormann J, Eugène F, Dennis EL, Gotlib IH. Neural correlates of rumination in depression. *Cognitive, Affective, & Behavioral Neuroscience*. 2010;10(4):470-478. doi:https://doi.org/10.3758/cabn.10.4.470

310. Martin-Soelch C. Is depression associated with dysfunction of the central reward system? *Biochemical Society Transactions*. 2009;37(1):313-317. doi:https://doi.org/10.1042/bst0370313

311. Mancini AD, Bonanno GA. Predictors and Parameters of Resilience to Loss: Toward an Individual Differences Model. *Journal of Personality*. 2009;77(6):1805-1832. doi:https://doi.org/10.1111/j.1467-6494.2009.00601.x

312. Coccurello R. Anhedonia in depression symptomatology: Appetite dysregulation and defective brain reward processing. *Behavioural Brain Research*. 2019;372:112041. doi:https://doi.org/10.1016/j.bbr.2019.112041

313. Albert PR. Adult neuroplasticity: A new "cure" for major depression?. *Journal of Psychiatry & Neuroscience*. 2019;44(3):147-150. doi:https://doi.org/10.1503/jpn.190072

314. News-Medical. Norepinephrine and Mental Health. News-Medical.net. Published January 24, 2019. https://www.news-medical.net/health/Norepinephrine-and-Mental-Health.aspx

315. Chou T, Deckersbach T, Dougherty DD, Hooley JM. The default mode network and rumination in individuals at risk for depression. *Social Cognitive and Affective Neuroscience*. 2023;18(1):nsad032. doi:https://doi.org/10.1093/scan/nsad032

316. Hamilton JP, Farmer M, Fogelman P, Gotlib IH. Depressive Rumination, the Default-Mode Network, and the Dark Matter of Clinical Neuroscience. *Biological Psychiatry*. 2015;78(4):224-230. doi:https://doi.org/10.1016/j.biopsych.2015.02.020

317. Osimo EF, Pillinger T, Rodriguez IM, Khandaker GM, Pariante CM, Howes OD. Inflammatory markers in depression: A meta-analysis of mean differences and variability in 5,166 patients and 5,083 controls. *Brain, Behavior, and Immunity*. 2020;87. doi:https://doi.org/10.1016/j.bbi.2020.02.010

318. Jia Y, Liu L, Sheng C, et al. Increased Serum Levels of Cortisol and Inflammatory Cytokines in People With Depression. *The Journal of Nervous and Mental Disease*. 2019;207(4):271-276. doi:https://doi.org/10.1097/NMD.0000000000000957

319. Rădulescu I, Drăgoi A, Trifu S, Cristea M. Neuroplasticity and depression: Rewiring the brain's networks through pharmacological therapy (Review). *Experimental and Therapeutic Medicine*. 2021;22(4). doi:https://doi.org/10.3892/etm.2021.10565

320. Olders H. Mourning and Grief as Healing Processes in Psychotherapy. *The Canadian Journal of Psychiatry*. 1989;34(4):271-278. doi:https://doi.org/10.1177/070674378903400402

321. Garland EL, Fredrickson B, Kring AM, Johnson DP, Meyer PS, Penn DL. Upward spirals of positive emotions counter downward spirals of negativity: Insights from the broaden-and-build theory and affective neuroscience on the treatment of emotion dysfunctions and deficits in psychopathology. *Clinical Psychology Review*. 2010;30(7):849-864. doi:https://doi.org/10.1016/j.cpr.2010.03.002

322. Curtis V, de Barra M, Aunger R. Disgust as an adaptive system for disease avoidance behaviour. *Philosophical Transactions of the Royal Society B: Biological Sciences*. 2011;366(1563):389-401. doi:https://doi.org/10.1098/rstb.2010.0117

323. Rottman J. Evolution, Development, and the Emergence of Disgust. *Evolutionary Psychology*. 2014;12(2):147470491401200. doi:https://doi.org/10.1177/147470491401200209

324. Verstaen A, Eckart JA, Muhtadie L, et al. Insular atrophy and diminished disgust reactivity. *Emotion*. 2016;16(6):903-912. doi:https://doi.org/10.1037/emo0000195

325. Woolley JD, Strobl EV, Sturm VE, et al. Impaired Recognition and Regulation of Disgust Is Associated with Distinct but Partially Overlapping Patterns of Decreased Gray Matter Volume in the Ventroanterior Insula. *Biological Psychiatry*. 2015;78(7):505-514. doi:https://doi.org/10.1016/j.biopsych.2014.12.031

326. Pochedly JT, Widen SC, Russell JA. What emotion does the "facial expression of disgust" express?. *Emotion*. 2012;12(6):1315-1319. doi:https://doi.org/10.1037/a0027998

327. Davey GCL. Disgust: the disease-avoidance emotion and its dysfunctions. *Philosophical Transactions of the Royal Society B: Biological Sciences*. 2011;366(1583):3453-3465. doi:https://doi.org/10.1098/rstb.2011.0039

328. Sapolsky R. The Yuck Factor. Walsworth.com. Published May 31, 2017. Accessed July 23, 2025. https://digitaleditions.walsworth.com/publication/?i=413226&article_id=2801184&view=articleBrowser

329. Moll J, de Oliveira-Souza R, Moll FT, et al. The Moral Affiliations of Disgust. *Cognitive and Behavioral Neurology*. 2005;18(1):68-78. doi:https://doi.org/10.1097/01.wnn.0000152236.46475.a7

330. Terrizzi JA, Pond RS, Shannon TCJ, Koopman ZK, Reich JC. How does disgust regulate social rejection? a mini-review. *Frontiers in Psychology*. 2023;14:1141100. doi:https://doi.org/10.3389/fpsyg.2023.1141100

331. Tao D, Leng Y, Huo J, Peng S, Xu J, Deng H. Effects of Core Disgust and Moral Disgust on Moral Judgment: An Event-Related Potential Study. *Frontiers in Psychology*. 2022;13. doi:https://doi.org/10.3389/fpsyg.2022.806784

332. Lim J, Kurnianingsih YA, Ong HH, Mullette-Gillman OA. Moral judgment modulation by disgust priming via altered fronto-temporal functional connectivity. *Scientific Reports*. 2017;7(1). doi:https://doi.org/10.1038/s41598-017-11147-7

333. aan het Rot M, Friederici C, Krause SC, de Jong PJ. Interpersonal responses to facial expressions of disgust, anger, and happiness in individuals with varying levels of social anxiety. Pavlova MA, ed. *PLOS ONE*. 2022;17(4):e0263990. doi:https://doi.org/10.1371/journal.pone.0263990

334. Liu D, Giner-Sorolla R. Bad People Alert: The Expression of Disgust Signals Its Target's Bad Moral Character. *Collabra Psychology*. 2024;10(1). doi:https://doi.org/10.1525/collabra.116193

335. McFarlane JM. EM.2: Deep Dive – How Our Feeling of Disgust Can Be Used to Reinforce Racial, Gender, Sexual and Other Prejudices. Opentextbc.ca. Published August 22, 2024. Accessed July 23, 2025. https://opentextbc.ca/psychologymtdisupplement/chapter/how-our-feeling-of-disgust-can-be-used-to-reinforce-racial-gender-sexual-and-other-prejudices/

336. Kringelbach ML, Berridge KC. The Neuroscience of Happiness and Pleasure. *Social research*. 2024;77(2):659. https://pmc.ncbi.nlm.nih.gov/articles/PMC3008658/

337. Berridge KC, Kringelbach ML. Building a neuroscience of pleasure and well-being. *Psychology of Well-Being: Theory, Research and Practice*. 2011;1(1):3. doi:https://doi.org/10.1186/2211-1522-1-3

338. Dfarhud D, Malmir M, Khanahmadi M. Happiness & Health: The Biological Factors- Systematic Review Article. *Iranian Journal of Public Health*. 2014;43(11):1468. https://pmc.ncbi.nlm.nih.gov/articles/PMC4449495/

339. Whiteman H. Laughter releases "feel good hormones" to promote social bonding. www.medicalnewstoday.com. Published June 3, 2017. https://www.medicalnewstoday.com/articles/317756

340. Akimbekov NS, Razzaque MS. Laughter therapy: A humor-induced hormonal intervention to reduce stress and anxiety. *Current Research in Physiology*. 2021;4(4):135-138. doi:https://doi.org/10.1016/j.crphys.2021.04.002

341. Yim J. Therapeutic benefits of laughter in mental health: A theoretical review. The Tohoku journal of experimental medicine. Published July 1, 2016. https://pubmed.ncbi.nlm.nih.gov/27439375/

342. Fredrickson BL. The Broaden-and-Build Theory of Positive Emotions. *Philosophical Transactions of the Royal Society of London Series B: Biological Sciences*. 2004;359(1449):1367-1377. doi:https://doi.org/10.1098/rstb.2004.1512

343. Blood AJ, Zatorre RJ. Intensely Pleasurable Responses to Music Correlate with Activity in Brain Regions Implicated in Reward and Emotion. *Proceedings of the National Academy of Sciences*. 2001;98(20):11818-11823. doi:https://doi.org/10.1073/pnas.191355898

344. University of Turku. Social laughter releases endorphins in the brain. ScienceDaily. Published 2017. https://www.sciencedaily.com/releases/2017/06/170601124121.htm

345. Scott E. How Hedonic Adaptation Robs You of Happiness—and How to Change That. Verywell Mind. Published 2019. https://www.verywellmind.com/hedonic-adaptation-4156926

346. ScienceDirect. Hedonic Adaptation - an overview | ScienceDirect Topics. www.sciencedirect.com. Published 2018. https://www.sciencedirect.com/topics/psychology/hedonic-adaptation

347. Warren S, Warren S. The Science of Gratitude: How it Changes Your Brain and Body. Somatic Movement Center. Published November 21, 2019. Accessed July 23, 2025. https://www.somaticmovementcenter.com/gratitude/

348. From. Selfless acts of kindness activate brain's reward regions. The New Indian Express. Published September 30, 2018. Accessed July 23, 2025. https://www.newindianexpress.com/lifestyle/health/2018/Sep/30/selfless-acts-of-kindness-activate-brains-reward-regions-1879161.html

349. Simon-Thomas ER. Is Kindness Really Its Own Reward? Greater Good. Published 2008. https://greatergood.berkeley.edu/article/item/is_kindness_really_its_own_reward

350. Guan F, Zhao S, Chen S, Lu S, Chen J, Xiang Y. The Neural Correlate Difference Between Positive and Negative Awe. *Frontiers in Human Neuroscience*. 2019;13. doi:https://doi.org/10.3389/fnhum.2019.00206

351. Steptoe A, Wardle J, Marmot M. Positive affect and health-related neuroendocrine, cardiovascular, and inflammatory processes. *Proceedings of the National Academy of Sciences*. 2005;102(18):6508-6512. doi:https://doi.org/10.1073/pnas.0409174102

352. Shao R, Man ISC, Yau SY, et al. The interplay of acute cortisol response and trait affectivity in associating with stress resilience. *Nature Mental Health*. 2023;1(2):114-123. doi:https://doi.org/10.1038/s44220-023-00016-0

353. Kozlowska K, Walker P, McLean L, Carrive P. Fear and the Defense Cascade. *Harvard Review of Psychiatry*. 2015;23(4):263-287. doi:https://doi.org/10.1097/hrp.0000000000000065

354. Mindscape. Fight, Flight, or Freeze. Harvard.edu. Published 2025. Accessed July 23, 2025. https://www.health.harvard.edu/mindscape/for-young-people/brain-body-connection/fight-flight-or-freeze

355. Rajbhandari AK, Bakshi VP. Repeated norepinephrine receptor stimulation in the BNST induces sensorimotor gating deficits via corticotropin releasing factor. *Neuropharmacology*. 2020;172:108090. doi:https://doi.org/10.1016/j.neuropharm.2020.108090

356. Sinclair AH, Manalili GM, Brunec IK, R. Alison Adcock, Barense MD. Prediction errors disrupt hippocampal representations and update episodic memories. *PNAS*. 2021;118(51). doi:https://doi.org/10.1073/pnas.2117625118

357. Plikat V, Grassi PR, Frack J, Bartels A. Hierarchical surprise signals in naturalistic violation of expectations. *Imaging Neuroscience*. 2025;3. doi:https://doi.org/10.1162/imag_a_00459

358. Lousiana EDU. Chap2. userweb.ucs.louisiana.edu. https://userweb.ucs.louisiana.edu/~cgc2646/LRN/Chap2.html

359. News N. How New Experiences Boost Memory Formation - Neuroscience News. Neuroscience News. Published September 8, 2016. Accessed July 23, 2025. https://neurosciencenews.com/experience-memory-neuroscience-4991/

360. Metternich B, Spanhel K, Schoendube A, et al. Flashbulb memory recall in healthy adults – a functional magnetic resonance imaging study. *Memory*. 2020;28(4):461-472. doi:https://doi.org/10.1080/09658211.2020.1733022

361. Schliephake LM, Trempler I, Roehe MA, Heins N, Schubotz RI. Positive and negative prediction error signals to violated expectations of face and place

stimuli distinctively activate FFA and PPA. *NeuroImage*. 2021;236:118028. doi:https://doi.org/10.1016/j.neuroimage.2021.118028

362. Chen KH, Okerstrom KL, Kingyon JR, Anderson SW, Cavanagh JF, Narayanan NS. Startle Habituation and Midfrontal Theta Activity in Parkinson Disease. *Journal of Cognitive Neuroscience*. 2016;28(12):1923-1932. doi:https://doi.org/10.1162/jocn_a_01012
363. Beppi C, Beringer G, Straumann D, Bögli SY. Light-stimulus intensity modulates startle reflex habituation in larval zebrafish. *Scientific Reports*. 2021;11(1). doi:https://doi.org/10.1038/s41598-021-00535-9
364. Marzola P, Melzer T, Pavesi E, Gil-Mohapel J, Brocardo PS. Exploring the role of neuroplasticity in development, aging, and neurodegeneration. *Brain Sciences*. 2023;13(12):1-32. doi:https://doi.org/10.3390/brainsci13121610
365. Tworek G. What Is Neuroplasticity? How It Works. Cleveland Clinic. Published December 12, 2023. https://health.clevelandclinic.org/neuroplasticity
366. Burklund LJ, Creswell JD, Irwin MR, Lieberman MD. The common and distinct neural bases of affect labeling and reappraisal in healthy adults. *Frontiers in Psychology*. 2014;5. doi:https://doi.org/10.3389/fpsyg.2014.00221
367. Brain First Institute. Labeling Our Emotions: Benefits, Neuroscience, And Strategies. Brainfirstinstitute.com. Published 2024. https://www.brainfirstinstitute.com/blog/labeling-our-emotions-benefits-neuroscience-and-strategies
368. Cutuli D. Cognitive reappraisal and expressive suppression strategies role in the emotion regulation: an overview on their modulatory effects and neural correlates. *Frontiers in Systems Neuroscience*. 2014;8(175). doi:https://doi.org/10.3389/fnsys.2014.00175
369. Fuchs E, Flügge G. Adult Neuroplasticity: More Than 40 Years of Research. *Neural Plasticity*. 2014;2014(541870):1-10. doi:https://doi.org/10.1155/2014/541870
370. Sagendorf C. The intersection of resilience and neuroplasticity: Rewiring the mind for wellness | Mental Health America. Mental Health America. Published 2025. https://mhanational.org/blog/resilience-and-neuroplasticity/
371. Raypole C. How to Rewire Your Brain: 6 Neuroplasticity Exercises. Healthline. Published November 1, 2024. https://www.healthline.com/health/rewiring-your-brain
372. Kong F, Ma X, You X, Xiang Y. The resilient brain: psychological resilience mediates the effect of amplitude of low-frequency fluctuations in orbitofrontal cortex on subjective well-being in young healthy adults. *Social Cognitive and Affective Neuroscience*. 2018;13(7):755-763. doi:https://doi.org/10.1093/scan/nsy045
373. Moore M, Culpepper S, Phan KL, Strauman TJ, Dolcos F, Dolcos S. Neurobehavioral Mechanisms of Resilience Against Emotional Distress: An Integrative Brain-Personality-Symptom Approach Using Structural

Equation Modeling. *Personality Neuroscience*. 2018;1. doi:https://doi.org/10.1017/pen.2018.11

374. Zhang W, Wang X, Feng T. Identifying the Neural Substrates of Procrastination: a Resting-State fMRI Study. *Scientific Reports*. 2016;6(1). doi:https://doi.org/10.1038/srep33203

375. Basten U, Biele G, Heekeren HR, Fiebach CJ. How the brain integrates costs and benefits during decision making. *Proceedings of the National Academy of Sciences*. 2010;107(50):21767-21772. doi:https://doi.org/10.1073/pnas.0908104107

376. Hosokawa T, Kennerley SW, Sloan J, Wallis JD. Single-Neuron Mechanisms Underlying Cost-Benefit Analysis in Frontal Cortex. *Journal of Neuroscience*. 2013;33(44):17385-17397. doi:https://doi.org/10.1523/jneurosci.2221-13.2013

377. Liu T, Ji RR. New insights into the mechanisms of itch: are pain and itch controlled by distinct mechanisms? *Pflügers Archiv - European Journal of Physiology*. 2013;465(12):1671-1685. doi:https://doi.org/10.1007/s00424-013-1284-2

378. Sun S, Xu Q, Guo C, Guan Y, Liu Q, Dong X. Leaky Gate Model: Intensity-Dependent Coding of Pain and Itch in the Spinal Cord. *Neuron*. 2017;93(4):840-853.e5. doi:https://doi.org/10.1016/j.neuron.2017.01.012

379. Chen XJ, Sun YG. Central circuit mechanisms of itch. *Nature Communications*. 2020;11(1). doi:https://doi.org/10.1038/s41467-020-16859-5

380. Xiao X, Ding M, Zhang YQ. Role of the Anterior Cingulate Cortex in Translational Pain Research. *Neuroscience Bulletin*. 2021;37(3):405-422. doi:https://doi.org/10.1007/s12264-020-00615-2

381. Ko HG, Jung H, Han S, et al. Processing of pain and itch information by modality-specific neurons within the anterior cingulate cortex in mice. *Nature Communications*. 2025;16(1):1-16. doi:https://doi.org/10.1038/s41467-025-57041-z

382. Zeidan F, Emerson NM, Farris SR, et al. Mindfulness Meditation-Based Pain Relief Employs Different Neural Mechanisms Than Placebo and Sham Mindfulness Meditation-Induced Analgesia. *Journal of Neuroscience*. 2015;35(46):15307-15325. doi:https://doi.org/10.1523/jneurosci.2542-15.2015

383. Carstens E, Akiyama T. Central Mechanisms of Itch. *Current problems in dermatology*. Published online January 1, 2016:11-17. doi:https://doi.org/10.1159/000446011

384. Lipshetz B, Khasabov SG, Truong H, Netoff TI, Simone DA, Giesler GJ. Responses of thalamic neurons to itch- and pain-producing stimuli in rats. *Journal of Neurophysiology*. 2018;120(3):1119-1134. doi:https://doi.org/10.1152/jn.00264.2018

385. Arain M, Haque M, Johal L, et al. Maturation of the Adolescent Brain. *Neuropsychiatric Disease and Treatment*. 2013;9(9):449-461. doi:https://doi.org/10.2147/ndt.s39776

386. Jones T. Brain Development During Adolescence | Lifespan Development. courses.lumenlearning.com. Published 2020. https://courses.

lumenlearning.com/wm-lifespandevelopment/chapter/brain-development-during-adolescence/

387. Somerville LH, Casey B. Developmental neurobiology of cognitive control and motivational systems. *Current Opinion in Neurobiology*. 2010;20(2):236-241. doi:https://doi.org/10.1016/j.conb.2010.01.006
388. Perlman SB, Pelphrey KA. Regulatory brain development: Balancing emotion and cognition. *Social Neuroscience*. 2010;5(5-6):533-542. doi:https://doi.org/10.1080/17470911003683219
389. Salamone JD, Correa M. The Neurobiology of Activational Aspects of Motivation: Exertion of Effort, Effort-Based Decision Making, and the Role of Dopamine. *Annual Review of Psychology*. 2023;75(1). doi:https://doi.org/10.1146/annurev-psych-020223-012208
390. Ford BQ, Mauss IB. Culture and emotion regulation. *Current Opinion in Psychology*. 2015;3(1):1-5. doi:https://doi.org/10.1016/j.copsyc.2014.12.004
391. Nagulendran A, Jobson L. Exploring cultural differences in the use of emotion regulation strategies in posttraumatic stress disorder. *European Journal of Psychotraumatology*. 2020;11(1):1729033. doi:https://doi.org/10.1080/20008198.2020.1729033
392. Trommsdorff G, Heikamp T. Socialization of emotions and emotion regulation in cultural context. Uni-konstanz.de. Published 2025. Accessed July 24, 2025. https://kops.uni-konstanz.de/entities/publication/6f30567e-6c38-4f29-9960-e559aa896e24
393. Alinajimi F, Deldar Z, Dehghani M, Khatibi A. Emotion regulation mediates the relationship between family caregivers' pain-related beliefs and patients' coping strategies. *Frontiers in Behavioral Neuroscience*. 2023;17. doi:https://doi.org/10.3389/fnbeh.2023.983350
394. Kang G. Cultural Influences on Regulating Emotion. *Intuition: The BYU Undergraduate Journal of Psychology*. 2018;13. https://scholarsarchive.byu.edu/cgi/viewcontent.cgi?article=1229&context=intuition
395. for A. Emotion regulation mediates the relationship between family caregivers' pain-related beliefs and patients' coping strategies. - International Association for the Study of Pain (IASP). International Association for the Study of Pain (IASP). Published July 13, 2021. Accessed July 24, 2025. https://www.iasp-pain.org/publications/pain-research-forum/papers-of-the-week/paper/emotion-regulation-mediates-the-relationship-between-family-caregivers-pain-related-beliefs-and-patients-coping-strategies/
396. Cosio D. Family: Their Role and Impact on Pain Management. www.medcentral.com. Published December 12, 2019. https://www.medcentral.com/pain/alternative-therapies/family-their-role-impact-pain-management
397. Wadley J. Dopamine: New theory integrates its role in learning, motivation. University of Michigan News. Published November 23, 2015. https://news.umich.edu/dopamine-new-theory-integrates-its-role-in-learning-motivation/

398. Berridge KC, Robinson TE, Aldridge JW. Dissecting components of reward: "liking", "wanting", and learning. *Current Opinion in Pharmacology*. 2009;9(1):65-73. doi:https://doi.org/10.1016/j.coph.2008.12.014

399. Covey DP, Cheer JF. Accumbal Dopamine Release Tracks the Expectation of Dopamine Neuron-Mediated Reinforcement. *Cell Reports*. 2019;27(2):481-490.e3. doi:https://doi.org/10.1016/j.celrep.2019.03.055

400. Berridge Lab. Neuroscience of Liking and Wanting – BERRIDGE LAB. sites.lsa.umich.edu. https://sites.lsa.umich.edu/berridge-lab/research-overview/neuroscience-of-linking-and-wanting/

401. De Martino B, Strange BA, Dolan RJ. Noradrenergic neuromodulation of human attention for emotional and neutral stimuli. *Psychopharmacology*. 2007;197(1):127-136. doi:https://doi.org/10.1007/s00213-007-1015-5

402. Mather M, Clewett D, Sakaki M, Harley CW. Norepinephrine ignites local hotspots of neuronal excitation: How arousal amplifies selectivity in perception and memory. *Behavioral and Brain Sciences*. 2015;39. doi:https://doi.org/10.1017/s0140525x15000667

403. Dahl MJ, Mather M, Sander MC, Werkle-Bergner M. Noradrenergic Responsiveness Supports Selective Attention across the Adult Lifespan. *The Journal of Neuroscience*. 2020;40(22):4372-4390. doi:https://doi.org/10.1523/jneurosci.0398-19.2020

404. Wahis J, Holt MG. Astrocytes, Noradrenaline, α1-Adrenoreceptors, and Neuromodulation: Evidence and Unanswered Questions. *Frontiers in Cellular Neuroscience*. 2021;15. doi:https://doi.org/10.3389/fncel.2021.645691

405. Marks R. Overwhelmed? Your Astrocytes Can Help with That. Overwhelmed? Your Astrocytes Can Help with That | UC San Francisco. Published April 6, 2023. Accessed July 24, 2025. https://www.ucsf.edu/news/2023/03/425036/overwhelmed-your-astrocytes-can-help

406. Eskenazi D, Malave L, Mingote S, et al. Dopamine Neurons That Cotransmit Glutamate, From Synapses to Circuits to Behavior. *Frontiers in Neural Circuits*. 2021;15. doi:https://doi.org/10.3389/fncir.2021.665386

407. GSU EDU. Glutamic Acid. Gsu.edu. Published 2025. Accessed July 24, 2025. http://hyperphysics.phy-astr.gsu.edu/hbase/Organic/glutamicacid.html

408. Cleveland Clinic. Glutamate: What it is & function. Cleveland Clinic. Published April 25, 2022. https://my.clevelandclinic.org/health/articles/22839-glutamate

409. Batten SR, Pomerleau F, Quintero J, Gerhardt GA, Beckmann JS. The role of glutamate signaling in incentive salience: second-by-second glutamate recordings in awake Sprague-Dawley rats. *Journal of Neurochemistry*. 2018;145(4):276-286. doi:https://doi.org/10.1111/jnc.14298

410. Broussard JI. Co-transmission of dopamine and glutamate. *Journal of General Physiology*. 2011;139(1):93-96. doi:https://doi.org/10.1085/jgp.201110659

411. LeCocq MR, Amélie Mainville-Berthiaume, Laplante I, Samaha AN. Activating Group II Metabotropic Glutamate Receptors in the Basolateral Amygdala Inhibits Increases in Reward Seeking Triggered by Discriminative Stimuli in Rats. *The International Journal of*

Neuropsychopharmacology. 2025;28(6). doi:https://doi.org/10.1093/ijnp/pyaf030

412. Onaolapo AY, Onaolapo OJ. Glutamate and depression: Reflecting a deepening knowledge of the gut and brain effects of a ubiquitous molecule. *World Journal of Psychiatry*. 2021;11(7):297-315. doi:https://doi.org/10.5498/wjp.v11.i7.297
413. Khoodoruth MAS, Estudillo-Guerra MA, Pacheco-Barrios K, Nyundo A, Chapa-Koloffon G, Ouanes S. Glutamatergic System in Depression and Its Role in Neuromodulatory Techniques Optimization. *Frontiers in Psychiatry*. 2022;13. doi:https://doi.org/10.3389/fpsyt.2022.886918
414. Demuyser T, Femenía T, Niels Danbolt, et al. The glutamate hypothesis of depression: a possible role for glutamate transporters in the pathophysiology of MDD. Vrije Universiteit Brussel. Published 2025. Accessed July 24, 2025. https://researchportal.vub.be/en/publications/the-glutamate-hypothesis-of-depression-a-possible-role-for-glutam
415. Wei X. The glutamatergic system in the development of stress-induced depression. *Annals of Medicine & Surgery*. 2024;86(10):5930-5937. doi:https://doi.org/10.1097/ms9.0000000000002487
416. Filho RVT. Phineas Gage's great legacy. *Dementia & Neuropsychologia*. 2020;14(4):419-421. doi:https://doi.org/10.1590/1980-57642020dn14-040013
417. Washington Edu. Neuroscience for Kids - In the News - Moral Brains. faculty.washington.edu. Published 1999. https://faculty.washington.edu/chudler/moral.html
418. Neylan TC. Frontal Lobe Function. *The Journal of Neuropsychiatry and Clinical Neurosciences*. 1999;11(2):280-281. doi:https://doi.org/10.1176/jnp.11.2.280
419. Kvetnansky R, Sabban EL, Palkovits M. Catecholaminergic Systems in Stress: Structural and Molecular Genetic Approaches. *Physiological Reviews*. 2009;89(2):535-606. doi:https://doi.org/10.1152/physrev.00042.2006
420. Cerritelli F, Frasch MG, Antonelli MC, et al. A Review on the Vagus Nerve and Autonomic Nervous System During Fetal Development: Searching for Critical Windows. *Frontiers in Neuroscience*. 2021;15:721605. doi:https://doi.org/10.3389/fnins.2021.721605
421. Wang T, Avedis Tufenkjian, Ajijola OA, Oka Y. Molecular and functional diversity of the autonomic nervous system. *Nature reviews Neuroscience*. Published online July 3, 2025. doi:https://doi.org/10.1038/s41583-025-00941-2
422. Xingchao Wang, Qiong Wu, Egan L, et al. Anterior insular cortex plays a critical role in interoceptive attention. eLife. Published April 15, 2019. https://elifesciences.org/articles/42265
423. Marasco PD, de Nooij JC. Proprioception: A New Era Set in Motion by Emerging Genetic and Bionic Strategies? *Annual Review of Physiology*. 2022;85(1). doi:https://doi.org/10.1146/annurev-physiol-040122-081302
424. Sugawara A, Ruri Katsunuma, Terasawa Y, Sekiguchi A. Interoceptive training impacts the neural circuit of the anterior insula cortex. *Translational Psychiatry*. 2024;14(1). doi:https://doi.org/10.1038/s41398-024-02933-9

425. Okonogi T, Kuga N, Yamakawa M, Tasuku Kayama, Yuji Ikegaya, Sasaki T. Stress-induced vagal activity influences anxiety-relevant prefrontal and amygdala neuronal oscillations in male mice. *Nature communications*. 2024;15(1). doi:https://doi.org/10.1038/s41467-023-44205-y
426. Hafez OA, Chang RB. Regulation of Cardiac Function by the Autonomic Nervous System. *Physiology*. 2025;40(3). doi:https://doi.org/10.1152/physiol.00018.2024
427. Duk Su Koh, Hille B. Modulation by neurotransmitters of catecholamine secretion from sympathetic ganglion neurons detected by amperometry. *Proceedings of the National Academy of Sciences of the United States of America*. 1997;94(4):1506-1511. doi:https://doi.org/10.1073/pnas.94.4.1506
428. Diehl MM, Bravo-Rivera C, Rodriguez-Romaguera J, et al. Active avoidance requires inhibitory signaling in the rodent prelimbic prefrontal cortex. *eLife*. 2018;7. doi:https://doi.org/10.7554/elife.34657
429. Wang KS, Delgado MR. Corticostriatal Circuits Encode the Subjective Value of Perceived Control. *Cerebral Cortex*. 2019;29(12):5049-5060. doi:https://doi.org/10.1093/cercor/bhz045
430. Muhammad Badarnee, Wen Z, Hammoud MZ, Glimcher P, Cain CK, Milad MR. Intersect between brain mechanisms of conditioned threat, active avoidance, and reward. *Communications Psychology*. 2025;3(1). doi:https://doi.org/10.1038/s44271-025-00197-7
431. Boeke EA, Moscarello JM, LeDoux JE, Phelps EA, Hartley CA. Active Avoidance: Neural Mechanisms and Attenuation of Pavlovian Conditioned Responding. *The Journal of Neuroscience*. 2017;37(18):4808-4818. doi:https://doi.org/10.1523/jneurosci.3261-16.2017
432. Ehret B, Boehringer R, Amadei EA, et al. Population-level coding of avoidance learning in medial prefrontal cortex. *Nature Neuroscience*. Published online July 29, 2024. doi:https://doi.org/10.1038/s41593-024-01704-5
433. Dundon NM, Shapiro AD, Babenko V, Okafor GN, Grafton ST. Ventromedial Prefrontal Cortex Activity and Sympathetic Allostasis During Value-Based Ambivalence. *Frontiers in Behavioral Neuroscience*. 2021;15. doi:https://doi.org/10.3389/fnbeh.2021.615796
434. McEwen BS, Bowles NP, Gray JD, et al. Mechanisms of stress in the brain. *Nature Neuroscience*. 2015;18(10):1353-1363. doi:https://doi.org/10.1038/nn.4086
435. Lakoff G, Johnson M. Metaphors We Live By. Bibliovault.org. Published 2025. https://www.bibliovault.org/BV.landing.epl?ISBN=9780226468013
436. Kapoor A. "Knowing yourself is the beginning of all wisdom." — Aristotle. Medium. Published May 10, 2020. https://medium.com/@ankushskapoor/knowing-yourself-is-the-beginning-of-all-wisdom-aristotle-d4a99843be1b
437. Friedrich Nietzsche Quote. A-Z Quotes. Published 2024. https://www.azquotes.com/quote/563942
438. A quote by Michael Bassey Johnson. Goodreads.com. Published 2024. https://www.goodreads.com/quotes/4442124-your-real-self-may-be-hiding-somewhere-look-for-it

439. Bridie. Painting is self-discovery. Every good artist paints what he is – Jackson Pollock. Pentreath & Hall. Published December 31, 2015. Accessed July 24, 2025. https://pentreath-hall.com/blogs/inspiration/painting-is-self-discovery-every-good-artist-paints-what-he-is-jackson-pollock?srsltid=AfmBOoq09eDyT3IuWlZfEteZVwvXrMSRImNvF6W-x2KQpDgnvh0gBKQI
440. Jesuit Resource - Character Quotes. www.xavier.edu. https://www.xavier.edu/jesuitresource/online-resources/quote-archive1/character-quotes
441. Cavanna AE, Trimble MR. The precuneus: a review of its functional anatomy and behavioural correlates. *Brain*. 2006;129(3):564-583. doi:https://doi.org/10.1093/brain/awl004
442. Utevsky AV, Smith DV, Huettel SA. Precuneus Is a Functional Core of the Default-Mode Network. *The Journal of Neuroscience*. 2014;34(3):932-940. doi:https://doi.org/10.1523/jneurosci.4227-13.2014
443. Vatansever D, Menon DK, Stamatakis EA. Default mode contributions to automated information processing. *Proceedings of the National Academy of Sciences*. 2017;114(48):12821-12826. doi:https://doi.org/10.1073/pnas.1710521114
444. The Times Driving. Research Reveals Top Distractions for Drivers. The Times Driving - Motoring news, reviews, guides and tips. Published 2024. Accessed July 24, 2025. https://www.driving.com.au/motoring/39296-research-reveals-top-distractions-for-drivers
445. Zhou C, Ding L, Skibniewski MJ, Luo H, Jiang S. Characterizing time series of near-miss accidents in metro construction via complex network theory. *Safety Science*. 2017;98:145-158. doi:https://doi.org/10.1016/j.ssci.2017.06.012
446. Haas B, Doumouras AG, Gomez D, et al. Close to home: An analysis of the relationship between location of residence and location of injury. *The journal of trauma and acute care surgery*. 2015;78(4):860-865. doi:https://doi.org/10.1097/TA.0000000000000595
447. Fletcher PC, Frith CD, Baker SC, Shallice T, Frackowiak RSJ, Dolan RJ. The Mind's Eye—Precuneus Activation in Memory-Related Imagery. *NeuroImage*. 1995;2(3):195-200. doi:https://doi.org/10.1006/nimg.1995.1025
448. Zhang S, Li CR. Functional connectivity mapping of the human precuneus by resting state fMRI. *NeuroImage*. 2012;59(4):3548-3562. doi:https://doi.org/10.1016/j.neuroimage.2011.11.023
449. Petrides M, Lefebvre S, Novek J, Zlatkina V. Interaction of the dorsolateral prefrontal cortex with the precuneal medial parietal cortex for the monitoring of information in working memory in the macaque monkey. *Cerebral Cortex*. 2024;34(8). doi:https://doi.org/10.1093/cercor/bhae315
450. Ren Y, Nguyen VT, Sonkusare S, et al. Effective connectivity of the anterior hippocampus predicts recollection confidence during natural memory retrieval. *Nature Communications*. 2018;9(1). doi:https://doi.org/10.1038/s41467-018-07325-4
451. Herbet G, Lemaitre AL, Moritz-Gasser S, Cochereau J, Duffau H. The antero-dorsal precuneal cortex supports specific aspects of bodily

awareness. *Brain*. 2019;142(8):2207-2214. doi:https://doi.org/10.1093/brain/awz179

452. Whitfield-Gabrieli S, Moran JM, Nieto-Castañón A, Triantafyllou C, Saxe R, Gabrieli JDE. Associations and dissociations between default and self-reference networks in the human brain. *NeuroImage*. 2011;55(1):225-232. doi:https://doi.org/10.1016/j.neuroimage.2010.11.048
453. Harrison BJ, Pujol J, Lopez-Sola M, et al. Consistency and functional specialization in the default mode brain network. *Proceedings of the National Academy of Sciences*. 2008;105(28):9781-9786. doi:https://doi.org/10.1073/pnas.0711791105
454. Denny BT, Kober H, Wager TD, Ochsner KN. A Meta-analysis of Functional Neuroimaging Studies of Self- and Other Judgments Reveals a Spatial Gradient for Mentalizing in Medial Prefrontal Cortex. *Journal of Cognitive Neuroscience*. 2012;24(8):1742-1752. doi:https://doi.org/10.1162/jocn_a_00233
455. Terneusen A, Winkens I, van Heugten C, et al. Neural Correlates of Impaired Self-awareness of Deficits after Acquired Brain Injury: A Systematic Review. *Neuropsychology Review*. Published online February 3, 2022. doi:https://doi.org/10.1007/s11065-022-09535-6
456. Zheng S, Zhang FX, Hubert, et al. Unraveling the brain dynamics of Depersonalization-Derealization Disorder: a dynamic functional network connectivity analysis. *BMC Psychiatry*. 2024;24(1). doi:https://doi.org/10.1186/s12888-024-06096-1
457. Filho RVT. Phineas Gage's great legacy. *Dementia & Neuropsychologia*. 2020;14(4):419-421. doi:https://doi.org/10.1590/1980-57642020dn14-040013
458. Norman S, Maguen S. Moral Injury in the Context of War - PTSD: National Center for PTSD. U.S. Department of Veterans Affairs. Published 2014. https://www.ptsd.va.gov/professional/treat/cooccurring/moral_injury.asp
459. Jia Y, Song N, Ning Y, et al. Altered Self-Referential-Related Brain Regions in Depersonalization-Derealization Disorder. *Brain and Behavior*. 2025;15(2). doi:https://doi.org/10.1002/brb3.70314
460. Goldman B. Where in the brain is my sense of self? News Center. Published 2023. Accessed July 24, 2025. https://med.stanford.edu/news/insights/2023/06/where-in-the-brain-is-my-sense-of-self.html
461. Gogtay N, Giedd JN, Lusk L, et al. Dynamic mapping of human cortical development during childhood through early adulthood. *Proceedings of the National Academy of Sciences*. 2004;101(21):8174-8179. doi:https://doi.org/10.1073/pnas.0402680101
462. Li R, Utevsky AV, Huettel SA, et al. Developmental Maturation of the Precuneus as a Functional Core of the Default Mode Network. *Journal of Cognitive Neuroscience*. 2019;31(10):1506-1519. doi:https://doi.org/10.1162/jocn_a_01426
463. Brewer JA, Worhunsky PD, Gray JR, Tang YY ., Weber J, Kober H. Meditation experience is associated with differences in default mode network activity and connectivity. *Proceedings of the National Academy of*

Sciences. 2011;108(50):20254-20259. doi:https://doi.org/10.1073/pnas.1112029108

464. Rahrig H, Vago DR, Passarelli MA, Auten A, Lynn NA, Brown KW. Meta-analytic evidence that mindfulness training alters resting state default mode network connectivity. *Scientific Reports*. 2022;12(1). doi:https://doi.org/10.1038/s41598-022-15195-6

465. Why the Octopus Brain is so Extraordinary | Smithsonian Ocean. ocean.si.edu. https://ocean.si.edu/ocean-life/invertebrates/why-octopus-brain-so-extraordinary

466. Fabian P, Sven G, Braun W, Raoul-Martin M. From single neurons to behavior in the jellyfish Aurelia aurita. *ProQuest*. Published online 2019. doi:https://doi.org/10.7554/eLife.50084

467. Keeping A Nose Out. Defenders of Wildlife. https://defenders.org/blog/2012/10/keeping-nose-out

468. Pfeiffenberger JA, Hsieh ST. Autotomy-induced effects on the locomotor performance of the ghost crab Ocypode quadrata. *Journal of Experimental Biology*. 2021;224(10). doi:https://doi.org/10.1242/jeb.233536

469. Sadiq M. How Elephants Remember Friends After Decades. Animals Around The Globe. Published June 20, 2025. Accessed July 24, 2025. https://www.animalsaroundtheglobe.com/how-elephants-remember-friends-after-decades-1-345099/

470. Prior H, Schwarz A, Güntürkün O. Mirror-Induced Behavior in the Magpie (Pica pica): Evidence of Self-Recognition. de Waal F, ed. *PLoS Biology*. 2008;6(8):e202. doi:https://doi.org/10.1371/journal.pbio.0060202

471. Plotnik JM, de Waal FBM, Reiss D. Self-recognition in an Asian elephant. *Proceedings of the National Academy of Sciences*. 2006;103(45):17053-17057. doi:https://doi.org/10.1073/pnas.0608062103

472. Ekman P. Darwin's contributions to our understanding of emotional expressions. *Philosophical Transactions of the Royal Society B: Biological Sciences*. 2009;364(1535):3449-3451. doi:https://doi.org/10.1098/rstb.2009.0189

473. Darwin C. Darwin Online: The Descent of Man. Darwin-online.org.uk. Published 2023. https://darwin-online.org.uk/EditorialIntroductions/Freeman_TheDescentofMan.html

474. Bruner E, Preuss TM, Chen X, Rilling JK. Evidence for expansion of the precuneus in human evolution. *Brain Structure and Function*. 2016;222(2):1053-1060. doi:https://doi.org/10.1007/s00429-015-1172-y

475. Pereira-Pedro AS, Bruner E, Gunz P, Neubauer S. A morphometric comparison of the parietal lobe in modern humans and Neanderthals. *Journal of Human Evolution*. 2020;142:102770. doi:https://doi.org/10.1016/j.jhevol.2020.102770

476. Viganò S, Bayramova R, Doeller CF, Bottini R. Mental search of concepts is supported by egocentric vector representations and restructured grid maps. *Nature communications*. 2023;14(1). doi:https://doi.org/10.1038/s41467-023-43831-w

477. Brosch T, Sander D. Neurocognitive mechanisms underlying value-based

decision-making: from core values to economic value. *Frontiers in Human Neuroscience*. 2013;7. doi:https://doi.org/10.3389/fnhum.2013.00398

478. Marshall L, Born J. The contribution of sleep to hippocampus-dependent memory consolidation. *Trends in Cognitive Sciences*. 2007;11(10):442-450. doi:https://doi.org/10.1016/j.tics.2007.09.001

479. Squire LR, Stark CEL, Clark RE. THE MEDIAL TEMPORAL LOBE. *Annual Review of Neuroscience*. 2004;27(1):279-306. doi:https://doi.org/10.1146/annurev.neuro.27.070203.144130

480. Alberini CM, Travaglia A. Infantile Amnesia: A Critical Period of Learning to Learn and Remember. *The Journal of Neuroscience*. 2017;37(24):5783-5795. doi:https://doi.org/10.1523/jneurosci.0324-17.2017

481. Cleveland Clinic . Hippocampus. Cleveland Clinic. Published May 14, 2024. https://my.clevelandclinic.org/health/body/hippocampus

482. Josselyn SA, Tonegawa S. Memory engrams: Recalling the past and imagining the future. *Science*. 2020;367(6473). doi:https://doi.org/10.1126/science.aaw4325

483. Hall SA, Rubin DC, Miles A, et al. The Neural Basis of Involuntary Episodic Memories. *Journal of Cognitive Neuroscience*. 2014;26(10):2385-2399. doi:https://doi.org/10.1162/jocn_a_00633

484. Psychology Today. Semantic Memory. Psychology Today. Published 2025. https://www.psychologytoday.com/us/basics/subpage/semantic-memory

485. Procedural Memory. Psychology Today. Published 2025. https://www.psychologytoday.com/us/basics/subpage/procedural-memory

486. Bostan AC, Strick PL. The Cerebellum and Basal Ganglia are Interconnected. *Neuropsychology Review*. 2010;20(3):261-270. doi:https://doi.org/10.1007/s11065-010-9143-9

487. Emotional Memory - an overview | ScienceDirect Topics. www.sciencedirect.com. https://www.sciencedirect.com/topics/neuroscience/emotional-memory

488. Rodriguez-Ortiz CJ, Bermúdez-Rattoni F. Memory Reconsolidation or Updating Consolidation? Nih.gov. Published 2017. https://www.ncbi.nlm.nih.gov/books/NBK3905/

489. Euston David R, Gruber Aaron J, McNaughton Bruce L. The Role of Medial Prefrontal Cortex in Memory and Decision Making. *Neuron*. 2012;76(6):1057-1070. doi:https://doi.org/10.1016/j.neuron.2012.12.002

490. Payne JD. Sleep, dreams, and memory consolidation: The role of the stress hormone cortisol. *Learning & Memory*. 2004;11(6):671-678. doi:https://doi.org/10.1101/lm.77104

491. Wamsley EJ. Dreaming and offline memory consolidation. *Current Neurology and Neuroscience Reports*. 2014;14(3). doi:https://doi.org/10.1007/s11910-013-0433-5

492. Blomkvist A. Shaping the Space: A Role for the Hippocampus in Mental Imagery Formation. *Vision*. 2025;9(1):2. doi:https://doi.org/10.3390/vision9010002

493. Pearson J. The human imagination: The cognitive neuroscience of visual mental imagery. *Nature Reviews Neuroscience*. 2019;20(10):624-634. doi:https://doi.org/10.1038/s41583-019-0202-9
494. Boccia M, Piccardi L, Palermo L, Nori R, Palmiero M. Where do bright ideas occur in our brain? Meta-analytic evidence from neuroimaging studies of domain-specific creativity. *Frontiers in Psychology*. 2015;6. doi:https://doi.org/10.3389/fpsyg.2015.01195
495. Milton F, Fulford J, Dance C, et al. Behavioral and Neural Signatures of Visual Imagery Vividness Extremes: Aphantasia vs. Hyperphantasia. *Cerebral Cortex Communications*. 2021;2(2). doi:https://doi.org/10.1093/texcom/tgab035
496. Keogh R, Pearson J, Zeman A. Aphantasia: The science of visual imagery extremes. *Handbook of Clinical Neurology*. 2021;178:277-296. doi:https://doi.org/10.1016/B978-0-12-821377-3.00012-X
497. Keogh R, Bergmann J, Pearson J. Cortical excitability controls the strength of mental imagery. *eLife*. 2020;9. doi:https://doi.org/10.7554/elife.50232
498. Press Pack . Study finds link between functional brain connectivity and aphantasia. eLife. Published February 27, 2024. https://elifesciences.org/for-the-press/7ead8959/study-finds-link-between-functional-brain-connectivity-and-aphantasia
499. Robson D. "Like a film in my mind": hyperphantasia and the quest to understand vivid imaginations. *The Observer*. https://www.theguardian.com/science/2024/apr/20/like-a-film-in-my-mind-hyperphantasia-and-the-quest-to-understand-vivid-imaginations. Published April 20, 2024.
500. Zeman A. Aphantasia and hyperphantasia: Exploring imagery vividness extremes. *Trends in Cognitive Sciences (Regular ed)*. 2024;28(5). doi:https://doi.org/10.1016/j.tics.2024.02.007
501. Wendelpublished J. What happens in our brains when we "hear" our own thoughts?. livescience.com. Published May 28, 2022. https://www.livescience.com/how-hear-inner-thoughts
502. Stephane M, Dzemidzic M, Yoon G. Keeping the inner voice inside the head, a pilot fMRI study. *Brain and Behavior*. 2021;11(4). doi:https://doi.org/10.1002/brb3.2042
503. Isaac AR, Marks DF. Individual differences in mental imagery experience: Developmental changes and specialization. *British Journal of Psychology*. 1994;85(4):479-500. doi:https://doi.org/10.1111/j.2044-8295.1994.tb02536.x
504. Lu J, Riecke L, Ryan BE, Gelder B de. The contribution of body perception to self-identity. An ERP study. *Social Cognitive and Affective Neuroscience*. Published online February 27, 2025. doi:https://doi.org/10.1093/scan/nsaf020
505. Holt-Lunstad J, Smith TB, Layton JB. Social Relationships and Mortality Risk: a Meta-analytic Review. *PLoS Medicine*. 2010;7(7). doi:https://doi.org/10.1371/journal.pmed.1000316
506. Darwin C. Darwin Online: The Descent of Man. Darwin-online.org.uk. Published 2023. https://darwin-online.org.uk/EditorialIntroductions/Freeman_TheDescentofMan.html

507. Uchii S. Darwin on the Evolution of Morality. philsci-archive.pitt.edu. Published 1999. Accessed November 12, 2023. https://philsci-archive.pitt.edu/137/1/DonM-text.html

508. Steptoe A, Shankar A, Demakakos P, Wardle J. Social Isolation, Loneliness, and All-Cause Mortality in Older Men and Women. *Proceedings of the National Academy of Sciences*. 2013;110(15):5797-5801. doi:https://doi.org/10.1073/pnas.1219686110

509. Aristotle. A quote from Politics. Goodreads.com. Published 2019. https://www.goodreads.com/quotes/183896-man-is-by-nature-a-social-animal-an-individual-who

510. Atterton P. Levinas and Buber: Dialogue and Difference. Notre Dame Philosophical Reviews. Published 2025. Accessed July 25, 2025. https://ndpr.nd.edu/reviews/levinas-and-buber-dialogue-and-difference/

511. Edelstein B. The I-Thou Relationship and Unconditional Positive Regard | Psychology Today. www.psychologytoday.com. Published August 21, 2022. https://www.psychologytoday.com/us/blog/authentic-engagement/202208/the-i-thou-relationship-and-unconditional-positive-regard

512. Reynolds J, Renaudie PJ. Jean-Paul Sartre. Stanford Encyclopedia of Philosophy. Published March 26, 2022. https://plato.stanford.edu/entries/sartre/

513. Dores AR, Peixoto M, Fernandes C, Marques A, Barbosa F. The Effects of Social Feedback Through the "Like" Feature on Brain Activity: A Systematic Review. *Healthcare*. 2025;13(1):89-89. doi:https://doi.org/10.3390/healthcare13010089

514. Maza MT, Fox KA, Kwon SJ, et al. Association of Habitual Checking Behaviors on Social Media With Longitudinal Functional Brain Development. *JAMA Pediatrics*. 2023;177(2):160-167. doi:https://doi.org/10.1001/jamapediatrics.2022.4924

515. Op de Macks ZA, Bunge SA, Bell ON, Kriegsfeld LJ, Kayser AS, Dahl RE. The effect of social rank feedback on risk taking and associated reward processes in adolescent girls. *Social Cognitive and Affective Neuroscience*. 2016;12(2):240-250. doi:https://doi.org/10.1093/scan/nsw125

516. Montag C, Markowetz A, Blaszkiewicz K, et al. Facebook usage on smartphones and gray matter volume of the nucleus accumbens. *Behavioural Brain Research*. 2017;329:221-228. doi:https://doi.org/10.1016/j.bbr.2017.04.035

517. De D, El Jamal M, Aydemir E, Khera A. Social Media Algorithms and Teen Addiction: Neurophysiological Impact and Ethical Considerations. *Cureus*. 2025;17(1):1-7. doi:https://doi.org/10.7759/cureus.77145

518. Dolan EW. Does TikTok really cause brain rot? New study links short video addiction to brain abnormalities. PsyPost - Psychology News. Published January 17, 2025. https://www.psypost.org/does-tiktok-really-cause-brain-rot-new-study-links-short-video-addiction-to-brain-abnormalities/

519. Liu D, Rahman M, Johnson A, et al. A hypothalamic circuit underlying the dynamic control of social homeostasis. *Nature*. Published online February 26, 2025. doi:https://doi.org/10.1038/s41586-025-08617-8

520. Finley AJ, Schaefer SM. Affective Neuroscience of Loneliness: Potential Mechanisms underlying the Association between Perceived Social Isolation, Health, and Well-Being. *Journal of Psychiatry and Brain Science*. 2022;7(6). doi:https://doi.org/10.20900/jpbs.20220011

521. Paré D, Headley DB. The amygdala mediates the facilitating influence of emotions on memory through multiple interacting mechanisms. *Neurobiology of Stress*. 2023;24:100529. doi:https://doi.org/10.1016/j.ynstr.2023.100529

522. Alves H, Koch A, Unkelbach C. Why Good Is More Alike Than Bad: Processing Implications. *Trends in Cognitive Sciences*. 2017;21(2):69-79. doi:https://doi.org/10.1016/j.tics.2016.12.006

523. Institute of Medicine (US) and National Research Council (US) Committee on the Science of Adolescence. Biobehavioral Processes. Nih.gov. Published 2011. https://www.ncbi.nlm.nih.gov/books/NBK53414/

524. Salvato G, Richter F, Sedeño L, Bottini G, Paulesu E. Building the bodily self-awareness: Evidence for the convergence between interoceptive and exteroceptive information in a multilevel kernel density analysis study. *Human Brain Mapping*. Published online October 14, 2019. doi:https://doi.org/10.1002/hbm.24810

525. Dewall CN, Macdonald G, Webster GD, et al. Acetaminophen reduces social pain: behavioral and neural evidence. *Psychological science*. 2010;21(7):931-937. doi:https://doi.org/10.1177/0956797610374741

526. Harris E. Meta-Analysis: Social Isolation, Loneliness Tied to Higher Mortality. *JAMA*. 2023;330(3):211-211. doi:https://doi.org/10.1001/jama.2023.11958

527. Schreuders E, Braams BR, Crone EA, Güroğlu B. Friendship stability in adolescence is associated with ventral striatum responses to vicarious rewards. *Nature Communications*. 2021;12(1). doi:https://doi.org/10.1038/s41467-020-20042-1

528. Graham L. The Neuroscience of Attachment. Linda Graham. Published September 6, 2008. https://lindagraham-mft.net/the-neuroscience-of-attachment/

529. Carr L, Iacoboni M, Dubeau MC ., Mazziotta JC, Lenzi GL. Neural mechanisms of empathy in humans: A relay from neural systems for imitation to limbic areas. *Proceedings of the National Academy of Sciences*. 2003;100(9):5497-5502. doi:https://doi.org/10.1073/pnas.0935845100

530. Šimić G, Tkalčić M, Vukić V, et al. Understanding Emotions: Origins and Roles of the Amygdala. *Biomolecules*. 2021;11(6):823. doi:https://doi.org/10.3390/biom11060823

531. Krause L, Enticott PG, Zangen A, Fitzgerald PB. The role of medial prefrontal cortex in theory of mind: A deep rTMS study. *Behavioural Brain Research*. 2012;228(1):87-90. doi:https://doi.org/10.1016/j.bbr.2011.11.037

532. Gu X, Gao Z, Wang X, et al. Anterior insular cortex is necessary for empathetic pain perception. *Brain*. 2012;135(9):2726-2735. doi:https://doi.org/10.1093/brain/aws199

533. Hillis AE. Inability to empathize: brain lesions that disrupt sharing and understanding another's emotions. *Brain*. 2013;137(4):981-997. doi:https://doi.org/10.1093/brain/awt317

534. Acharya S, Shukla S. Mirror neurons: Enigma of the metaphysical modular brain. *Journal of Natural Science, Biology and Medicine*. 2012;3(2):118-124. doi:https://doi.org/10.4103/0976-9668.101878

535. Lesley University. The Psychology of Emotional and Cognitive Empathy. Lesley.edu. Published 2024. https://lesley.edu/article/the-psychology-of-emotional-and-cognitive-empathy

536. Ciaramelli E, Bernardi F, Moscovitch M. Individualized Theory of Mind (iToM): When Memory Modulates Empathy. *Frontiers in Psychology*. 2013;4(4). doi:https://doi.org/10.3389/fpsyg.2013.00004

537. Riess H. The Science of Empathy. *Journal of Patient Experience*. 2017;4(2):74-77. doi:https://doi.org/10.1177/2374373517699267

538. de Sousa A, McDonald S, Rushby J, Li S, Dimoska A, James C. Why don't you feel how I feel? Insight into the absence of empathy after severe Traumatic Brain Injury. *Neuropsychologia*. 2010;48(12):3585-3595. doi:https://doi.org/10.1016/j.neuropsychologia.2010.08.008

539. Hiser J, Koenigs M. The Multifaceted Role of the Ventromedial Prefrontal Cortex in Emotion, Decision Making, Social Cognition, and Psychopathology. *Biological Psychiatry*. 2018;83(8):638-647. doi:https://doi.org/10.1016/j.biopsych.2017.10.030

540. de Sousa A, McDonald S, Rushby J, Li S, Dimoska A, James C. Understanding deficits in empathy after traumatic brain injury: The role of affective responsivity. *Cortex*. 2011;47(5):526-535. doi:https://doi.org/10.1016/j.cortex.2010.02.004

541. Filho RVT. Phineas Gage's great legacy. *Dementia & Neuropsychologia*. 2020;14(4):419-421. doi:https://doi.org/10.1590/1980-57642020dn14-040013

542. Baird AD, Scheffer IE, Wilson SJ. Mirror neuron system involvement in empathy: A critical look at the evidence. *Social Neuroscience*. 2011;6(4):327-335. doi:https://doi.org/10.1080/17470919.2010.547085

543. Banissy MJ, Kanai R, Walsh V, Rees G. Inter-individual differences in empathy are reflected in human brain structure. *NeuroImage*. 2012;62(3):2034-2039. doi:https://doi.org/10.1016/j.neuroimage.2012.05.081

544. Cao R, Dubois J, Mamelak AN, Adolphs R, Wang S, Rutishauser U. Domain-specific representation of social inference by neurons in the human amygdala and hippocampus. *Science Advances*. 2024;10(49). doi:https://doi.org/10.1126/sciadv.ado6166

545. Brown EC, Brüne M. Evolution of Social Predictive Brains? *Frontiers in Psychology*. 2012;3. doi:https://doi.org/10.3389/fpsyg.2012.00414

546. Charles D. Darwinism stated by Darwin himself Characteristic passages from the writings of Charles Darwin. Gutenberg.org. Published 2022. https://www.gutenberg.org/cache/epub/69147/pg69147-images.html

547. Rozzi R. The Reciprocal Links between Evolutionary-Ecological Sciences and Environmental Ethics. *BioScience*. 1999;49(11):911-921. doi:https://doi.org/10.2307/1313650

548. Salzman CD, Fusi S. Emotion, Cognition, and Mental State Representation in Amygdala and Prefrontal Cortex. *Annual Review of Neuroscience*. 2010;33(1):173-202. doi:https://doi.org/10.1146/annurev.neuro.051508.135256

549. Pierce K, Redcay E. Fusiform Function in Children with an Autism Spectrum Disorder Is a Matter of "Who." *Biological Psychiatry*. 2008;64(7):552-560. doi:https://doi.org/10.1016/j.biopsych.2008.05.013

550. *Reading 22: I CAN SEE IT ALL over YOUR FACE!* https://solomonr1.weebly.com/uploads/1/7/5/0/17505523/psy_22_-_i_can_see_it_all_over_your_face.pdf

551. Ekman P. Universal Emotions | What are Emotions? | Paul Ekman Group. Paul Ekman Group. Published 2019. https://www.paulekman.com/universal-emotions/

552. Coppini S, Lucifora C, Vicario CM, Gangemi A. Experiments on real-life emotions challenge Ekman's model. *Scientific Reports*. 2023;13(1):9511. doi:https://doi.org/10.1038/s41598-023-36201-5

553. Yu H, Lin C, Sun S, Cao R, Kar K, Wang S. Multimodal investigations of emotional face processing and social trait judgment of faces. *Annals of the New York Academy of Sciences*. Published online November 15, 2023. doi:https://doi.org/10.1111/nyas.15084

554. Preston Alison R, Eichenbaum H. Interplay of Hippocampus and Prefrontal Cortex in Memory. *Current Biology*. 2013;23(17):R764-R773. doi:https://doi.org/10.1016/j.cub.2013.05.041

555. Foreman P. *"IT'S JUST THAT for the FIRST TIME, I FEEL… WICKED": A RHETORICAL ANALYSIS of WICKED'S ELPHABA USING KENNETH BURKE'S GUILT-PURIFICATION-REDEMPTION CYCLE.*; 2013. https://digitalcommons.liberty.edu/cgi/viewcontent.cgi?article=1267&context=masters

556. Psychology Today. Jealousy | Psychology Today. Psychology Today. Published 2019. https://www.psychologytoday.com/us/basics/jealousy

557. Eisenberger NI, Lieberman MD, Williams KD. Does Rejection Hurt? An fMRI Study of Social Exclusion. *Science*. 2003;302(5643):290-292. doi:https://doi.org/10.1126/science.1089134

558. Office of the Surgeon General (OSG). *Our Epidemic of Loneliness and Isolation: The U.S. Surgeon General's Advisory on the Healing Effects of Social Connection and Community*. US Department of Health and Human Services; 2023. https://www.ncbi.nlm.nih.gov/books/NBK595227/

559. Ramachandran VS, Jalal B. The Evolutionary Psychology of Envy and Jealousy. *Frontiers in Psychology*. 2017;8. doi:https://doi.org/10.3389/fpsyg.2017.01619

560. Takahashi H, Matsuura M, Yahata N, Koeda M, Suhara T, Okubo Y. Men and women show distinct brain activations during imagery of sexual and emotional infidelity. *NeuroImage*. 2006;32(3):1299-1307. doi:https://doi.org/10.1016/j.neuroimage.2006.05.049

561. Lenroot RK, Giedd JN. The changing impact of genes and environment on brain development during childhood and adolescence: Initial findings from

a neuroimaging study of pediatric twins. *Development and Psychopathology*. 2008;20(4):1161-1175. doi:https://doi.org/10.1017/s0954579408000552

562. Kelley NJ, Eastwick PW, Harmon-Jones E, Schmeichel BJ. Jealousy increased by induced relative left frontal cortical activity. *Emotion*. 2015;15(5):550-555. doi:https://doi.org/10.1037/emo0000068
563. Some People Truly Don't Feel Jealousy. Psychology Today. Published 2017. Accessed July 25, 2025. https://www.psychologytoday.com/us/blog/the-polyamorists-next-door/201711/some-people-truly-don-t-feel-jealousy
564. Zheng X, Luo L, Li J, et al. A dimensional approach to jealousy reveals enhanced fronto-striatal, insula and limbic responses to angry faces. *Brain Structure and Function*. 2019;224(9):3201-3212. doi:https://doi.org/10.1007/s00429-019-01958-x
565. Dvash J, Gilam G, Ben-Ze'ev A, Hendler T, Shamay-Tsoory SG. The envious brain: The neural basis of social comparison. *Human Brain Mapping*. 2010;31(11):NA-NA. doi:https://doi.org/10.1002/hbm.20972
566. Eisenberger NI. The neural bases of social pain: Evidence for shared representations with physical pain. *Psychosomatic Medicine*. 2012;74(2):126-135. doi:https://doi.org/10.1097/psy.0b013e3182464dd1
567. Sun Y, Yu H, Chen J, et al. Neural substrates and behavioral profiles of romantic jealousy and its temporal dynamics. *Scientific Reports*. 2016;6(1). doi:https://doi.org/10.1038/srep27469
568. Dolan EW. Neuroscientists shed new light on the roots of interpersonal neural synchrony during social interactions. PsyPost - Psychology News. Published July 28, 2023. Accessed July 25, 2025. https://www.psypost.org/neuroscientists-shed-new-light-on-the-roots-of-interpersonal-neural-synchrony-during-social-interactions/
569. Levy J, Lankinen K, Hakonen M, Feldman R. The integration of social and neural synchrony: a case for ecologically valid research using MEG neuroimaging. *Social Cognitive and Affective Neuroscience*. 2020;16(1-2):143-152. doi:https://doi.org/10.1093/scan/nsaa061
570. Rogers JF, Morgane Vandendoren, Prather JF, Landen JG, Bedford NL, Nelson AC. Neural Cell-types and Circuits Linking Thermoregulation and Social Behavior. *Neuroscience & biobehavioral reviews/Neuroscience and biobehavioral reviews*. 2024;161:105667-105667. doi:https://doi.org/10.1016/j.neubiorev.2024.105667
571. Robinson GE, Fernald RD, Clayton DF. Genes and Social Behavior. *Science*. 2008;322(5903):896-900. doi:https://doi.org/10.1126/science.1159277
572. Haas BW, Filkowski MM, Cochran RN, et al. Epigenetic modification of OXT and human sociability. *Proceedings of the National Academy of Sciences*. 2016;113(27):E3816-E3823. doi:https://doi.org/10.1073/pnas.1602809113
573. Chen FS, Kumsta R, von Dawans B, Monakhov M, Ebstein RP, Heinrichs M. Common oxytocin receptor gene (OXTR) polymorphism and social support interact to reduce stress in humans. *Proceedings of the National Academy of Sciences*. 2011;108(50):19937-19942. doi:https://doi.org/10.1073/pnas.1113079108

574. NIH. Scientists map unprecedented detail of connections and visual perception in the mouse brain. National Institutes of Health (NIH). Published April 9, 2025. https://www.nih.gov/news-events/news-releases/scientists-map-unprecedented-detail-connections-visual-perception-mouse-brain

575. Trafton A. How the brain processes emotions. MIT News | Massachusetts Institute of Technology. Published March 31, 2016. https://news.mit.edu/2016/brain-processes-emotions-mental-illness-depression-0331

576. Berns GS, Atran S. The biology of cultural conflict. *Philosophical Transactions of the Royal Society B: Biological Sciences*. 2012;367(1589):633-639. doi:https://doi.org/10.1098/rstb.2011.0307

577. Vitale EM, Smith AS. Neurobiology of Loneliness, Isolation, and Loss: Integrating Human and Animal Perspectives. *Frontiers in Behavioral Neuroscience*. 2022;16. doi:https://doi.org/10.3389/fnbeh.2022.846315

578. Ressler KJ. Amygdala activity, fear, and anxiety: Modulation by stress. *Biological Psychiatry*. 2020;67(12):1117-1119. doi:https://doi.org/10.1016/j.biopsych.2010.04.027

579. Kenwood MM, Kalin NH, Barbas H. The prefrontal cortex, pathological anxiety, and anxiety disorders. *Neuropsychopharmacology*. 2021;47(1). doi:https://doi.org/10.1038/s41386-021-01109-z

580. Watson S. Feel-good hormones: How They Affect Your mind, Mood and Body. Harvard Health. Published April 18, 2024. https://www.health.harvard.edu/mind-and-mood/feel-good-hormones-how-they-affect-your-mind-mood-and-body

581. Voss JL, Bridge DJ, Cohen NJ, Walker JA. A Closer Look at the Hippocampus and Memory. *Trends in Cognitive Sciences*. 2017;21(8):577-588. doi:https://doi.org/10.1016/j.tics.2017.05.008

582. Cacioppo JT, Hawkley LC, Crawford LE, et al. Loneliness and health: potential mechanisms. *Psychosomatic medicine*. 2002;64(3):407-417. doi:https://doi.org/10.1097/00006842-200205000-00005

583. mckensied. How Loneliness Disrupts the Brain and the Body - Texas A&M Biology. Texas A&M Biology. Published July 2, 2025. Accessed July 25, 2025. https://www.bio.tamu.edu/how-loneliness-disrupts-the-brain-and-the-body/

584. Cherry K. How neuroplasticity works. Verywell Mind. Published 2024. https://www.verywellmind.com/what-is-brain-plasticity-2794886

585. Puderbaugh M, Emmady PD. Neuroplasticity. National Library of Medicine. Published 2023. https://www.ncbi.nlm.nih.gov/books/NBK557811/

586. Sheffler ZM, Pillarisetty LS, Reddy V. Physiology, Neurotransmitters. Nih.gov. Published May 1, 2023. https://www.ncbi.nlm.nih.gov/books/NBK539894/

587. Lovinger DM. Neurotransmitter roles in synaptic modulation, plasticity and learning in the dorsal striatum. *Neuropharmacology*. 2010;58(7):951-961. doi:https://doi.org/10.1016/j.neuropharm.2010.01.008

588. Purves D, Augustine GJ, Fitzpatrick D, et al. Long-Term Synaptic Potentiation. *Neuroscience 2nd edition*. 2001;2. https://www.ncbi.nlm.nih.gov/books/NBK10878/
589. Wiegert JS, Oertner TG. Long-term depression triggers the selective elimination of weakly integrated synapses. *Proceedings of the National Academy of Sciences*. 2013;110(47):E4510-E4519. doi:https://doi.org/10.1073/pnas.1315926110
590. Bliss TVP, Cooke SF. Long-term potentiation and long-term depression: a clinical perspective. *Clinics*. 2011;66(1):3-17. doi:https://doi.org/10.1590/s1807-59322011001300002
591. Kempermann G, Song H, Gage FH. Neurogenesis in the Adult Hippocampus. *Cold Spring Harbor Perspectives in Biology*. 2015;7(9):a018812. doi:https://doi.org/10.1101/cshperspect.a018812
592. McEwen Bruce S, Morrison John H. The Brain on Stress: Vulnerability and Plasticity of the Prefrontal Cortex over the Life Course. *Neuron*. 2013;79(1):16-29. doi:https://doi.org/10.1016/j.neuron.2013.06.028
593. Ackerman S. Major Structures and Functions of the Brain. Nih.gov. Published 1992. https://www.ncbi.nlm.nih.gov/books/NBK234157/
594. Ilg R, Wohlschlager AM, Gaser C, et al. Gray Matter Increase Induced by Practice Correlates with Task-Specific Activation: A Combined Functional and Morphometric Magnetic Resonance Imaging Study. *Journal of Neuroscience*. 2008;28(16):4210-4215. doi:https://doi.org/10.1523/jneurosci.5722-07.2008
595. Khanal P, Hotulainen P. Dendritic Spine Initiation in Brain Development, Learning and Diseases and Impact of BAR-Domain Proteins. *Cells*. 2021;10(9):2392. doi:https://doi.org/10.3390/cells10092392
596. Runge K, Cardoso C, de Chevigny A. Dendritic Spine Plasticity: Function and Mechanisms. *Frontiers in Synaptic Neuroscience*. 2020;12. doi:https://doi.org/10.3389/fnsyn.2020.00036
597. White Matter Matters. Scientific American. https://www.scientificamerican.com/article/white-matter-matters/
598. Sampaio-Baptista C, Vallès A, Khrapitchev AA, et al. White matter structure and myelin-related gene expression alterations with experience in adult rats. *Progress in Neurobiology*. 2020;187:101770. doi:https://doi.org/10.1016/j.pneurobio.2020.101770
599. Wang S, Young KM. White matter plasticity in adulthood. *Neuroscience*. 2014;276:148-160. doi:https://doi.org/10.1016/j.neuroscience.2013.10.018
600. Donald Hebb - The Decision Lab. The Decision Lab. https://thedecisionlab.com/thinkers/neuroscience/donald-hebb
601. Hebbian Theory - an overview | ScienceDirect Topics. www.sciencedirect.com. https://www.sciencedirect.com/topics/neuroscience/hebbian-theory
602. Brewer B. Neuroplasticity After Stroke: How the Brain Overcomes Injury. Flint Rehab. Published January 10, 2020. https://www.flintrehab.com/neuroplasticity-after-stroke/

603. Aderinto N, AbdulBasit MO, Olatunji G, Adejumo T. Exploring the transformative influence of neuroplasticity on stroke rehabilitation: a narrative review of current evidence. *Annals of Medicine and Surgery*. 2023;85(9):4425-4432. doi:https://doi.org/10.1097/MS9.0000000000001137

604. Singh B, Murphy A, Maher C, Smith AE. Time to Form a Habit: A Systematic Review and Meta-Analysis of Health Behaviour Habit Formation and Its Determinants. *Healthcare*. 2024;12(23):2488. doi:https://doi.org/10.3390/healthcare12232488

605. Divine A, Astill S. Reinforcing implementation intentions with imagery increases physical activity habit strength and behaviour. *British Journal of Health Psychology*. 2025;30(2). doi:https://doi.org/10.1111/bjhp.12795

606. Ryan Zofay Author Coach & Speaker. Ryan Zofay. Published April 4, 2025. Accessed July 25, 2025. https://ryanzofay.com/power-of-a-good-intention/

607. Decoding Craving Through the Science of Habit. Psychology Today. Published 2025. Accessed July 25, 2025. https://www.psychologytoday.com/us/blog/sober-curiosity/202506/decoding-craving-through-the-science-of-habit

608. Ibrahim N. The Effectiveness Of A Persuasive Mobile App To Influence Habit Change. Published online June 10, 2021. doi:https://doi.org/10.15405/epsbs.2021.06.02.62

609. Ciotti G. The Best Way to Change Your Habits? Control Your Environment. NBC News. Published July 9, 2014. Accessed July 25, 2025. https://www.nbcnews.com/id/wbna55607628

610. Sustainability Directory. Conscious Desire Redirection → Term. Lifestyle → Sustainability Directory. Published April 20, 2025. Accessed July 25, 2025. https://lifestyle.sustainability-directory.com/term/conscious-desire-redirection/

611. Wein H. Mindfulness for Your Health. NIH News in Health. Published June 2021. https://newsinhealth.nih.gov/2021/06/mindfulness-your-health

612. Schwartz JM, Stapp HP, Beauregard M. Quantum physics in neuroscience and psychology: a neurophysical model of mind–brain interaction. *Philosophical Transactions of the Royal Society B: Biological Sciences*. 2005;360(1458):1309-1327. doi:https://doi.org/10.1098/rstb.2004.1598

613. Calderone A, Latella D, Impellizzeri F, et al. Neurobiological Changes Induced by Mindfulness and Meditation: A Systematic Review. *Biomedicines*. 2024;12(11):2613-2613. doi:https://doi.org/10.3390/biomedicines12112613

614. Sadeghi S, Schmidt SNL, Mier D, Hass J. Effective connectivity of the human mirror neuron system during social cognition. *Social Cognitive and Affective Neuroscience*. 2022;17(8). doi:https://doi.org/10.1093/scan/nsab138

615. Braadbaart L, de Grauw H, Perrett DI, Waiter GD, Williams JHG. The shared neural basis of empathy and facial imitation accuracy. *NeuroImage*. 2014;84:367-375. doi:https://doi.org/10.1016/j.neuroimage.2013.08.061

616. Wang S. Contagious Behavior. *APS Observer*. 2016;19(2). https://www.psychologicalscience.org/observer/contagious-behavior

617. Davidson RJ, McEwen BS. Social influences on neuroplasticity: stress and interventions to promote well-being. *Nature Neuroscience*. 2012;15(5):689-695. doi:https://doi.org/10.1038/nn.3093
618. Reeck C, Ames DR, Ochsner KN. The Social Regulation of Emotion: An Integrative, Cross-Disciplinary Model. *Trends in Cognitive Sciences*. 2016;20(1):47-63. doi:https://doi.org/10.1016/j.tics.2015.09.003
619. Bromberg-Martin ES, Matsumoto M, Hikosaka O. Dopamine in motivational control: Rewarding, aversive, and alerting. *Neuron*. 2010;68(5):815-834. doi:https://doi.org/10.1016/j.neuron.2010.11.022
620. Ciletti N. How Does Social Pressure Impact Our Choices? | Betterhelp. www.betterhelp.com. Published 2023. https://www.betterhelp.com/advice/general/how-does-social-pressure-impact-our-choices/
621. Worley SL. The Extraordinary Importance of Sleep: The Detrimental Effects of Inadequate Sleep on Health and Public Safety Drive an Explosion of Sleep Research. *Pharmacy and Therapeutics*. 2018;43(12):758-763. https://pmc.ncbi.nlm.nih.gov/articles/PMC6281147/
622. Huhta J. Sleep Traditions Across Cultures. American Mattress. Published December 9, 2024. https://www.americanmattress.com/blogs/learn/sleep-traditions-across-cultures
623. Backman I. Poor Sleep May Increase Markers of Poor Brain Health, New Study Finds. medicine.yale.edu. Published January 29, 2024. https://medicine.yale.edu/news-article/poor-sleep-may-increase-markers-of-poor-brain-health-new-study-finds/
624. Billones R, Liwang JK, Butler K, Graves L, Saligan LN. Dissecting the fatigue experience: A scoping review of fatigue definitions, dimensions, and measures in non-oncologic medical conditions. *Brain, Behavior, & Immunity - Health*. 2021;15(100266):100266. doi:https://doi.org/10.1016/j.bbih.2021.100266
625. Born J, Wilhelm I. System consolidation of memory during sleep. *Psychological Research*. 2012;76(2):192-203. doi:https://doi.org/10.1007/s00426-011-0335-6
626. Klinzing JG, Niethard N, Born J. Mechanisms of systems memory consolidation during sleep. *Nature Neuroscience*. 2019;22(10):1598-1610. doi:https://doi.org/10.1038/s41593-019-0467-3
627. Zhang MQ, Li R, Wang YQ, Huang ZL. Neural Plasticity Is Involved in Physiological Sleep, Depressive Sleep Disturbances, and Antidepressant Treatments. *Neural Plasticity*. 2017;2017:1-16. doi:https://doi.org/10.1155/2017/5870735
628. Gorgoni M, D'Atri A, Lauri G, Rossini PM, Ferlazzo F, De Gennaro L. Is Sleep Essential for Neural Plasticity in Humans, and How Does It Affect Motor and Cognitive Recovery? *Neural Plasticity*. 2013;2013(103949):1-13. doi:https://doi.org/10.1155/2013/103949
629. Havekes R, Abel T. The tired hippocampus: the molecular impact of sleep deprivation on hippocampal function. *Current Opinion in Neurobiology*. 2017;44:13-19. doi:https://doi.org/10.1016/j.conb.2017.02.005

630. Muzur A, Pace-Schott EF, Hobson JAllan. The prefrontal cortex in sleep. *Trends in Cognitive Sciences*. 2002;6(11):475-481. doi:https://doi.org/10.1016/s1364-6613(02)01992-7

631. Kaur H, Spurling BC, Bollu PC. Chronic Insomnia. PubMed. Published 2023. https://www.ncbi.nlm.nih.gov/books/NBK526136/

632. Minkel J, Moreta M, Muto J, et al. Sleep deprivation potentiates HPA axis stress reactivity in healthy adults. *Health Psychology*. 2014;33(11):1430-1434. doi:https://doi.org/10.1037/a0034219

633. Hanifin JP, Lockley SW, Cecil K, et al. Randomized trial of polychromatic blue-enriched light for circadian phase shifting, melatonin suppression, and alerting responses. *Physiology & Behavior*. 2019;198:57-66. doi:https://doi.org/10.1016/j.physbeh.2018.10.004

634. West KE, Jablonski MR, Warfield B, et al. Blue light from light-emitting diodes elicits a dose-dependent suppression of melatonin in humans. *Journal of Applied Physiology*. 2011;110(3):619-626. doi:https://doi.org/10.1152/japplphysiol.01413.2009

635. Newman MG, Basterfield C, Erickson TM, Caulley E, Przeworski A, Llera SJ. Psychotherapeutic treatments for generalized anxiety disorder: Cognitive and behavioral therapies, enhancement strategies, and emerging efforts. *Expert Review of Neurotherapeutics*. 2022;22(9):751-770. doi:https://doi.org/10.1080/14737175.2022.2125800

636. Månsson KNT, Salami A, Frick A, et al. Neuroplasticity in response to cognitive behavior therapy for social anxiety disorder. *Translational Psychiatry*. 2016;6(2):e727-e727. doi:https://doi.org/10.1038/tp.2015.218

637. Yuan S, Wu H, Wu Y, et al. Neural Effects of Cognitive Behavioral Therapy in Psychiatric Disorders: A Systematic Review and Activation Likelihood Estimation Meta-Analysis. *Frontiers in Psychology*. 2022;13(13). doi:https://doi.org/10.3389/fpsyg.2022.853804

638. Kang HS, Exworthy M. Wearing the Future—Wearables to Empower Users to Take Greater Responsibility for Their Health and Care: Scoping Review. *JMIR mHealth and uHealth*. 2022;10(7). doi:https://doi.org/10.2196/35684

639. Varma N, Cygankiewicz I, Turakhia MP, et al. 2021 ISHNE/HRS/EHRA/APHRS Collaborative Statement on mHealth in Arrhythmia Management: Digital Medical Tools for Heart Rhythm Professionals. *Cardiovascular Digital Health Journal*. 2021;2(1):4-54. doi:https://doi.org/10.1016/j.cvdhj.2020.11.004

640. Kyu Sik Kim, Joon Seok Park, Hwang E, et al. GLP-1 increases preingestive satiation via hypothalamic circuits in mice and humans. *Science*. 2024;385(6707):438-446. doi:https://doi.org/10.1126/science.adj2537

641. Bloemendaal L van, IJzerman RG, Kulve JS ten, et al. GLP-1 Receptor Activation Modulates Appetite- and Reward-Related Brain Areas in Humans. *Diabetes*. 2014;63(12):4186-4196. doi:https://doi.org/10.2337/db14-0849

642. Calder AE, Hasler G. Towards an understanding of psychedelic-induced neuroplasticity. *Neuropsychopharmacology*. 2022;48(48):1-9. doi:https://doi.org/10.1038/s41386-022-01389-z

643. Psychology Today. Motivation. Psychology Today. Published 2019. https://www.psychologytoday.com/us/basics/motivation
644. Change B. Nurturing Intrinsic Motivation Through Health Technology. Omadahealth.com. Published September 4, 2019. Accessed July 25, 2025. https://resourcecenter.omadahealth.com/blog/behavior-change-part-i-autonomy-intrinsic-motivation-5
645. Cherry K. Understanding Intrinsic Motivation. Verywell Mind. Published May 3, 2023. https://www.verywellmind.com/what-is-intrinsic-motivation-2795385
646. Bavelier D, Savulescu J, Fried LP, et al. Rethinking human enhancement as collective welfarism. *Nature Human Behaviour*. 2019;3(3):204-206. doi:https://doi.org/10.1038/s41562-019-0545-2
647. Read J. Feeling Machines that Think - Dr. Joshua Read. Dr. Joshua Read. Published August 20, 2018. Accessed July 28, 2025. https://drjoshuaread.com/feeling-machines-that-think/
648. Catani M, Dell'Acqua F, Thiebaut de Schotten M. A revised limbic system model for memory, emotion and behaviour. *Neuroscience & Biobehavioral Reviews*. 2013;37(8):1724-1737. doi:https://doi.org/10.1016/j.neubiorev.2013.07.001
649. AbuHasan Q, Siddiqui W, Reddy V. Neuroanatomy, Amygdala. Nih.gov. Published July 17, 2023. https://www.ncbi.nlm.nih.gov/books/NBK537102/
650. Kinaan Javed, Forshing Lui. Neuroanatomy, Cerebral Cortex. Nih.gov. Published 2019. https://www.ncbi.nlm.nih.gov/books/NBK537247/
651. Precuneus - an overview | ScienceDirect Topics. www.sciencedirect.com. https://www.sciencedirect.com/topics/neuroscience/precuneus
652. Dhikav V, Anand KS. Hippocampus in Health and disease: an Overview. *Annals of Indian Academy of Neurology*. 2012;15(4):239-246. doi:https://doi.org/10.4103/0972-2327.104323
653. Winn HR. Prefrontal Cortex - an overview | ScienceDirect Topics. Sciencedirect.com. Published 2013. https://www.sciencedirect.com/topics/medicine-and-dentistry/prefrontal-cortex
654. CDC. Loneliness | How Right Now. www.cdc.gov. https://www.cdc.gov/howrightnow/emotion/loneliness/index.html
655. CDC. Health Effects of Social Isolation and Loneliness. Social Connection. Published May 15, 2024. https://www.cdc.gov/social-connectedness/risk-factors/index.html
656. LeWine H. Oxytocin: The love hormone. Harvard Health. Published June 13, 2023. https://www.health.harvard.edu/mind-and-mood/oxytocin-the-love-hormone
657. Vilella RC, Reddivari AKR. Empathy. PubMed. Published 2021. https://www.ncbi.nlm.nih.gov/books/NBK549810/
658. Kilner JM, Lemon RN. What We Know Currently about Mirror Neurons. *Current Biology*. 2013;23(23):R1057-R1062. doi:https://doi.org/10.1016/j.cub.2013.10.051

659. Puderbaugh M, Emmady PD. Neuroplasticity. National Library of Medicine. Published 2023. https://www.ncbi.nlm.nih.gov/books/NBK557811/

Image References

1. Blaus B. WikiJournal of Medicine/Medical gallery of Blausen Medical 2014 - Wikiversity. Wikiversity.org. Published August 5, 2014. https://en.wikiversity.org/wiki/WikiJournal_of_Medicine/Medical_gallery_of_Blausen_Medical_2014
2. Macrovector. Human nervous system infographics | Free Vector. Freepik. Published 2022. Accessed July 28, 2025. https://www.freepik.com/free-vector/human-nervous-system-infographics_26762570.htm#fromView=search&page=1&position=6&uuid=e431e62a-e250-4c91-95c4-8e8b5b7e37d8&query=central+nervous+system
3. Macrovector. Human body nervous system sympathetic parasympathetic charts with realistic organs depiction and anatomical terminology vector illustration | Free Vector. Freepik. Published 2022. Accessed July 28, 2025. https://www.freepik.com/free-vector/human-body-nervous-system-sympathetic-parasympathetic-charts-with-realistic-organs-depiction-anatomical-terminology-vector-illustration_26762666.htm#from_element=cross_selling__vector
4. Hall GB. File:MRI anterior cingulate.png - Wikimedia Commons. Wikimedia.org. Published September 8, 2011. https://commons.wikimedia.org/wiki/File:MRI_anterior_cingulate.png
5. Jkwchui. File:Recurrent laryngeal nerve.svg - Wikimedia Commons. Wikimedia.org. Published February 5, 2014. Accessed July 28, 2025. https://commons.wikimedia.org/wiki/File:Recurrent_laryngeal_nerve.svg
6. Blaus B. Hypothalamus location. Wikiversity.org. Published August 5, 2014. Accessed July 28, 2025. https://en.wikiversity.org/wiki/WikiJournal_of_Medicine/Medical_gallery_of_Blausen_Medical_2014#/media/File:Blausen_0536_HypothalamusLocation.png
7. Rieder A, Traynor J, Hall GB. File:MRI Location Amygdala up.png - Wikimedia Commons. Wikimedia.org. Published September 8, 2011. https://commons.wikimedia.org/wiki/File:MRI_Location_Amygdala_up.png
8. Genesis12. File:Nucleus accumbens MRI.PNG - Wikimedia Commons. Wikimedia.org. Published December 18, 2009. Accessed July 28, 2025. https://commons.wikimedia.org/wiki/File:Nucleus_accumbens_MRI.PNG
9. Danielsabinasz. File:Hippocampus sagittal sections.gif - Wikimedia Commons. Wikimedia.org. Published April 5, 2021. Accessed July 28, 2025. https://commons.wikimedia.org/wiki/File:Hippocampus_sagittal_sections.gif
10. Blaus B. File:Blausen 0076 BasalGanglia.png - Wikimedia Commons.

Wikimedia.org. Published March 12, 2014. Accessed July 28, 2025. https://commons.wikimedia.org/wiki/File:Blausen_0076_BasalGanglia.png

11. Schappelle. File:Insula structure.png - Wikimedia Commons. Wikimedia.org. Published August 11, 2017. https://commons.wikimedia.org/wiki/File:Insula_structure.png
12. Blaus B. Types of neuroglia cells. Wikiversity.org. Published August 5, 2014. Accessed July 28, 2025. https://en.wikiversity.org/wiki/WikiJournal_of_Medicine/Medical_gallery_of_Blausen_Medical_2014#/media/File:Blausen_0870_TypesofNeuroglia.png
13. Wilgus J, Wilgus B, Harvard Medical School. Photograph of cased-daguerreotype studio portrait of brain-injury survivor Phineas P. Gage (1823–1860) shown holding the tamping iron which injured him. Wikimedia Commons. Published August 2, 2009. https://commons.wikimedia.org/wiki/File:Phineas_Gage_Daguerreotype_WilgusPhoto2008-12-19_CroppedInsideMat_Unretouched_BW.jpg
14. Moraes C. A Aproximação Facial e a Dinâmica do Acidente de Phineas Gage (1848) — documentação OrtogOnLineMag #7. Ortogonline.com. Published 2023. Accessed July 28, 2025. https://ortogonline.com/doc/pt_br/OrtogOnLineMag/7/Phineas.html
15. Hall GB. File:Precuneus.png - Wikimedia Commons. Wikimedia.org. Published September 8, 2011. Accessed July 28, 2025. https://commons.wikimedia.org/wiki/File:Precuneus.png
16. Graner J. File:Default mode network-WRNMMC.jpg - Wikimedia Commons. Wikimedia.org. Published July 23, 2010. https://commons.wikimedia.org/wiki/File:Default_mode_network-WRNMMC.jpg
17. Finereach. File:Ventromedial prefrontal cortex.png - Wikimedia Commons. Wikimedia.org. Published November 25, 8AD. Accessed July 28, 2025. https://commons.wikimedia.org/wiki/File:Ventromedial_prefrontal_cortex.png

www.ingramcontent.com/pod-product-compliance
Lightning Source LLC
LaVergne TN
LVHW052251200926
848481LV00002B/335
* 9 7 9 8 2 3 3 2 4 7 5 7 6 *